WebDoctor

Finding the Best Health Care Online

WebDoctor

Finding the Best Health Care Online

RICHARD M. SHARP, ED.D.
VICKI F. SHARP, PH.D.

St. Martin's Griffin ⚹ New York

ISBN 0-312-19536-2

First published in the United States by Quality Medical Publishing, Inc.

First St. Martin's Griffin/Quality Medical Publishing Home Health Library
Edition: September 1998

10 9 8 7 6 5 4 3 2 1

To

Bobbie E. Friedman
the late Paul Friedman

and

our son, David

Preface

WebDoctor: Your Online Guide to Health Care and Wellness provides consumers, medical doctors, and health care professionals with Web sites that will enrich and expand their medical knowledge.

What sets this book apart from other medical Web books is its currency, ease of use, comprehensiveness, and organization. The sites have been updated frequently and have the latest information. To simplify, we have intentionally avoided long explanations. Each site has an address (the uniform resource locator [URL]), a picture of the Web page, and a brief description with navigational shortcuts. For example, a mega-site such as the National Institutes of Health has been dissected so that it pinpoints the most useful information to save countless hours of time and fruitless effort and keep the reader from being lost in cyperspace. Furthermore, the reader never has to type in the Web site address because they are included on the CD-ROM that accompanies this book in the form of HTML files. *WebDoctor* covers topics ranging from alternative health to women's health. Finally, the book's organization is straightforward. It is divided into 23 categories without confusing subdivisions. An introductory chapter presents useful information to help you get started with your browser and suggests tips and tricks for finding inaccessible addresses or URLs.

We examined thousands of sites and included only those that met specific criteria. Because anyone with access to the Web can establish a Web page, many medical sites contain little useful information, even though they may be visually appealing. Other sites with relevant information for doctors and consumers may contain graphics that take too long to download. Still other sites are poorly organized or have hard-to-read screens and finding information is very difficult. We have selected sites that, in general, fulfill the following criteria:

- The site contains appropriate, relevant, and timely health care information.
- The site is organized effectively on a stable Internet location with good connectivity so that consumers, doctors, and health care professionals can easily find the information they are seeking.

- The site can be downloaded in a reasonable time period.

- The site is updated on a regular basis.

- The site is an award winner and has been cited as a valuable site for its authoritative and reliable information.

The following are a few examples of the sites featured in this book.

KidsHealth.org

http://kidshealth.org/

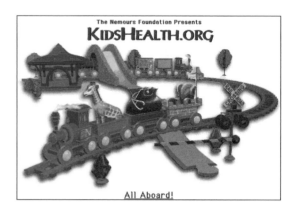

KidsHealth.org (in Chapter 4, You and Your Children), a premier site for kids and parents created by the Nemours Foundation, provides a comprehensive collection of resources and accurate up-to-date information on growth, food and fitness, childhood infections, immunizations, laboratory tests, medical and surgical conditions, and the most recent treatments.

Family and Cosmetic Dentistry

http://www.familyinternet.com/dentist/

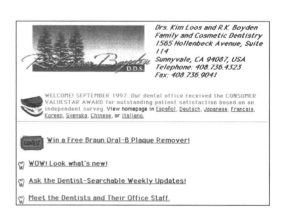

If you are looking for dental information, the Family and Cosmetic Dentistry home page of Dr. Kim Loos and Dr. R.K. Boyden (in Chapter 18, Dental Care) contains a plethora of dental resources. Among the resources are an ask the dentist feature with an archive of previous questions, what's new updates, online articles by dental experts, family tips for a better smile, and related dental links.

Cells Alive

http://www.cellsalive.com/

Cells Alive (in Chapter 11, Biomedical Education) is a primer on cellular biology. It features a fascinating collection of pictures and animations with clear explanations. You can see how penicillin destroys bacteria, how cells keep their shape and how they communicate, you can view microscopic parasites, and learn much more.

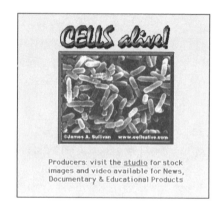

Producers: visit the studio for stock images and video available for News, Documentary & Educational Products

Information for Patients

http://www.aafp.org/patientinfo/

A must for exploring a particular disease is Information for Patients (in Chapter 3, Health Topics for Everyone, and Chapter 12, Diseases and Conditions) from the American Academy of Family Physicians. The site contains a collection of handouts covering more than 200 health topics. The handout categories consist of the body, common conditions/diseases/disorders, treatments, and healthy living.

Mental Health Net

http://mhnet.org/

If you have a question about mental illness visit Mental Health Net (in Chapter 8, Mental Health), a comprehensive guide to mental health online. It features over 6300 resources for disorders such as depression, anxiety, panic attacks, chronic fatigue syndrome, and substance abuse. Each category includes an annotated list of top-rated sites. In addition, the site has access to professional resources in psychology and psychiatry.

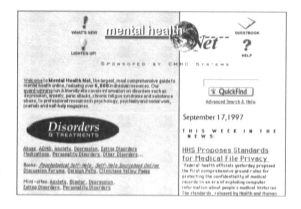

Achoo

http://www.achoo.com

One of our favorite directories is Achoo (in Chapter 23, Health Directories). It is one of the most comprehensive health care databases on the Internet with over 7000 indexed and searchable health care sites. The site is organized by categories that include Human Life, Practice of Medicine, Business of Health, and What's New.

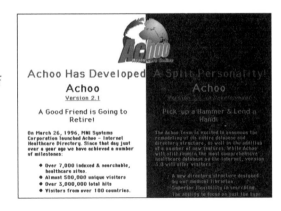

Femina

http://femina.cybergrrl.com/femina/ HealthandWellness/

Finally, for those interested in women's health problems, Femina (in Chapter 5, Women's Health) provides a collection of women's health and wellness sites categorized by topic. Topics range from AIDS/HIV to weight. The site also includes links to other women's health resources.

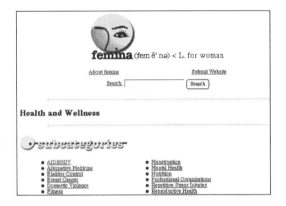

The material contained in this book is from our personal research on the Internet. Unfortunately, not all the information found on the Web is current or authoritative. We are not medical professionals and any decision regarding your health should not be based solely on the information you find on the Web. There is no substitute for professional medical care, but the Web is an excellent place to begin your exploration. Good Surfing!

Richard M. Sharp, Ed.D.
Vicki F. Sharp, Ph.D.

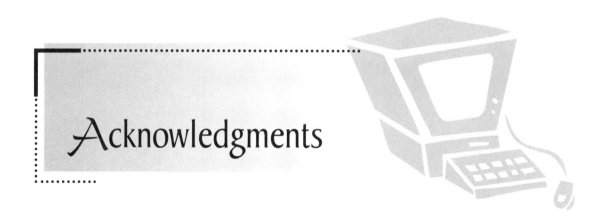

Acknowledgments

We want to express our special appreciation to Karen Berger for her advice and invaluable assistance and direction. We could not have written this book without her and the wonderful personnel at Quality Medical Publishing. Katherine Spakowski, Susan Trail, Cindy Meilink, Doug Wilmsmeyer, and David Berger all contributed their ideas and talents to this project.

Thanks to Dave Pola, Creative Marketing Director of Equilibrium for DeBabelizer, a real time saver. DeBabelizer was used to batch produce the screen shots and enhance the images. Equilibrium can be reached by phone at 415-332-4343 or on the Web at

    http://www.equilibrium.com/

Thanks also to Marc Weiss and Michael Radonic for Dragnet from TikiSoft, Inc. Dragnet was used to organize and create the bookmarks found on the *WebDoctor* CD-ROM disk. A sample copy of Dragnet and other connectivity software can be found on this CD-ROM disk. TikiSoft, Inc. can be reached by phone at 714-829-8585 or on the Web at

    http://www.tikisoft.com/

Finally, a very special thank you to Dr. Nathan Gittleman and Dr. Gary Dosik. These knowledgeable medical doctors saved Vicki Sharp's life!

Contents

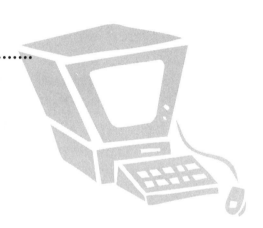

For ready access to topics of particular interest to you, consult the comprehensive index. If you do not locate the specific subject you are searching for there, consult one of the directories or A to Z guides.

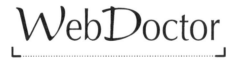

WebDoctor

Finding the Best Health Care Online

CHAPTER 1

Getting Started

The World Wide Web and the Internet

The World Wide Web (the Web) is an invaluable resource for anyone interested in finding medical information. Users are only a mouse click away from this vast reservoir. Consumers and health care professionals can access a giant library with millions of sites that are increasing at a phenomenal rate each week. The Web is the multimedia part of the Internet—that huge worldwide network of connected computers with no single master control center or authority. The Web consists of a collection of electronic documents called home pages or Web sites, complete with text, pictures, sounds, and even video. Thousands of Web sites take advantage of the Web's multimedia capabilities. Web users can get information on any medical problem, talk to an expert, explore the human body, participate in online discussion groups, and download chapters from books or lecture notes.

Web sites or home pages have their own unique addresses called Uniform Resource Locators (URLs), which make Web sites easy to find. URLs begin with http://. For example, the URL for the Web site for the publisher of this book, Quality Medical Publishing, is

http://www.qmp.com

Once connected to a site, users will see certain items on the Web pages underlined. These underlined items, called links, are like threads in a spider's web and give the Web its name. By clicking on these links with a mouse, the user can jump from one page on the Web to any other, whether it is a page on the same computer or a page on the other side of the world. One document is linked to another, which is linked to another, and so forth.

Connecting to the World Wide Web

To access the Web, you need a connection to the Internet. Two of the most popular services are America Online (800-827-6364) and CompuServe (800-848-8990). An Internet connection can also be obtained through an Internet Service Provider (ISP). Several places can

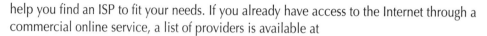

help you find an ISP to fit your needs. If you already have access to the Internet through a commercial online service, a list of providers is available at

> http://thelist.com/

Information about ISPs can also be found in your local Yellow Pages or from a local computer user group.

Web surfing also requires software called a browser that enables the user to take advantage of the Web's multimedia capabilities. Netscape Navigator and Internet Explorer are examples of Web browsers. Both the commercial online services and the ISPs provide users with the appropriate software.

To connect to the Web, your computer must be able to run MS-DOS or Windows with at least a 386 processor and 8 megabytes (MB) of RAM, or a Macintosh computer must run System 7.0 or higher with at least 8 MB of memory. Because of the memory requirements for most browsers, at least 16 MB of RAM is advisable. You also need a modem, which, if possible, should have a transfer speed of at least 28.8 bits per second (bps) or higher. A 14.4 bps modem will work, but it operates at a much slower speed.

Getting Started With Your Browser

All Web pages displayed in this book can be opened using either Internet Explorer or Netscape. They both work in a similar way, although the display of the home page on your monitor may look different. The following instructions tell you how to enter a URL to display a home page.

NETSCAPE NAVIGATOR

After you launch Netscape, you will see a toolbar at the top of its window. The toolbar has commands such as Print, Back, and Open.

1. Click Open on the Tool Bar.

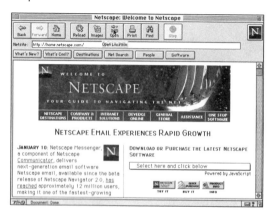

2. Type the following URL in the Open Location dialog box: http://www.qmp.com

3. Click Open.

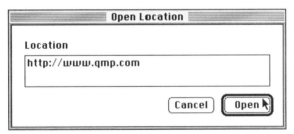

INTERNET EXPLORER

After launching Internet Explorer, you will see a toolbar with commands such as Stop, Back, and Forward.

1. Under the File menu, click Open.

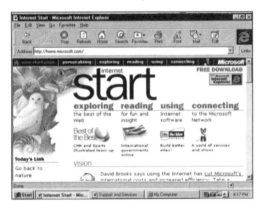

2. Type the following URL in the Open dialog box: http://www.qmp.com

3. Click OK.

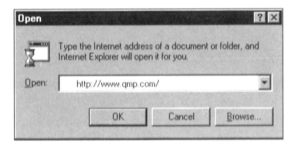

NETSCAPE NAVIGATOR AND INTERNET EXPLORER

4. After a few seconds, the home page corresponding to the URL will appear.

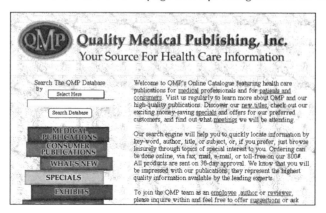

5. Wait until the page is fully loaded on your screen. You will see the word Done or the words Document: Done at the bottom of the screen.

6. You are now ready to explore links, or connections, to other Web pages. Links are words that are underlined or displayed in a different color or are pictures that have a colored border around them. (In the *WebDoctor: Your Online Guide to Health Care and Wellness* the links are set in **boldface** type.)

7. Click on a word link

> Welcome to QMP's Online Catalogue featuring health care publications for medical professionals and for patients and consumers. Visit us regularly to learn more about QMP and our high-quality publications. Discover our new titles, check out our exciting money-saving specials and offers for our preferred customers, and find out what meetings we will be attending.

or picture link.

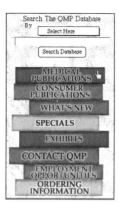

Note: When you click on a live link, the pointer (or arrow) becomes a hand.

Tips for Both Netscape Navigator and Internet Explorer Users
(other browsers work in a similar way so these tips are also applicable)

1   When you type a URL in the Open Location or Open box, omit the http:// part of the URL.

2   Use the Back button or arrow to return to the previous site or page.

3   If you cannot open a site with a given URL, use a search tool such as InfoSeek, Yahoo!, Lycos, Magellan, or Alta Vista. Type in the title of the site exactly as it appears, not its URL, and the search tool might pick up the new URL in the title entered. The All-In-One Search Page features a compilation of the various search tools that you can use to help you find things on the Internet. The URL is

> http://www.albany.net/allinone/

4   When using a search engine, you can narrow your search and avoid thousands of unnecessary hits. For example, when using Yahoo!, click on the Options button and try "an exact phrase match." In Yahoo! you can also scroll to the bottom of the page and click on other search engines that are listed.

5   When searching, avoid generic or commonly used words. For example, a search for "basketball" is too general and will deliver a tremendous number of matches. A search for "1970 World Series" is much better. The best searches have terms or words or phrases that are found in the documents you want.

6   Most search engines let you link your search terms such as "and," "or," and "minus" (–), as well as search for phrases, by placing the words in quotation marks (" "). For example, you might search for "Stan Musial" and "World Series," which would give you information on both topics. If you replace "and" with "or," the search will be directed to one topic or the other. If you replace the "and" with the minus sign (no spaces), the engine will find the pages that contain references to Stan Musial, but not the World Series. The connectors vary with the search engines. Check your search engine's help page for more tips.

7   When you find a site you like, place it in your bookmarks so that you never have to enter the site again.

- Under Netscape's Bookmarks menu, select Add Bookmark. The site will now be listed under the Bookmarks menu and Netscape will take you to the site whenever you select it.

- Under Internet Explorer's Favorites menu, click Add to Favorites. Type the name for the site or use the name supplied and then click OK. The site will now be listed under the Favorites List and the Internet Explorer will take you to the site whenever you select it.

8 The print size on a page may be too small for comfortable reading. However, most browsers let you change the size of the words displayed on the screen.

- With Netscape, go to General Preferences, then click on Fonts and choose a different size and shape font.

- With Internet Explorer, go under View Menu, then go to Fonts and choose a larger or smaller font for the text on that page.

9 If you just print the information from the site, you might get pages you do not need. Go to Print Preview and see how many pages are in the site and determine which pages you want. Next specify in your Print Dialog the pages you want printed.

10 Instead of printing pages, you can save them with the Save As feature on your browser. You have a choice of Source or Text. If you select Text, the pages will have no colors or formatting and can be opened with your word processor. If you select Source, the document is saved as an HTML document with color and formatting. The graphics must be saved separately.

- Using Netscape, press the mouse on a graphic and, when the dialog box pops up, save it.

- With Internet Explorer, right click on the graphic and then click Save Picture As on the short menu that appears.

11 Web pages that are long can be searched for a specific word or words.

- With Netscape, click Control then "f," on your keyboard. Type in the word in the dialog box. Then click Find Next in the dialog box or click Enter or return on your keyboard. The word will appear highlighted.

- With Internet Explorer, go under the Edit menu and click Find (On This Page). In the dialog box that appears, type in the word, then click Find Next in the dialog box. The word will appear highlighted.

Tips for Finding Inaccessible URLs

Be forewarned that Internet resources come and go with amazing speed. We cannot guarantee that all of the sites included in this book will be accessible when you try to open them. You might find messages such as "404 Not Found" or "No DNS entry exists for this server." The following tips might help you locate the site:

1 Try opening the site again, a few seconds later. The Internet computer serving the documents may be down temporarily or it may be so busy that you can't get in at the moment. Occasionally, your Internet Service Provider or commercial online service has problems with its Internet lines.

2 If you have waited more than 50 seconds for the site to load, click on the Stop Button and then reload.

3   Check to make sure you have spelled the URL exactly as it is printed in this book, using lower case and capital letters where appropriate. The Web is case sensitive and "Csun" is not the same as "csun."

4   If suddenly your sites do not load, it is a good idea to get offline and reboot your system.

5   For a faster loading of a site, turn off the graphics and sound options on your browser. Although graphics and audio files are great, they take forever to load. In most instances, you can make text only by loading your browser's default. After seeing the site, you can turn on these options and return to examine the site again.

6   When you can't find a site, sometimes you can physically modify your URL to get the page you desire. For example, when you try to dial up the Medical Matrix: Patient Education page at

> http://www.medmatrix.org/SPages/Patient_Education_and_Support.stm

and you get an error message, try deleting the "Patient_Education_and_Support.stm" and hitting Return or Enter. Continue removing segments from the URL up to the forward slashes until it works. The link http://www.medmatrix.org/ will work.

7   Since the Web is always changing, sites switch servers, change their names, or just disappear forever. In many cases the old location will point you to the site's new location. If this is not the case, try the company's name or product names. For instance, to find information about Apple Computing, type

> <http://www.apple.com>

If this procedure doesn't work, go to a search engine and type Apple Computing.

8   Many sites maintain numerous servers to accommodate high volume. To make sure the servers don't become overloaded, most Webmasters limit the number of users. To overcome this difficulty, try another server. For example, Netscape numbers its servers. If you can't access

> ftp://ftp3.netscape.com/

try

> ftp://ftp4.netscape.com/   and so forth.

9   Finally, instead of looking through one search engine at a time, try using the search tool MetaCrawler which allows you to search several engines at the same time. MetaCrawler can be found at

> <http://www.metacrawler.com>

Another choice is Search, which can be found at

> Search.com <http://www.search.com>

Shortcut for Using this Book

On the CD ROM that accompanies this book the Web site addresses are in the form of HTML files. Use these files so you don't have to type in an address for the Web site. For example, if you want to see the children's health links:

1. Under the File menu, open the document, in this example, Children's Health.

2. A list of links will appear on your browser's page.

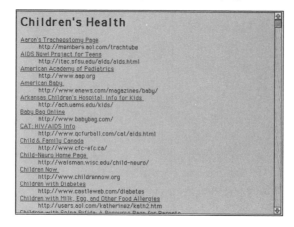

Tip: Drag the document (Children's Health) to an open active page on your browser.

3. Bookmark that page so that the addresses of the links or URLs do not have to be typed in each time.

Starting Point

As a quick introduction to finding health information on the Internet, we recommend the following sites as a starting point.

Your Health IS Your Business
http://www.siu.edu/departments/bushea/

Your Health IS Your Business, developed at the University of Southern Illinois, offers everything from health news, online journals, search tools, and topics ranging from alternative medicine to women's health. Each link has a brief description to help decide whether you want to visit it.

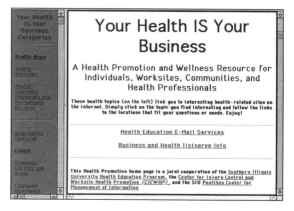

Mayo Health O@sis

http://www.mayohealth.org/

Mayo Health O@sis, sponsored by the Mayo Clinic and IVI Publishing, is an online service providing reliable, up-to-date health and wellness information on a wide variety of topics, including O@sis Library, Cancer Center, Diet & Nutrition, Heart Center, and Pregnancy & Children. Other features are Newsstand, with the most current breakthroughs and stories, and Ask Mayo, a place to talk with the experts. The site is updated daily.

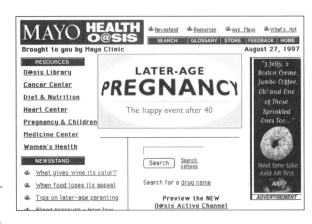

Your Comments and Suggestions

We hope that this book will enrich your Web experience and will translate into more productive time on the Internet. If you have comments or wish to add some of your favorite medical Web sites to the next edition, please let us know. Our e-mail addresses are:

vicki.sharp@csun.edu   and   richard.sharp@csun.edu

Staying Fit and Eating Right

CHAPTER 2

5-A-Day

http://www.dole5aday.com/

5-A-Day is a national nutrition program that encourages Americans to eat five or more servings of fruits and vegetables everyday. The site contains a list of recipes and tips, in addition to state programs with numerous classroom activities.

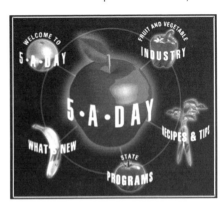

Amazing World

http://www.bupa.co.uk/

Amazing World, created by British United Provident Association (BUPA), provides consumer information on health and fitness, a MediCall medical information service, and a health quiz.

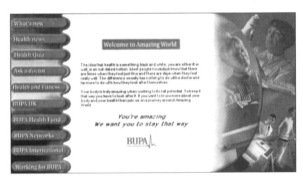

American Cancer Society Cookbook

The American Cancer Society Cookbook contains over 200 recipes reflecting the newest research on the simple nutritional guidelines that can reduce your risk of developing cancer. Each month the site features a new recipe from the cookbook and a recipe archive on the bottom of the **Recipe of the Month** page.

http://www.ca.cancer.org/services/nutrition/cook.html

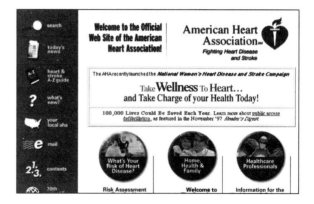

American Heart Association

The official Web site of the American Heart Association offers a wealth of information about heart disease and stroke. Click on **Home, Health, & Family** for invaluable information about healthy living and nutrition and fitness. In addition, the site includes a **Stroke Connection** section with information and access to support groups and reference materials, an online risk assessment test for heart disease, an enormous A to Z heart and stroke guide, and daily news about cardiovascular disease and cardiology. For an overview of the site, click on **Contents.**

http://207.211.141.25/

Arbor Nutrition Guide

http://arborcom.com/frame/arb_nutr.htm

The Arbor Nutrition Guide provides a wealth of information for dietitians and consumers alike. The site includes an efficient search engine and sections on the patient, public health, and school nutrition.

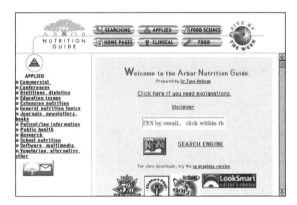

Ask the Dietitian

http://www.dietitian.com/

Ask the Dietitian provides sound nutrition advice in over 80 informative articles, arranged alphabetically from alcohol to zinc. Another feature is the Healthy Body Calculator, an interactive survey that helps you determine a healthy weight.

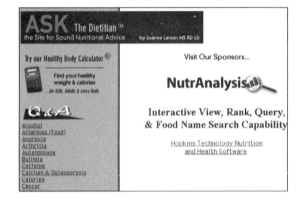

Aunt Edna's Kitchen

http://www.cei.net/~terry/auntedna/

Aunt Edna's Kitchen contains information on nutrition, a recipe file, and related links ranging from healthy eating to nutrition. Aunt Edna even offers cooking utensils to help you with your culinary pursuits.

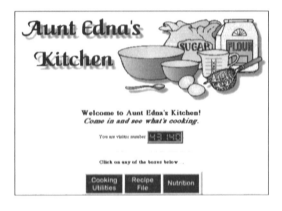

Austin Nutritional Research

http://www.realtime.net/anr/

Austin Nutritional Research provides a variety of online reference guides for health and nutrition, including vitamins, minerals, herbs, amino acids, and others. The site also lists other health and nutrition resources.

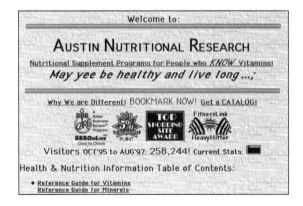

Balance

http://www.balance.net/

Balance is a monthly magazine offering a variety of online fitness articles ranging from exercise tips to burning fat. The site includes articles from the current issue, as well as back issues. In addition, automatic updates on the latest issue are available.

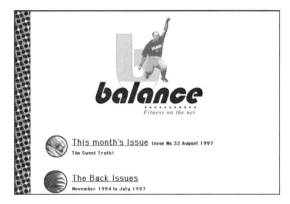

Basal Metabolism

http://www.room42.com/nutrition/basalcgi.html

Basal Metabolism features a metabolic calculator. After you enter your age, height, weight, gender, and activity level (be honest!), the program returns an estimate of your daily caloric requirements, including fat, protein, and carbohydrate recommendations.

Best Health and Fitness Web Sites

http://infotrek.simplenet.com/health.html

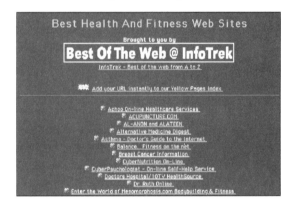

Best Health and Fitness Web Sites provides a compendium of online fitness and nutrition resources for the consumer.

The Blonz Guide

http://www.wenet.net/blonz/

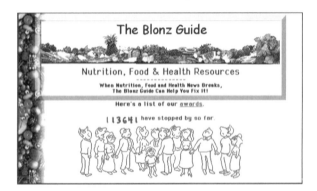

The Blonz Guide is an index to other Web sites: health and medical resources and associations, nutrition, online newspapers, magazines, government resources, networks, food resource companies and associations, and health, medical, and wellness publications. Many searchable databases are available for additional inquiry.

Body Stuff

http://www.healthink.com/bodystuff/body.html

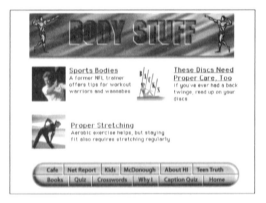

Body Stuff provides exercise tips for workout warriors and wanna-bes, information about the back, discs, and the spine, and aerobic exercise suggestions for staying fit.

Body Trends Online

http://www.bodytrends.com/article.htm

Body Trends Online offers a variety of health and fitness articles. Articles include "Are You Overweight?," "About Your Heart," "What to Look For in a Personal Trainer," "Set Up Your Own Home Gym," and "Treadmill Maintenance Tips."

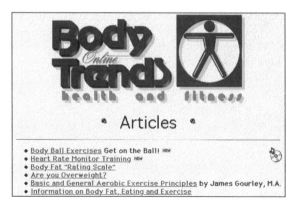

Boots

http://www.boots.co.uk/

Boots, a leading pharmacy house in Great Britain, provides a variety of health and nutrition resources. The site includes a vitamin database, a section on your health with exercise tips, and an extensive library with information on homeopathy, immunization, and sugar in drinks.

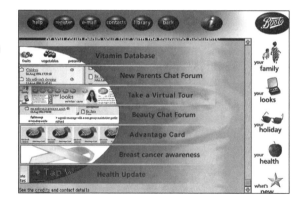

Calorie Control Council

http://www.caloriecontrol.org/

Calorie Control Council provides information on cutting calories and fat in your diet, achieving and maintaining a healthy weight, and a listing of your favorite low-calorie, reduced-fat foods and beverages. The site includes an online calorie counter calculator, low-fat recipes, and 2000 calories-a-day meal plans for one week.

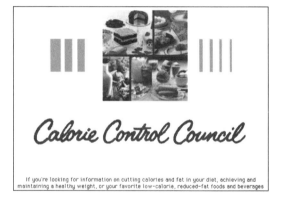

Center for Science in the Public Interest

http://www.cspinet.org/

The Center for Science in the Public Interest is a smorgasbord of delights on health and fitness. The site includes *Nutrition Action Healthletter,* nutrition quizzes, cool sites, and booze news.

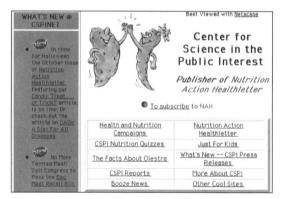

Cholesterol How-Low-Can-U-Go Quizsite

http://www.bev.net/health/lipid/

Cholesterol How-Low-Can-U-Go Quizsite is an online question-and-answer quiz designed to find out what you know and what you don't know about cholesterol and your heart. The site also includes related heart sites.

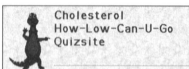

Christine

http://medialab.jmu.edu/christin/

Christine's home page is a one-stop collection of nutrition, health, and fitness resources. The **Links** page includes an alphabetical index with brief descriptions of each site, and the **Cooking** page contains Christine's healthy low-fat recipes such as black bean salad, jambalaya, and stuffed chicken.

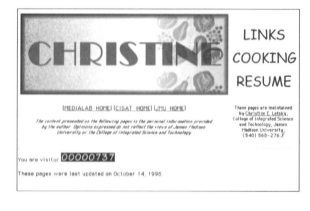

CNN Interactive Fitness and Health

http://cnnplus.cnn.com/consumer/health

CNN Interactive Fitness and Health contains a consumer medical library with information on a variety of health topics, including abortion, obesity, smoking, sleeping conditions, and many others. In addition, CNN's Allergy Report has daily updates on pollen levels across the United States.

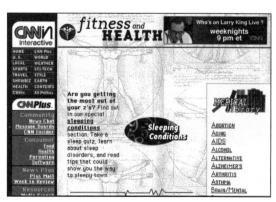

CNN Interactive Food

http://cnnplus.cnn.com/consumer/food/

CNN Interactive Food offers a wonderful array of interactive food and nutrition resources. The site contains a nutritional comparison of your favorite foods, quick facts and health information for alcohol, carbohydrates, fat, protein, and other items, and recipes for cooking light. In adddition, CNN provides the latest breaking news on a variety of topics, with related links, ranging from additives to vitamins and minerals.

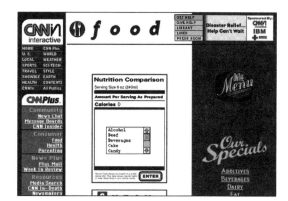

The Cook's Thesaurus

http://www.northcoast.com/~alden/cookhome.html

The Cook's Thesaurus, compiled by Lori Alden, suggests substitutions for thousands of cooking ingredients, including low-calorie and low-fat alternatives for dieters, inexpensive substitutes for gourmets on a budget, and innovative replacements for hard-to-find ethnic ingredients.

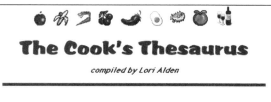

The Crazy Vegetarian

http://www.crazyveg.com/splash.html

The Crazy Vegetarian is a fun place for vegetarians, vegans, and wanna-bes. The site provides useful information, including recipes, facts, links, news and events, and a bookstore.

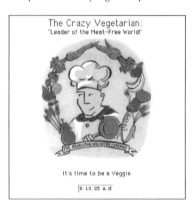

CyberDiet

http://www.cyberdiet.com/

CyberDiet provides information about diet, exercise, and nutrition. General categories include video exercise, nutrition, food facts, exercise tips, and eating right. A Daily Meal Planner features an interactive tool to help meet your nutritional needs.

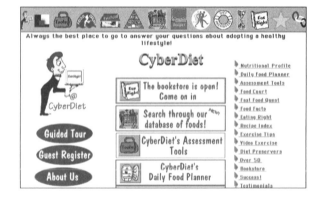

CyberNutrition On-Line

http://chd.syr.edu/CyberNutrition2.html

CyberNutrition On-Line, from the Syracuse University College for Human Development, answers your questions about food, nutrition, or diet. The site provides archives of questions and answers sorted into topics.

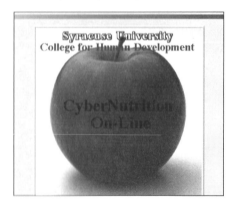

Diabetic Gourmet Magazine

http://gourmetconnection.com/diabetic/

The Diabetic Gourmet Magazine provides information and resources dedicated to diabetic dining and healthy living. The site includes exciting recipes, feature articles, and lots of diet-related reading. This magazine is also a great resource for nondiabetics looking for recipes and health information.

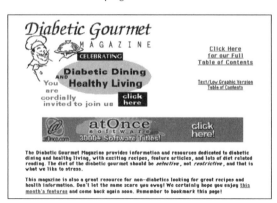

Diet & Weight Loss/Fitness

http://www1.mhv.net/~donn/diet.html

The Diet and Weight Loss/Fitness home page is a comprehensive resource of information, knowledge, and support for losing weight and keeping it off. Categories include new information, understanding what it's all about, eating the right stuff, moving and exercising, support and newsgroups, and meta-index links.

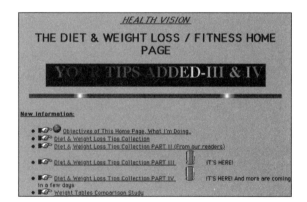

Dieting and Your Health

http://www.best.com/~westraw/Book.html

Dieting and Your Health provides chapter outlines of Dr. William E. Straw's book, *Stop Dieting Before It Kills You,* which explains why dieting doesn't work.

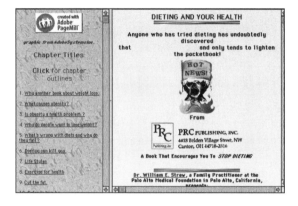

Dr. Pribut's Running Injuries Page

http://www.clark.net/pub/pribut/spsport.html

Dr. Pribut's Running Injuries Page provides advice from a podiatrist for treating and preventing any type of running injury. The site includes an online text for runners and athletes on training protocols and the treatment of common sports injuries and an exhaustive list of links to other sports pages.

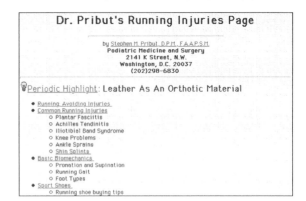

Eat Right America

http://www.eatright.org/

Eat Right America, the American Dietetic Association home page, contains a variety of online nutrition resources for the consumer. Click on **Tip for Today!** to find a health tip posted on weekdays and an archive of **previously posted tips.** You will also find a collection of nutrition **Fact Sheets** in the hot topics section and an alphabetical list of nutrition resources in the **gateway to nutrition** section.

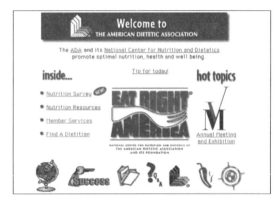

The Eat Well Calculator

http://homearts.com/helpers/calculators/ddiary.htm

The Eat Well Calculator is an interactive calculator. You tell the experts the servings you ate from each major food group and they in turn tell you how well you are doing.

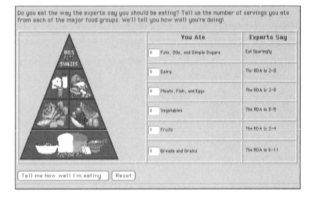

Eating in America Today

http://www.ncanet.org/industry_research/eat2_table.html

Eating in America Today, an online book sponsored by the National Livestock and Meat Board, covers a variety of nutrition topics, including the food pyramid, meat's role in America's diet, and dietary patterns of meat eaters.

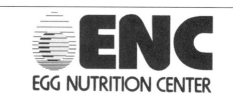

Egg Nutrition Center

http://www.enc-online.org/

The Egg Nutrition Center (ENC) offers a variety of online resources with information about eggs. The site includes newsletters and publications, news, information about eggs and cholesterol, and links to related sites.

Epicurious Food Menu

http://food.epicurious.com/

Epicurious Food Menu, presented by *Bon Appétit* and *Gourmet* magazines, offers a rich variety of resources for healthy eating, including over 6000 recipes, tips from great cooks, and many discussion forums. The site also includes a dictionary and reference guides for herbs and spices and metric conversions. The recipe file is updated monthly.

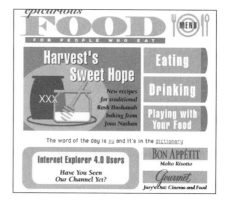

Family.com Food

http://www.family.com/Categories/Food/

Family.com Food contains thousands of recipes and menus for family healthy dining. The site includes a search feature for finding recipes and a shopping list to help you plan a week's menus.

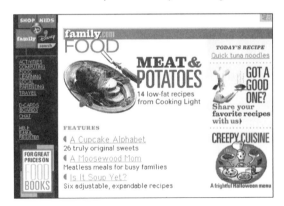

Fatfree: The Low Fat Vegetarian Archive

http://www.fatfree.com/

Fatfree: The Low Fat Vegetarian Archive contains over 2500 fat-free and low-fat vegetarian recipes, as well as information about healthy low-fat vegetarian diets. Click on the **searchable recipe archive** to find over 50 categories, including soups, casseroles, desserts, pasta, and pizza. New recipes are added on a regular basis.

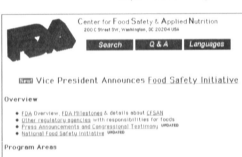

FDA Center for Food Safety & Applied Nutrition

http://vm.cfsan.fda.gov/list.html

FDA Center for Food Safety & Applied Nutrition contains a huge amount of useful information. Scroll to the section Special Interest Matters and click on **Consumer Advice from FDA** to find information about food and drug interactions, dietary guidelines for America, women's health, and much more.

FitLife

http://www.fitlife.com/

FitLife is an electronic resource of fitness, health promotion, wellness, and lifestyle with physical exercise guidelines and tips for getting and staying fit. The site includes information on health and wellness, nutrition, weight control, low-fat recipes, cooking tips, stress management, substance abuse, and related links. Many of the articles can be heard via RealAudio.

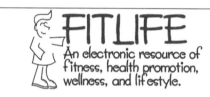

The Fitness Files

http://chitrib.webpoint.com/fitness

The *Chicago Tribune's* Fitness Files offers fitness fundamentrals at your fingertips. Click on **Get Active** and then browse the **Fitness Activity index.** This index includes workout tips, a list of required equipment, and advice on the benefits and risks of the activity. One of the most helpful sections is the **Injurenet,** which includes our favorite feature, Tell the Clickable Person Where It Hurts. Also worth looking into are the Injurenet's tips on how to make the office pain-free.

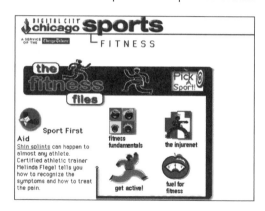

Fitness Partner Connection Jumpsite!

http://primusweb.com/fitnesspartner/

Fitness Partner Connection Jumpsite! is a giant Web site. It offers everything you could possibly want to know about fitness and nutrition and their relationship to health. Many articles are offered on a diverse range of topics, including aerobics, meditation, weight management, yoga, fitness clubs and gyms, and healthy vacations. A search tool is provided.

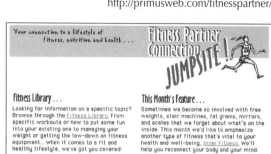

FitnessLink

http://www.fitnesslink.com/

FitnessLink discusses the ins and outs of regular exercise, including topics such as Why Should I Exercise?, Stretching Exercises, Changing to Low-Fat Cooking, and How Many Calories am I Burning When I Exercise? Links to related sites include those focusing on body building, aerobic exercise, exercise programs, and diet and nutrition.

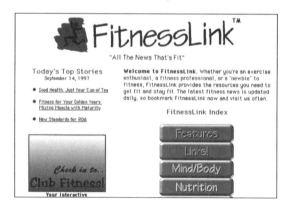

Fitnessonline.com

http://www.fitnessonline.com/

Fitnessonline.com provides a wide variety of fitness and nutrition resources. The Nutribase contains everything you need to know about nutrition; the Searchable Workouts is an excellent source for keeping workout routines exciting and fresh; Reuters Newswire gives the latest fitness and health headlines; and the magazine collection offers exercise tips, healthy recipes, and general health information.

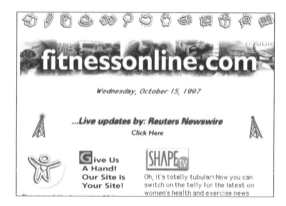

FitnessWorld

http://www.fitnessworld.com/

FitnessWorld offers fitness resources for professionals and enthusiasts. Features also include products, reference and news, chat forums, announcements, and events and programs.

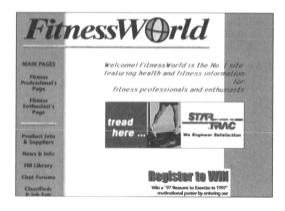

Flora's Recipe Hideout

http://www.deter.com/flora/recipes.html

Flora's Recipe Hideout contains thousands of recipes for low-fat food, desserts, cheesecakes, and chocolate.

Food & Nutrition

http://www.gsa.gov/staff/pa/cic/food.htm

Food & Nutrition, a part of the Consumer Information Catalog, offers a collection of health and nutrition articles, including "Action Guide for Healthy Living" and "Eat Right to Help Lower Your High Blood Pressure." To find a wealth of other articles, click on **More Publications About Food & Nutrition** and click on **Additional Resources** for the topics Food and Nutrition.

Food & Nutrition Newsletter

http://www.ext.vt.edu/news/periodicals/foods/

The Food & Nutrition Newsletter, from the Virginia Cooperative Extension, is a rich bibliographic index to other sources with topics such as dietary guidelines, food products, nutrition education, and package labeling. Its most commonly cited sources are *Consumer Reports* and the *Monthly Journal of the Food and Drug Administration.*

Food & Nutrition Solutions Series

http://www.ag.uiuc.edu/~robsond/solutions/nutrition.html

The Food & Nutrition Solutions Series, maintained by the Illinois Cooperative Extension Service, offers a great deal of information about food buying and preparation, food preservation and food safety, and food storage. In addition, a glossary, a nutritional analysis of selected foods, and a food substitution guide in recipes are provided.

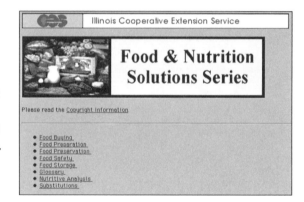

Food and Nutrition Information Center

http://www.nal.usda.gov/fnic/

The Food and Nutrition Information Center, maintained by the U.S. Department of Agriculture, provides a number of informational databases on food safety, general nutrition, nutrition education, foodborne illnesses, dietary guidelines, and food composition. The site also contains a healthy school meals resource and an index of food and nutrition resources with thousands of topics arranged alphabetically.

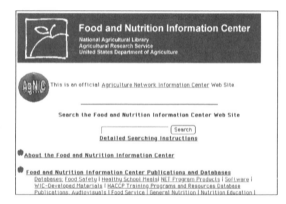

Food Finder

http://www.olen.com/food/

Food Finder, by Olen Publishing and based on the book, *Fast Food Facts,* is an interactive calorie and fat calculator for major fast food chains with a searchable database of nutrition information.

The Food Pyramid Guide

http://www.ganesa.com/food/

The Food Pyramid Guide presents a brief discussion of each of the different food groups. The site also offers links to related sites.

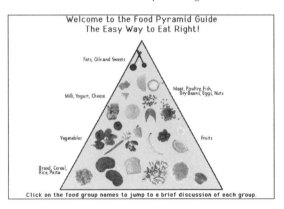

Frequently Asked Questions (FAQ) about Health and Fat People

http://www.comlab.ox.ac.uk/oucl/users/
sharon.curtis/BigFolks/health_FAQ.html

Frequently Asked Questions (FAQ) about Health and Fat People contains information about health issues for fat people. Many articles are offered that relate not only to being overweight as such, but also to those medical conditions often associated with being overweight. Numerous links to other resources, as well as bibliographic references, are available.

Get Healthy

http://www.rightfoods.com/

Dr. John McDougall, a nutrition expert and an internist, offers a diet program described as the "optimum way to health and weight." The site provides the basics of nutrition, current nutrition research findings, and the ways in which The McDougall Plan helps with certain maladies. In addition, there are tips on healthy ways of eating, vegetarian recipes, as well as the doctor's radio show broadcast in RealAudio.

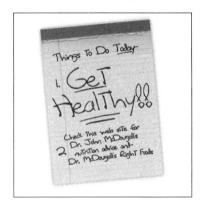

The Good Health Web

http://www.social.com/health/

The Good Health Web emphasizes prevention of illness through nutrition, exercise, and other practices related to a healthy lifestyle. It brings together a broad range of resources related to personal health. One of these is a U.S. government database of over 1000 health organizations throughout the country. The site includes a search tool and numerous links.

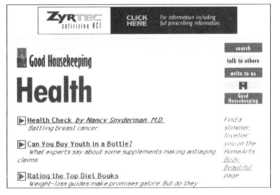

Good Housekeeping Health

http://homearts.com/gh/toc/oshealth.htm

Good Housekeeping Health contains a collection of short articles to help improve your lifestyle. Among the articles are "Improve Your Diet," "Secondhand Smoke," "The Fitness Connection" series, and "Nutritional Drinks."

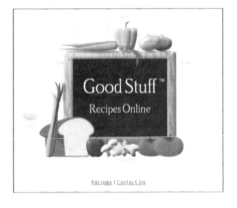

Good Stuff

http://www.goodstuffonline.com/

Good Stuff provides a collection of healthy recipes for entrees, breads, soups, and desserts. The site also includes a glossary with cooking terms, measurements, and conversion equivalents for the recipes.

Great Vegetarian Recipes!

http://members.aol.com/meadowscd/recipes/

Great Vegetarian Recipes!, collected by Debbie Meadows, contains an extensive list, including low-fact recipes.

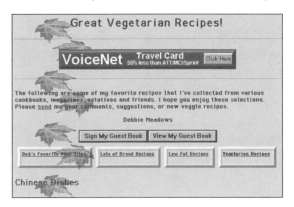

Guardian's Health and Fitness

http://pages.prodigy.com/guardian/fitness.htm

Guardian's Health and Fitness pages contain a collection of sites for overall fitness, aerobics, stretching, massage, and body building.

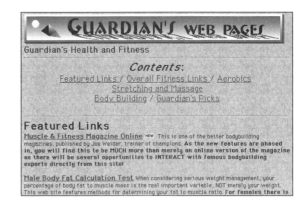

A Guide to Feeding Solid Food

http://www.beechnut.com/solid.htm

A Guide to Feeding Solid Food, from Beech-Nut, offers information about solid baby food in four categories: (1) starting solid foods, (2) feeding tips and other useful information, (3) FAQs about feeding solids, and (4) basic food groups for your baby.

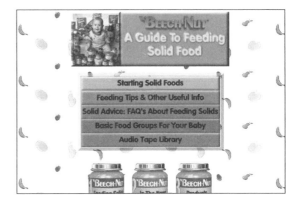

Health & Fitness

http://www.aisp.net/health.htm

The Health & Fitness home page is a collection of sites with information on a healthier lifestyle, environmental health, training and body building tips, fitness, nutrition, and vitamins.

Absolute Health	Many look , . Few See. . (Old Indian proverb.) . . . Philosophy pertaining to a healthier lifestyle
ATSDR (Agency for Toxic Substances and Disease Registry)	Science Corner is a simple guide to search the World Wide Web for environmental health information.
Body Mechanics	Training Tips, Nutrition hints and recipes, bodybuilding tips and information.
FITS Basics and Information	This Flexible Image Transport System (FITS) information is provided by the FITS Support Office, operated under the guidance of the Astrophysics Data Facility at the NASA Goddard Space Flight Center.

Health & Fitness

http://www.vonl.com/vtab12/health.htm

Health and Fitness, from Village Online, provides links to medical, expectant parents, fitness, and nutrition sites.

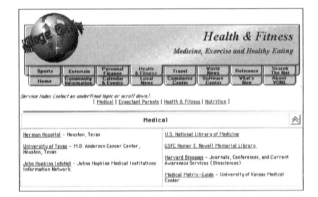

Health & Fitness
Worldguide Forum

http://www.worldguide.com/Fitness/hf.html

The Health & Fitness Worldguide Forum provides a wealth of information on a broad range of topics, including anatomy, weight training, cardiovascular exercise, eating well, and sports medicine.

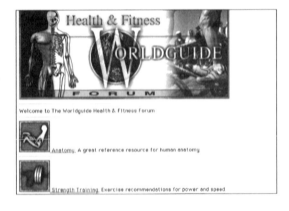

Health & You Online

http://www.ibx.com/healthnyou/

Health & You Online has nutrition resources, including food information on vegetables, fish, grains, and beverages, and a one-week program to low-fat eating with menus and recipes. The site also features a **Wellness** center with healthy lifestyles information, preventive health education brochures, and related links.

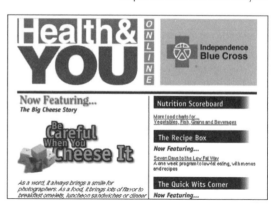

The Health Authority

http://www.healthauthority.com/

The Health Authority, edited by Dr. Albert Jerome, offers a large collection of articles, compiled from many sources, that discuss issues such as tobacco addiction, weight loss, cholesterol management, hypertension, and exercise.

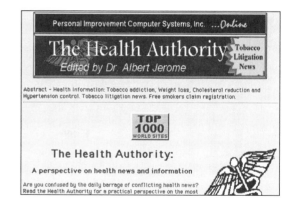

Health Spa

http://gourmetconnection.com/healt697.shtml

Health Spa, from the *Gourmet Connection* magazine, has information and resources related to nutrition, exercise, fitness, therapy, and other healthful things. The site also includes calorie and fat charts and a collection of related links.

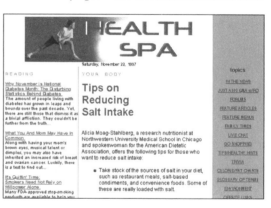

Healthy Choice

http://www.healthychoice.com/

Healthy Choice offers an assortment of online nutrition resources, including recipes, food information, menu planners, and related links. The site contains a rich array of features, including a healthy news archives of nutrition articles, a personal trainer with fitness tips, an FAQ section containing chat rooms, a nutrition test, and an online nutritionist.

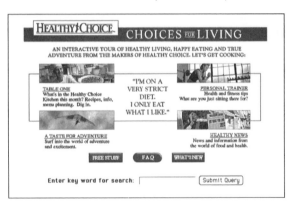

Healthy Ideas
Vitamin Dispenser

http://www.healthyideas.com/healing/vitamin/

Healthy Ideas Vitamin Dispenser provides a wealth of information and the correct vitamin dosage for over 75 conditions and ailments.

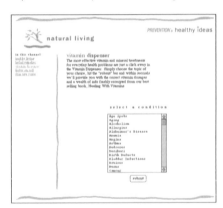

Healthy Nutrition

http://www.lbcommunity.com/family/yhnut.html

Healthy Nutrition, provided by the Long Beach Community Medical Center in Southern California, contains a variety of nutrition resources. Take an interactive quiz to test your nutrition quotient or read an informative article from a collection ranging from safe summers to keys to nutritional success. The site also offers healthy recipes.

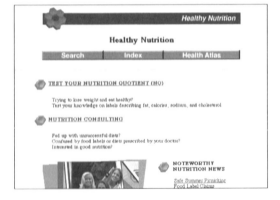

Healthy Recipes

http://www1.sympatico.ca/healthyway/HEALTHYWAY/hrecipes.html

Healthy Recipes, from HealthyWay, is a collection of links to over 2000 recipes organized by meal type and special diet. The site also provides a collection of nutritious recipes and drinks that can be accessed by clicking on **Incredible Edibles.** The site is updated weekly with new recipes, tips, and articles.

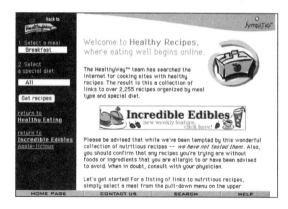

Healthy Weight

http://healthyweight.com/

Healthy Weight features an interactive body mass index (BMI) calculator to help you manage your weight. There is also news about weight management and information for a healthier lifestyle.

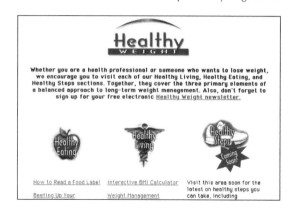

HomeArts Body & Soul

http://www.homearts.com/depts/health/00dphec1.htm

HomeArts Body & Soul provides a wide variety of consumer health resources that include sections on pregnancy and childbirth, health headlines, preventing or dealing with cancer, managing your weight, an ask the doctors feature, discussion forums, and special features such as the healthy traveler and managing menopause.

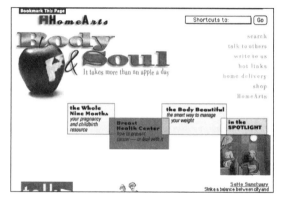

HomeArts Eats

http://homearts.com/depts/food/00dpfdc1.htm

HomeArts Eats offers an assortment of resources for nutrition and fitness. Among these are a recipe finder with thousands of healthy recipes, articles providing information and tips for making the body beautiful, the cook's corner, related links, and discussion groups.

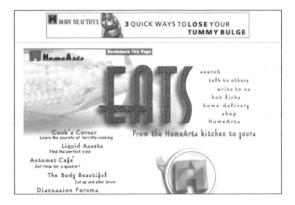

Human Kinetics

http://www.humankinetics.com/

Human Kinetics, an information leader in physical activities, contains a collection of over 2000 sites for every imaginable sports activity. To find this collection, click on **Links** in the InfoKinetics section.

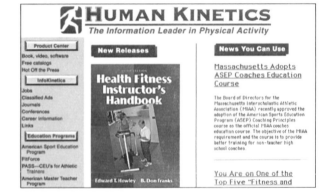

International Food Information Council

http://ificinfo.health.org/

The International Food Information Council provides guides and information on health and nutrition in the **Food Safety and Nutrition** section.

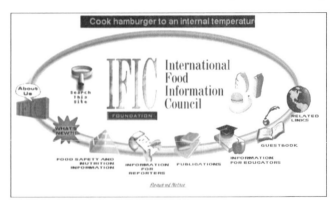

Internet Food Channel

http://www.foodchannel.com/

The Internet Food Channel features an assortment of food and nutrition resources. The site contains a food wire service that provides daily food headlines and past news stories. Other features include a daily food fact along with its archive, ethnic recipes, the food pyramid, restaurant reviews, a chat room, and newsgroups. To view the site's table of contents, click on **Index.**

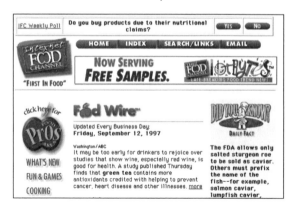

The Internet's Fitness Resource

http://rampages.onramp.net/~chaz/

The Internet's Fitness Resource offers a comprehensive listing of fitness-related sites, as well as a weekly editorial on nutrition, the fitness plan, and more!

Just Ask!

http://gourmetconnection.com/ezine/justask/

Just Ask!, a service of *Gourmet Connection* magazine, allows you to ask questions about nutrition, food science, and diet. Donna Handley, a registered dietician and an university health science professor, will post an answer within two weeks. You can also search and browse the archives of past questions and answers.

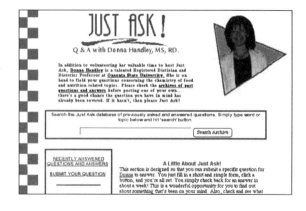

The Kitchen Link

http://www.kitchenlink.com/

The Kitchen Link, compiled by Betsy Couch, is a virtual recipe box filled with over 7000 links to food and cooking sites. To find recipes for kids, diets, food allergies, and other health-related topics, scroll to **TKL Site Index** and check out the Hot Topics area, or go to **On the Menu** to find healthy, fat-free or low-fat, or diabetic recipes, and thousands of others.

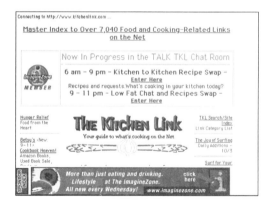

Krispin Komments on Nutrition and Health

http://www.krispin.com/

Krispin Komments on Nutrition and Health provides nutrition and health information on magnesium, potassium, proteins, and the thyroid.

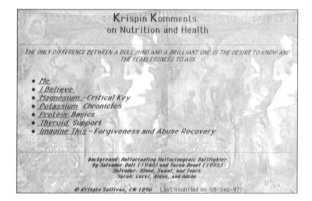

LifeLines @ Work

http://www.lifelines.com/

LifeLines @ Work presents monthly an online newsletter, *HealthStyle,* featuring articles on eating right, keeping fit, not smoking, staying well, and other topics. The site also includes a health science library with an A to Z index of articles on nutrition and prevention and links to many nutrition and fitness sites.

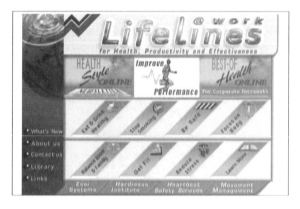

LifeMatters

http://lifematters.com/

LifeMatters offers counseling, biofeedback, physical education, and t'ai chi health care resources. The site is an interactive forum and features a variety of authors, interviews, and discussions relevant to the quest for well-being. To view the table of contents, click on **Site Map.** You can also post questions on fitness, health, nutrition, and other matters.

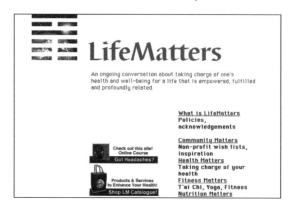

Light Cooking

http://www.lightcooking.com/

Light Cooking features low-fat, low-cholesterol cooking for a healthy lifestyle. The site includes recipes and tips, a kids page, and cooking and health questions and answers.

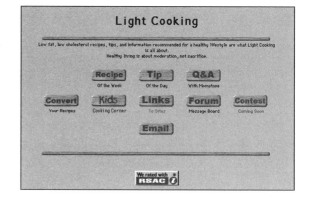

Low Fat 4 Life

http://www.lowfat4life.com/myframes.html

Low Fat 4 Life features articles and an index of recipe categories ranging from appetizers to vegetables. Each recipe includes preparation time.

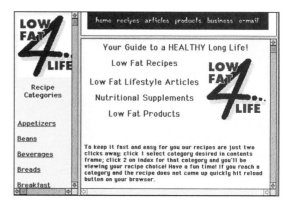

The Low-Fat Lifestyle Forum

http://www.wctravel.com/lowfat/

The Low-Fat Lifestyle Forum offers people a place to exchange ideas and tips for living a low-fat lifestyle. The site provides useful information on many healthier living topics, hundreds of low-fat recipes ranging from appetizers to soups and stews, and food-related links and newsgroups.

Welcome to the Low-Fat Lifestyle Forum

This forum is for people who are interested in adopting a low-fat lifestyle or for those who are already living a low-fat lifestyle. My husband and I currently consume 20-40 grams of fat each day. I count grams of fat rather than calculate the percentage of fat/calories because I find it much easier and less complicated. Our daily fat percentage of calories runs from 10% to 20%. Today we have lost a significant amount of weight and we are very healthy and full of energy. Living a low-fat lifestyle is not difficult, it just takes a little organization and a committment to change the way you eat as a lifestyle change, not as a diet. The problem with a diet is that when you think about going on a diet, you think of it as having a beginning and an end. The end is the problem. I have been on numerous diets in my lifetime and lost more weight than I care to think about, only to gain it all back in less time than it took to lose it! Making a commitment to living a low-fat lifestyle for the rest of your life is the key. All the recipes in this forum are 15

MasterCook Recipe Library

http://www.sierra.com/titles/mastercook4/library/

MasterCook Recipe Library contains thousands of quick, healthy, and gourmet recipes that can be viewed online. Recipe categories include appetizers, healthy and hearty, special diets, and vegetarian.

MASTERCOOK
recipe
library

▶ home
▶ search for recipes...
▶ help

Appetizers
Beverages
Breads
Breakfast
Desserts
Ethnic
Fish and Seafood
Fruits and Vegetables
Healthy and Hearty
Meats
Miscellaneous
Snacks
Soups and Salads
Southwestern
Special Diets
Vegetarian

welcome to the Recipe Library. Here you'll find an exciting variety of recipes to add to your collection — quick, healthy, gourmet, and everything in between. We add new recipes frequently, so come back often!

Whether looking for a particular recipe, trying to expand your recipe collection, or just browsing, our Recipe Library is the place to go. We offer thousands of recipes for viewing on-line, and if you're a MasterCook user, you can download entire cookbooks in MasterCook format or have the server send exported recipes to you in e-mail.

To begin browsing the library, click on a bookshelf at the left, a list of cookbooks on that "shelf" will appear. You can browse the recipes in each cookbook by selecting "View Recipes," or you can click on another category and/or cookbook to see its contents.

your own personal recipe box
When you search for recipes, our server stores a personal list of the recipes you find. This list is saved for one week from the time of your last access, so each time you come back to this site it will be waiting for you.

The MetaMetrix Nutrition Resource

http://www.metametrix.com/~nutrition/contents.htm

The MetaMetrix Nutrition Resource advises users of the latest research and technology related to nutritional science. For example, the category entitled Nutrition News contains information about nutritional supplements, anabolic steroids, chronic fatigue, and amino acids. Other categories consider topics such as products and the laboratory testing of blood and urine samples to determine individual nutritional needs.

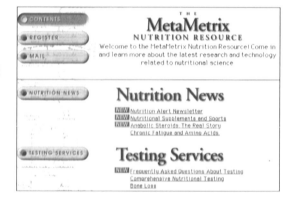

Mirkin Report for Healthier Living

htttp://www.wdn.com/mirkin

Dr. Gabe Mirkin presents an extensive index to topics of a broad medical interest. Based on Dr. Mirkin's CBS radio program, each article is a transcript that addresses some curious or interesting aspect of health or medicine. Every article is presented in clear language and is easily understood by the layperson. A search tool is provided for further inquiries.

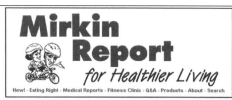

Breakthroughs in Health and Fitness by Dr. Gabe Mirkin

Last updated on July 22, 1997

This site has been rated among the top 5% of all web sites by Point Survey.

National Institute of Nutrition

http://www.nin.ca/conscorn.htm

National Institute of Nutrition, Canada's source of reliable nutrition information, contains tips and information on nutrition in its Consumer's Corner, which is updated weekly and includes an interactive quiz, healthy eating tips, and an online quarterly newsletter, *Healthy Bites,* with articles on nutrition.

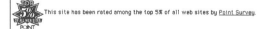

Consumers' Corner

Enjoy healthy eating year-round. We hope these tips help!

SPOTTING THE INVISIBLE FATS

You can't miss the fat in margarine or butter, or the fat around a steak – it's visible. But the fats in muffins or ice cream may escape you. Nutrition labels can help make that invisible fat "visible".

- Claims will highlight products that are "fat free" (almost no fat), "low in fat" (less than 3 grams per serving) or which have a major fat reduction.
- When a claim about fat is made, the amount of fat in a serving must be on the label; it is required by government.
- Note that a product that has been "reduced in fat" (at least 25% less fat) may not be low in fat.

National Pasta Association

http://www.ilovepasta.org/

The National Pasta Association Web site provides a variety of resources for pasta. Among these are facts and answers to FAQs, nutrition and pasta shapes information, and an assortment of pasta recipes.

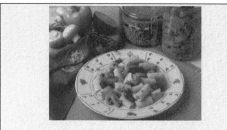

Welcome to the National Pasta Association's World Wide Web site!

Here, pasta lovers will find pasta recipes, pasta FAQs (Frequently Asked Questions) and Facts, pasta nutrition, and pasta shapes information.

NewTrition

http://newtrition.com/front.htm

The NewTrition site contains stories, recipes, columns, and issues of interest for anyone interested in nutrition and health.

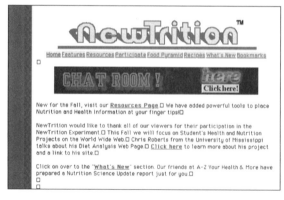

The No Milk Page

http://www.panix.com/~nomilk/

The No Milk Page provides resources for millions of people who must be cautious about consuming milk and milk by-products. The site contains nutritional fact sheets, essays, articles, recipes, charts, studies, and even poetry.

Non-Dairy: Something to Moo About

http://www.non-dairy.org/

Non-Dairy: Something to Moo About is an online magazine for non-dairy families. The site contains milk allergy basics FAQs, Moo News with monthly updates, shopping ideas for dairy-free substitutions, articles on cooking tips, parenting articles on how to help your allergic child live a happy dairy-free childhood at home and school, nutrition and medical articles, a product index of dairy-free food, and related links.

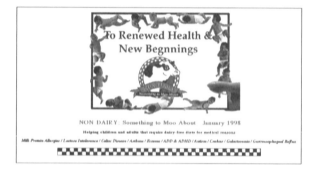

Notes on the World of Healthy Cooking

http://home1.gte.net/nigro/

Notes on the World of Healthy Cooking Web site is based on the book, *Companion Guide to Healthy Cooking: A Practical Introduction to Natural Ingredients.* The site provides practical information and "how-tos" about using healthy ingredients. There are links to **Changing Your Diet, Kitchen Tips,** and an **Ingredient Guide.**

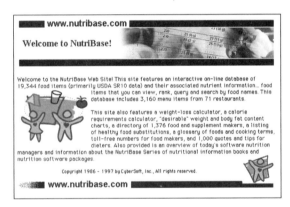

NutriBase

http://www.nutribase.com/

NutriBase features an interactive online database of over 19,000 food items and their associated nutrient information. The site also includes a weight loss calculator, a calorie requirements calculator, "desirable" weight and body fat content charts, a directory of 1376 food and supplement makers, a listing of healthy food substitutions, a glossary of foods and cooking terms, toll-free numbers for food makers, and 1000 quotes and tips for dieters.

NutriSite

http://www.nutrisite.com/

NutriSite contains information designed to help people improve their health and eating habits. The site includes the Canada Food Guide, shopping guide, serving sizes, common foods and their nutritional value, links to heath sites, and women's nutrition.

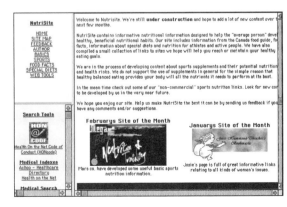

Nutrition Analysis Tool

http://www.ag.uiuc.edu/~food-lab/nat/

The Nutrition Analysis Tool is a Web-based program that allows you to analyze the foods you eat for various different nutrients.

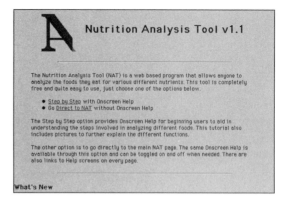

Nutrition and Health

http://www.medlib.arizona.edu/educ/nutrition.html

Nutrition and Health, from the Arizona Health Sciences Library, is a rich source of information about a great many areas related to health and nutrition. General categories include exercise and fitness, nutrition and foods industry, herbs and herbal medicine, diatetics sources, food safety, consumer information, and foods and recipes. A search tool is provided.

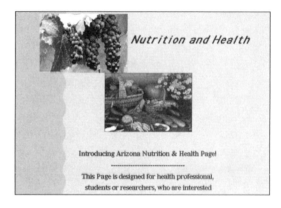

Nutrition and Your Health: Dietary Guidelines for Americans

http://www.nalusda.gov/fnic/dga/dguide95.html

Nutrition and Your Health: Dietary Guidelines for Americans offers advice about food choices that promote health and prevent disease. The site is an enormous resource to those who wish to know more about the specific elements of nutrition and how it relates to healthful living.

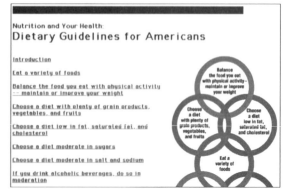

Nutrition Fact Sheets

http://www.eatright.org/nufactsheet.html

The American Dietetic Association offers approximately 65 Nutrition Fact Sheets on a wide range of topics about healthful eating. Sample articles include "Picking Snacks for Picky Eaters," "Good News for Nut Lovers," "Food Labels for Infants Under Two Years," "Facts About Olestra," "Focus on Fiber," and "For the Love of Chocolate."

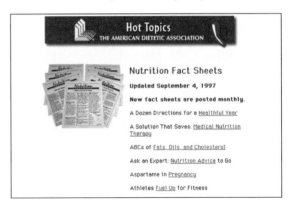

Nutrition, Food, and Health

http://www.mes.umn.edu/Nutrition/

Nutrition, Food, and Health, a service of the University of Minnesota Extension Service, assists people in making informed decisions to improve their health and quality of life. Articles attempt to put information about food, health, and disease into perspective. Access is provided to current and past issues of the *Minnesota Expanded Food and Nutrition Program Newsletter* and to a search tool.

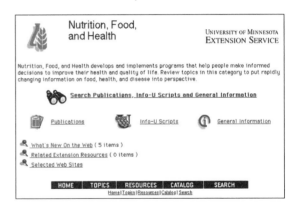

Nutrition Navigator

http://navigator.tufts.edu/

Nutrition Navigator, from Tufts University School of Nutrition, provides an online rating and review guide that helps you quickly find useful and accurate information on nutrition. The site covers topics such as general nutrition, women, kids, special dietary needs, health professionals, and other topics.

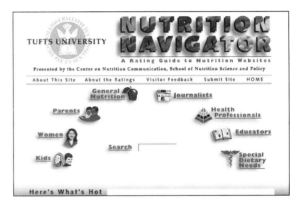

ParentsPlace.com

http://www.parentsplace.com/genobject.cgi/
readroom/recipes/recipes.html

Parentsplace.com offers a list of hundreds of healthy recipes for baby food, salads, soups, sauces, dips and spreads, chili, side dishes, breakfast, easy dinners, vegetables, and much more. Click on **Nutrition Center** to ask nutritionist Sue Gilbert a question or read Sue's large collection of past answers arranged by topic from starting solids to nutritional guidelines.

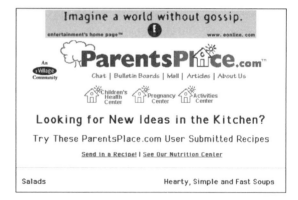

Personal Food & Nutrition Center

http://www.medilife.com/medilife/diabetes/culinary/

Personal Food & Nutrition Center, from MediLife, offers a database that analyzes the nutritional value of over 16,000 foods. It also gives tips for weight loss and presents help with meal planning, chiefly in the form of healthful recipes. Additional information considers the benefits of regular exercise and its overall relationship to general health and longevity.

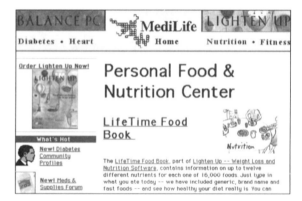

Phys Calculators

http://www.phys.com/c_tools/02calculator/calc_intro.htm

Phys Calculators is a collection of eight, easy-to-use online calculators that provide measurement information for staying fit and healthy. The calculators include a body mass index (BMI), ideal weight, and health risk assessment.

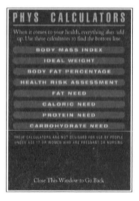

Phys Nutrition for Normal People

http://www.phys.com/

Phys Nutrition for Normal People, an online interactive magazine for health-conscious women in their twenties, thirties, and forties, has articles and information from a number of sources, including the U.S. Department of Agriculture. The site includes measuring tools for self-analysis, daily fat-fighting tips, an encyclopedia of nutrients and additives, and discussion boards. The site's personal nutritionist will also provide a customized diet plan and a sample menu.

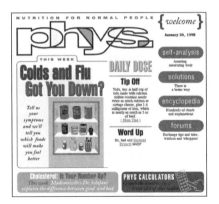

Physical Activity and Health

http://www.cdc.gov/nccdphp/sgr/sgr.htm

Physical Activity and Health, a 1996 report from the Surgeon General of the United States, stresses the importance of exercise in reducing the risk of developing or dying from hypertension, coronary heart disease, non-insulin–dependent diabetes, and colon cancer.

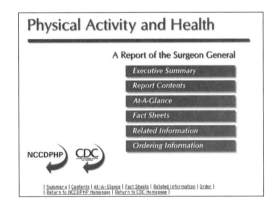

Professor Geoff Skurray's Food, Nutrition & Health Information Page

http://www.hawkesbury.uws.edu.au/~geoffs/

Professor Geoff Skurray's Food, Nutrition & Health Information Page, from the Centre for Advanced Food Research at the University of Western Sydney (Hawkesbury), provides extensive information about food composition, including proteins, carbohydrates, cholesterol, fiber energy, vitamins, minerals, and food additives. The site also has information on diet and disease, weight reduction, and toxins in foods.

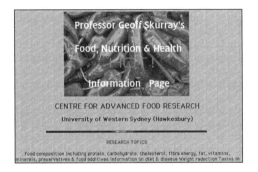

Recipe Archive Index

http://www.cs.cmu.edu/People/mjw/recipes/

The Recipe Archive Index contains a food and cooking recipe collection from Amy Gale's newsgroup. Recipe topics include pasta, salads, seafood, vegetable, and K. Young's special recipes for diabetics.

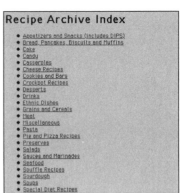

The Recipes Folder

http://eserver.org/recipes/

The Recipes Folder, part of the English Server Web site, contains vegetarian recipes and links to sites for healthy eating.

Redbook Diet & Health

http://homearts.com/rb/toc/00rbhec1.htm

Diet & Health, from *Redbook* magazine, offers selected articles on diet, health, and fitness.

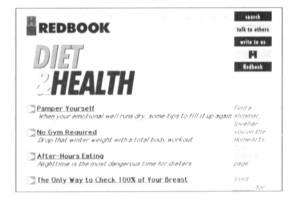

Runner's World Online

http://www.runnersworld.com/

Runner's World Online has a variety of health topics for runners, including first aid and home cures for 36 of the most common running injuries, nutrition information, and women's links.

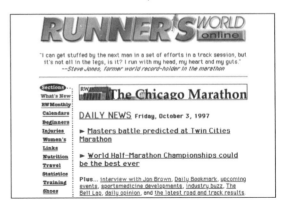

Sainsbury's Fresh Food, Fresh Ideas

http://www.sainsburys.co.uk/

Sainsbury's Fresh Food, Fresh Ideas provides nutrition and food safety advice to help you choose a healthy balanced diet, as well as offering tips and recommendations on the preparation and storage of food. The site also includes information for vegetarians and people with special dietary needs. For over 1000 of their mouthwatering recipes, click on **Recipes.**

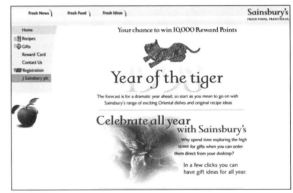

The Science of Obesity and Weight Control

http://www.loop.com/~bkrentzman/

The Science of Obesity and Weight Control, maintained by Dr. Ben Z. Krentzman, provides information about weight control. Scroll to the **Table of Contents** for current news about weight control medicines such as Phen-Fen. In addition, there is information about a *Weight Control Handbook* and medications, numerous articles, and hundreds of links to obesity sites.

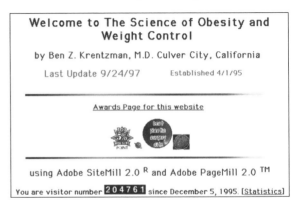

Searchable Online Archive of Recipes

http://soar.Berkeley.EDU/recipes/

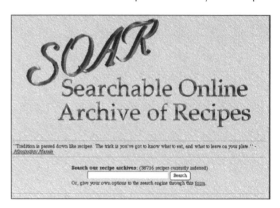

The Searchable Online Archive of Recipes, part of the Recipe Ring, is a searchable database of nearly 40,000 recipes for healthy eating. The recipes are sorted by main dishes; soups, stews, and chili; breads and baked goods; fruits, grains, and vegetables; on the side; sweets and desserts; snacks and appetizers; breakfast dishes; special occasions; and restricted and special diets. The site also offers nutrition information in the miscellaneous category.

Shape Up America!

http://www2.shapeup.org/sua/

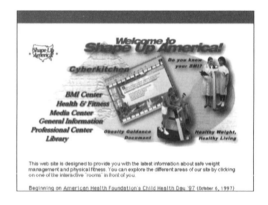

Shape Up America! provides the latest information about safe weight management and physical fitness. The site includes an online guide to healthy eating in the **Cyberkitchen** section, an interactive calculator in the **BMI Center** for determining body mass index (BMI), a health club in the **Health & Fitness Center** for assessing your fitness level and finding out about different types of physical activity, and a reading room in the **Library** with online publications such as *Eating Smart* and *99 Tips for Family Fitness Fun.*

Sportfit.com

http://www.sportfit.com/

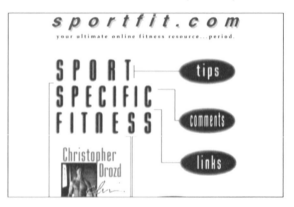

Sportfit.com is an online guide for improving your body fitness. The site features a large collection of body building tips and related links to health, fitness, and sports resources on the Web.

Stoutness Exercises

http://members.aol.com/rlauera/stoutnes.htm

Stoutness Exercises contains reprints from a newspaper column, "On the Go."

Stoutness exercises

and other health and fitness topics

Sadly, it's difficult to make a living as a Pooh fan. So, in real life, I work for Synaptx Worldwide writing and editing all sorts of fascinating stuff about the world of telecommunications. And then, just for grins, I do a bit of freelance journalism, including a pseudo-syndicated health and fitness column for Copley Newspapers here in Chicagoland. It pays next to nothing a week, but I get my picture in the paper, and, due to the subject matter, the attention of adoring fans who occasionally follow me around the grocery store to see if I ever buy junk food. (I do.)

I've got about five years' worth of columns stored up now, so if there's a fitness topic you're interested in, e-mail me your request, and I'll post it here (if I don't have a column on your topic, maybe I'll write one and dedicate it to you!). Meanwhile, here are some columns covering FAQs about fitness and weight loss. I'll change them periodically (hopefully weekly) or as requests come in. I'm always looking for topic ideas, so keep those virtual cards and letters coming!

Back To Pooh Page   Back To Main Index

Fitness Columns _On The Go_

Updated 3/3/96

• Top 5 tips for sound nutrition and weight loss

Stretching and Flexibility

http://www.mit.edu:8001/people/wchuang/health/stretching.html

Stretching and Flexibility is an online manual that provides a wealth of information about stretching and flexibility exercises. To find information on stretching, flexibility, types of stretching, and how to stretch, click on **Introduction.** The site also includes an A to Z topic index.

STRETCHING AND FLEXIBILITY

Version: 1.11, Last Modified 94/02/15 Copyright (C) 1993, 1994 by Bradford D. Appleton

Permission is granted to make and distribute verbatim copies of this document provided the copyright notice and this permission notice are preserved on all copies.

This document is available in ascii, texinfo, postscript, dvi, and html formats via anonymous ftp from the host 'cs.huji.ac.il' located under the directory '/pub/doc/faq/rec/martial_arts'. The file name matches the wildcard pattern 'stretching.*'. The file suffix indicates the format. For www and Mosaic users, the URL is in 'http://archie.ac.il:8001/papers/rma/stretching.html'.

Introduction

This document is a modest attempt to compile a wealth of information in order to answer some frequently asked questions about stretching and flexibility. It is organized into chapters covering the following topics:

1. Physiology (as it relates to stretching)
2. Flexibility
3. Types of Stretching
4. How to Stretch

Although each chapter may refer to sections in other chapters, it is not required that you read every chapter in the order presented. (It is important, however, that you read the disclaimer

Thrive

http://www.thriveonline.com/

Thrive, updated daily, is an online resource in the format of a contemporary health magazine. It features articles on nutrition, diet, vitamins, a healthy sex life, and other topics. The site also includes advice columns from a number of experts, interactive activities, a newsstand with the latest health headlines, healthy recipes, and a recipe finder. For an overview of this site, scroll and click on the **Table of Contents.**

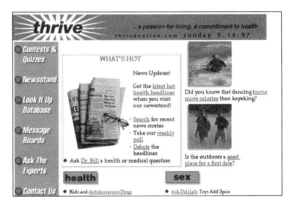

Tim's Fitness and Nutrition Page

http://plainfield.bypass.com/~twilbur/fitness.html

Tim's Fitness and Nutrition Page provides online *An Illustrated Guide to Exercises for Free Weights* with routines for the whole body. The site features a collection of easy-to-read articles on various nutrition and fitness topics ranging from terms used on food labels to body mass index (BMI). Quizzes test your knowledge of exercise and weight control and are offered for the aerobics, weight training, and vegetarian pages. The site also contains related links to nutrition and resources.

Tim's Fitness and Nutrition Page

The purpose of this page is to offer both general and specific information related to nutrition, fitness, and weightlifting. These articles and links are ones I have found useful and informative over the years. I am always looking for improvements, new material, etc. for this page. Please send your ideas, comments, and suggestions to twilbur@plainfield.bypass.com

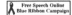
Free Speech Online
Blue Ribbon Campaign

General Fitness Articles:

- Guidelines for Beginning an Exercise Program
- More Information on Starting an Exercise Program
- Body Mass Index (BMI)
- Waist-to-Hip Ratio
- This is probably **NOT** the best way to lose excess body weight

Nutrition Articles:

- Timing Meals With Exercise
- Daily Calorie Needs
- The Risks of Eating Vegetarian
- Cholesterol Levels and How to Lower Them

Tough Turf

http://www.tinactin.com/

Tough Turf, from Tinactin, provides expert training tips for your favorite sports, information for treating injuries and preventing them, and a list of other sports-related sites.

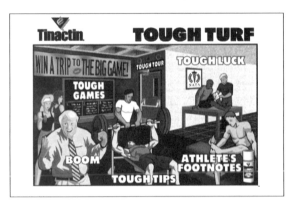

Training Nutrition

http://www.dgsys.com/~trnutr/

Training Nutrition is a mailing list that serves as a forum for hard-core natural body builders and other serious amateur (and professional) athletes to discuss nutritional and physiologic issues connected with training.

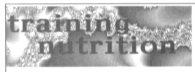

Breaking news from the top of the food chain

Hi and welcome.

I'm Paul Moses and I run the Training-Nutrition mailing list. It's intended to work in conjunction with Michael Sullivan's *weights* list. **trnutr** is a forum for hardcore natural bodybuilders and other serious amateur (and professional) athletes to discuss nutritional and physiological issues connected with training.

What's here.

- **The Training-Nutrition FAQs**
- **Latest issues**
- The Ten Commandments of Sports Nutrition
- Summer is on its way, so you might want to start thinking about getting cut up
- Having a tough time adding lean bodyweight?

Turnstep.com

http://www.turnstep.com/

Turnstep.com features a large collection of aerobic exercises. You can browse an online library for an exercise pattern by type or year.

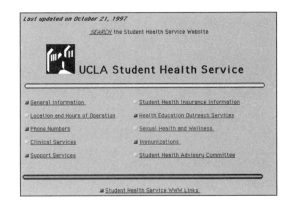

UCLA Student Health Service

http://www.saonet.ucla.edu/health.htm

UCLA Student Health Service contains a **Sexual Health and Wellness** section and an **Immunizations** section with health information and advice for college students. To find an A to Z index of health education handouts on topics ranging from acne to yeast infection, click on **Health Education Outreach Services.**

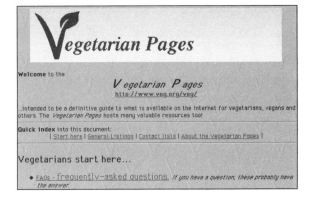

Vegetarian Pages

http://www.veg.org/veg/

Vegetarian Pages is an index to links of interest to vegetarians and vegans. FAQs are answered and links to another major index are offered. The site contains readers' recipes, articles about nutrition and health, and a worldwide list of vegetarian and vegetarian friendly restaurants.

Vegetarian Resource Center

http://www.tiac.net/users/vrc/

Vegetarian Resource Center contains links to vegetarian discussion groups, sites, and various information in the areas of vegetarian diet and lifestyle.

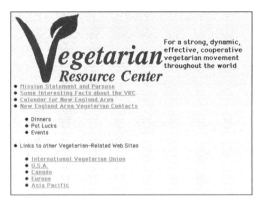

The Vegetarian Society of the United Kingdom

http://www.veg.org/veg/Orgs/VegSocUK/

The Vegetarian Society of the United Kingdom, established in 1847, provides a collection of online resources for healthy living. The site includes an index with hundreds of vegetarian recipes for every occasion, information sheets, a health and nutrition section, and youth pages.

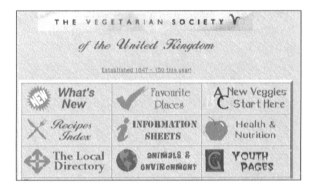

Veggie Heaven

http://www.webserve.co.uk/Veggie/

Veggie Heaven, created by Rosamond Richardson, furnishes over 160 vegetarian recipes, amazing facts and figures, and much more. There are tasty recipes for main dishes, salads, desserts, and other things.

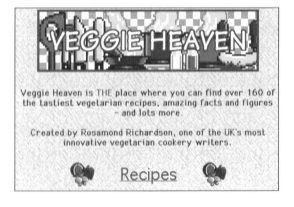

Veggies Unite!

http://www.vegweb.com/

Veggies Unite!, an online guide to vegetarian living, contains a directory of over 2000 vegan recipes. In addition, the site offers a grocery list maker, a weekly meal planner, and a monthly e-mail *VegWeb* newsletter.

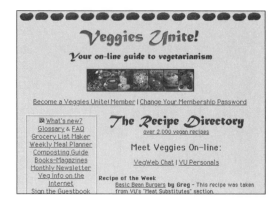

VegSource

http://www.vegsource.com/

VegSource offers news, recipes, information, and discussion boards related to vegetarianism and other topics. Two featured participants, Charles Atwood, M.D., and Ruth Heidrich, Ph.D., provide answers to health questions as well as fitness and nutrition information.

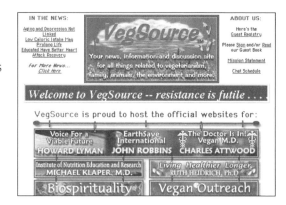

The Vitamin Index

http://www.users.zetnet.co.uk/prowland/vitframe.htm

The Vitamin Index lets you select a common vitamin and then provides you with a brief description, what it does, the best natural sources, and any possible toxic concerns.

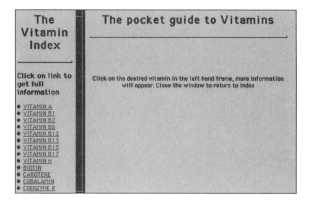

Vitamins Network

http://www.vitamins.net/

Vitamins Network offers manufacturer-direct prices on thousands of vitamin, mineral, and herb products. The site also includes dozens of forums with message boards, chat rooms, and online guides for consumer briefs, vitamins, and herbs.

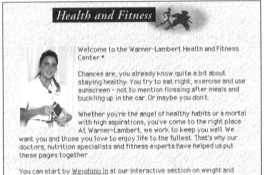

Warner-Lambert Health and Fitness Center

http://www.warner-lambert.com/info/healthintro.html

Warner-Lambert Company has provided an online Health and Fitness Center to help keep you fit and healthy. The Center is based on the collaborations of doctors, nutrition specialists, and fitness experts, and features an interactive scale for weighing yourself, a personal meal planner, and invaluable information on the weight-health connection.

WebRunner Running Page

http://www.gate.net/~wbrunner/running.htm

The WebRunner Running Page is a comprehensive fitness site organized in a question-and-answer format for all runners. The site includes a New Runners Part 1 section with practical information for people who want to start running and a New Runners Part 2 section with 28 topics on preventing running injuries.

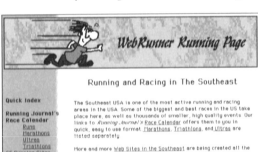

Wellness Shopper

http://planetwellness.com

The Wellness Shopper offers a variety of fitness and nutrition resources, including articles, a newsletter, news, and message boards. The library has hundreds of fitness articles and the menu planner helps find the nutritional value of a food item.

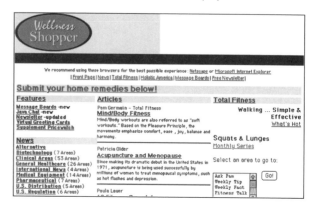

World of Vitality

http://www.vitality.com/

World of Vitality, an online version of *Vitality* magazine, contains a variety of health/nutrition resources, including articles for men and women, special reports, chat groups, daily health tips, and health games.

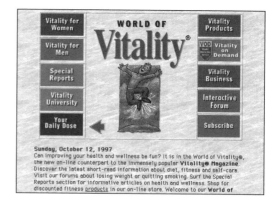

Yona's Health and Fitness

http://www.yona.com/fitness/

Yona's Health and Fitness contains a comprehensive collection of sites organized by categories ranging from aerobics to yoga.

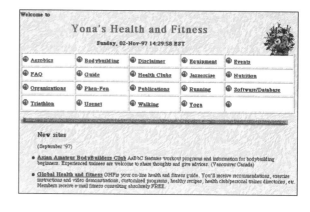

Health Topics
for Everyone

CHAPTER 3

Advocate Health Care

http://www.advocatehealth.com/

Advocate Health Care provides a variety of health resources, including **Your Health,** which gives useful information on staying well and managing your health, and an online health care magazine, *Health Advocate,* with extensive archives. For an overview of the site click on **Site Guide** at the top of the page.

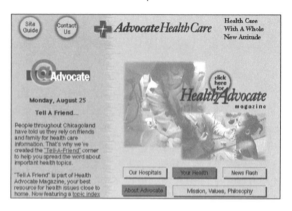

Agency for Health Care Policy and Research

http://www.ahcpr.gov/consumer/

The Agency for Health Care Policy and Research contains a growing list of online consumer health publications for a variety of medical conditions. Publications include "Recovering After a Stroke, No. 16," "You Can Quit Smoking, No. 18," and "Preventing Pressure Ulcers, No. 3."

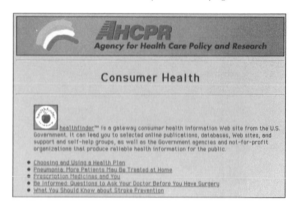

Agency for Toxic Substances and Disease Registry

http://atsdr1.atsdr.cdc.gov:8080/atsdrhome.html

Agency for Toxic Substances and Disease Registry, an agency of the U.S. Public Health Service, provides extensive information on the health effects associated with hazardous substances. Among the resources of interest to the consumer are **HazDat Database, ToxFAQs,** and **Top 20 Hazardous Substances.**

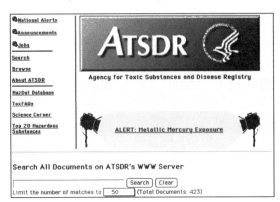

All Saints Healthcare System

http://www.execpc.com/~vbudzisz/

All Saints Healthcare System provides a health sciences library, including an interactive age-adjusted guide that recommends immunizations, examinations, and tests derived from the *Clinician's Handbook of Preventive Services.* Furthermore, there is information on staying fit, including exercises, drug abuse, safe sex, as well as a home health quiz.

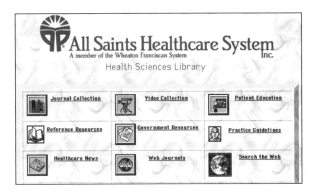

AMA Health Insight

http://www.ama-assn.org/insight/insight.htm

AMA Health Insight, from the American Medical Association, provides a wealth of consumer health resources. **Specific Conditions** gives information about such topics as migraine headaches and asthma, **General Health** focuses on news and atlases, **Health Focus** emphasizes kids', adolescents', and women's health, and **Interactive Health** gives online information on topics such as weight and the advice of a personal nutritionist.

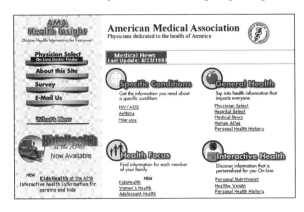

American Family Physician

http://www.aafp.org/family/afp/

American Family Physician is the official clinical bimonthly journal of the American Academy of Family Physicians. Each online issue contains a health article from the journal of interest to consumers. To find a list of these articles dating back to March 1993, scroll to the bottom of the page and click on **Patient Information Index.**

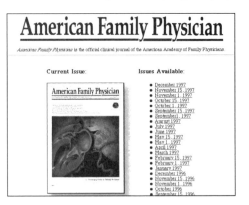

American Heart Association Heart & Stroke A-Z Guide

http://www.amhrt.org/Heart_and_Stroke_A_Z_Guide/

The American Heart Association site contains an enormous resource, the **Heart & Stroke A-Z Guide,** an index to hundreds of topics related to conditions and factors associated with heart problems and stroke. The Guide also includes a search tool.

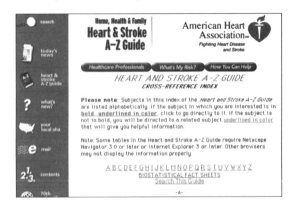

American Safety & Health Institute

http://www.ashinstitute.com/links.html

American Safety & Health Institute provides a wide variety of essential safety and health links ranging from **CPR-You CAN do it!** and **FireSafe-Fire and Safety Directory** to **Living With Heart Disease.**

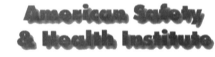

Ask An Expert: Health

http://www.askanexpert.com/askanexpert/cat/hea.html

Ask An Expert is a directory of health and medicine experts in over 40 different disciplines. An e-mail address and/or a link to the expert's Web site is provided for your query.

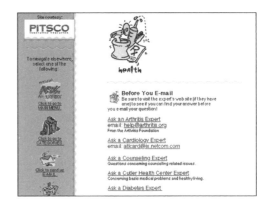

Ask Ken!

http://www.efn.org/~andrec/ask_ken.html

Ask Ken! is America's longest running advice column on the Internet. Ken has given daily tips and advice on any problem, including health, since 1994.

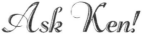

Ask NOAH About: Health Topics and Resources

http://www.noah.cuny.edu/qksearch.html

The New York Online Access to Health (NOAH) is the combined effort of the New York Public Library and other educational institutions. Ask NOAH About: Health Topics and Resources contains a wide assortment of health topics and consumer resources, including personal health, environmental health, and healthy living.

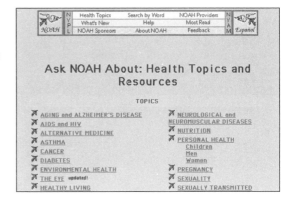

The Beth Israel Web Guide to Good Health

http://www.bimc.edu/

The Beth Israel Web Guide to Good Health, from Beth Israel Health Care System in New York, provides a wealth of consumer health resources, including an online **Physician & Referral Service** for the metropolitan New York City area and the **Ask the Doctor** feature with an extensive archive. In addition, the site offers **Health Information** on topics such as the heart and neurological disorders in children.

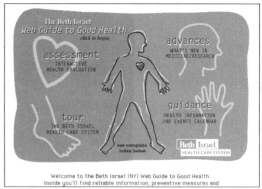

Better Health

http://www.betterhealth.com/

Better Health provides a database of easy-to-understand health information that is geared toward answering your questions and addressing your needs as a health consumer. The site includes an A to Z index of consumer health topics, mutual support chat groups, and message boards.

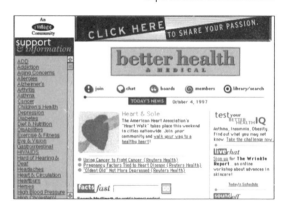

Bluestem Health for Kansans

http://www2.kumc.edu/bluestem/

Bluestem Health for Kansans contains a wealth of online consumer resources organized by categories. The categories include Disease and Disorders, Drugs, Surgeries, and Procedures, Health News and Issues, Health Organizations, Mental Health and Illness, Prevention, Wellness, and General Health.

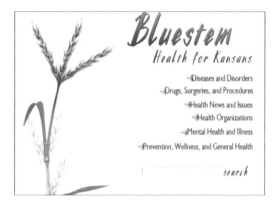

CDC Travel Information

http://www.cdc.gov/travel/travel.html

The Centers for Disease Control and Prevention (CDC) provides international travel information, including reference materials, disease outbreaks, and geographical health recommendations for vaccines, food, water, and other health concerns.

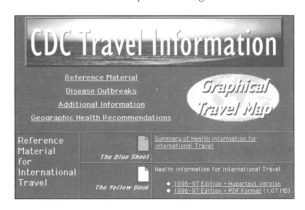

Chicago Tribune Nursing News

http://www.chicago.tribune.com/articles/n_news/

The Chicago Tribune Nursing News features personal stories of nurses and nursing health information of interest to consumers. The site includes archives of previous issues.

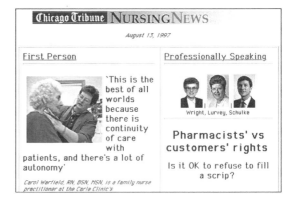

The Coalition for Consumer Health and Safety

http://www.healthandsafety.org/

The Coalition for Consumer Health and Safety Web site is part of an effort to educate the public about a broad range of health and safety threats, including motor vehicle safety, home and product safety, indoor air quality, nutrition, tobacco use, alcohol consumption, food and drinking water safety, and AIDS. The Coalition is a partnership of approximately 40 consumer, health, and insurer groups.

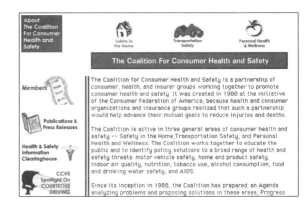

Common Ailments

http://www.virginia.edu/~std-hlth/ailment1.htm

Common Ailments, from the University of Virginia Department of Student Health, provides a guide to common medical illnesses, their symptoms, and their remedies. The ailments include stress, swimmer's ear, upset stomach, flu, ear wax, sinusitis, and many more.

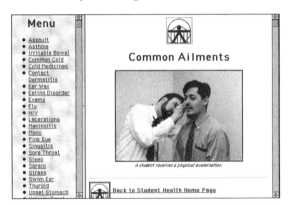

Commonly Requested Federal Services

http://www.whitehouse.gov/WH/Services/

Commonly Requested Federal Services, from the White House, presents an enormous amount of consumer health information about a variety of topics, including consumer health, Medicare and Medicaid, cancer, aging, food safety, and nutrition.

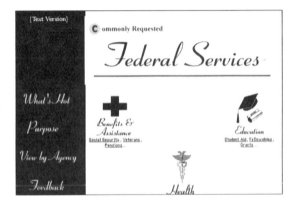

Community Outreach Health Information System

http://web.bu.edu/COHIS/

Community Outreach Health Information System (COHIS), from Boston University Medical Center, provides a variety of online health information resources. Topics range from AIDS and HIV to trauma and emergency medicine. For a complete catalog of resources, click on **HealthSource.** The site also features consumer information on diabetes in the notebook and drugs in the COHIS drugstore.

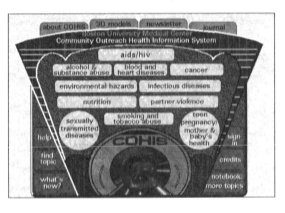

Congressional Email Directory

http://www.webslingerz.com/jhoffman/congress-email.html

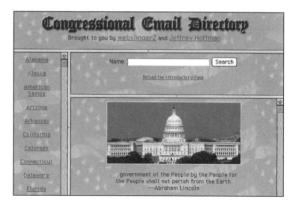

Congressional Email Directory provides e-mail addresses for the senators and representatives for each of the United States and its possessions. The search tool can also be used to find the e-mail address of a congress person.

Consumer Health Links

http://www.cheshire-med.com/medlinks/medlinks.shtml

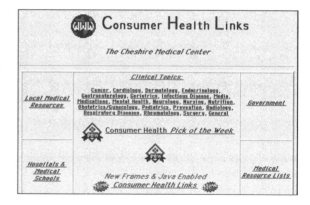

Consumer Health Links, from the Cheshire Medical Center in New Hampshire, provides links organized by topic. Among the topics are cardiology, dermatology, endocrinology, gastroenterology, geriatrics, and surgery.

Cyberspace Telemedical Office

http://www.telemedical.com/

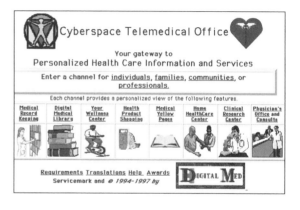

Cyberspace Telemedical Office provides a wealth of consumer and professional health information organized by topics, including a medical library, a wellness center, and others.

Department of Family Practice Information

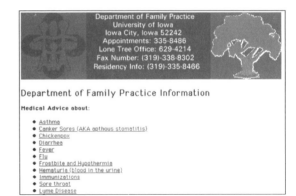

http://www.uiowa.edu/~famprac/med.html

The Department of Family Practice, at the University of Iowa, supplies medical advice for patients on topics such as asthma, flu, immunizations, sore throat, and urinary tract infections.

Doc in the Box

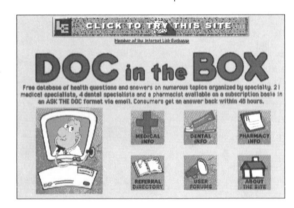

http://www.onlinedoc.com/

Doc in the Box provides a wide range of consumer information featuring 20 medical specialties, five dental specialties, and a pharmacist. The site also includes related links and specialty forums where medical information can be exchanged with others on the Internet.

Doctor's Guide to the Internet

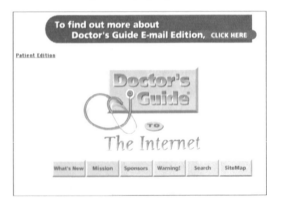

http://www.pslgroup.com/PTGUIDE.HTM

The Doctor's Guide to the Internet contains a variety of online resources. Scroll to **Of specific interest** to find a wealth of information and resources on topics such as AIDS/HIV, diabetes, insomnia, menopause, migraine headaches, and schizophrenia. In addition, the site offers the latest medical news from conferences, the literature, newswires, and the Internet.

DoctorNet

http://www.doctornet.com/

DoctorNet offers the consumer numerous health/medical resources, including information from physicians about their specialties and their practices. Among the other resources are aids to finding a specialist, an online doctor's magazine, *DoctorNet Public Health Journal,* and an index of medical sites.

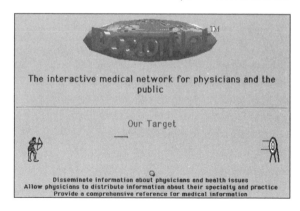

The Doctors' Page

http://members.aol.com/DrsPage/

The Doctors' Page, although designed by physicians, is a rich consumer resource with articles about diseases, search tools, and other health-related topics. Areas addressed are diverse, ranging from everyday medical concerns such as geriatrics to a comprehensive discussion of the PBS television special on managed care entitled, "Your Money & Your Life."

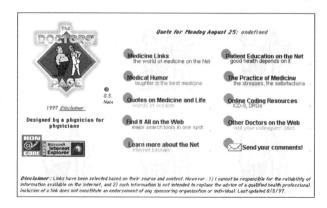

Dr. Schueler's On-line Medical Glossary

http://www.drschueler.com/glossary/glossary.htm

Dr. Schueler's On-line Medical Glossary is an easy-to-use, comprehensive, and reliable dictionary for finding definitions of medical terms.

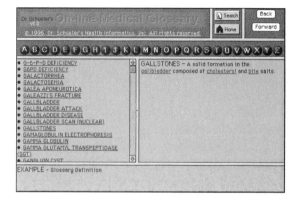

Ear, Nose, and Throat Information Center

http://www.netdoor.com/entinfo/

Ear, Nose, and Throat Information Center offers information on topics such as stuffy nose, the common cold, the effects of altitude and air travel on the ears, and other topics that are of interest to the consumer.

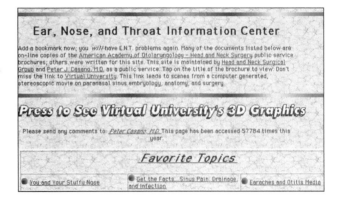

Emergency Services WWW Site List

http://pplant.uafadm.alaska.edu/www-911.htm

Emergency Services WWW Site List provides resources for known fire, rescue, and emergency services available on the Internet. The site is updated weekly.

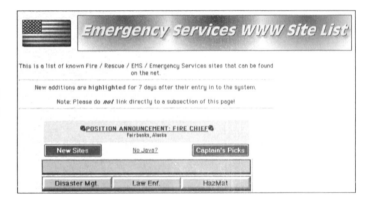

The Eyes Have It

http://www.aoanet.org/aoanet/

The Eyes Have It, presented by the American Optometric Association, includes a series of comprehensive, informative, and easy-to-read articles about eye care, vision conditions, lenses, and eye disease.

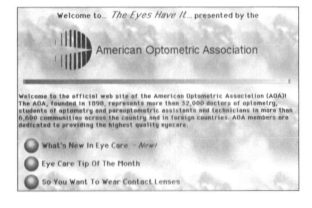

Fairview HealthWise

http://www.fairview.org/healthwise/

Fairview HealthWise is a consumer health information and physician referral service. The site offers two online publications, a quarterly newsletter and a monthly *Health Tips* magazine, with articles ranging from infant safety and diet and exercise to the ups and downs of menopause.

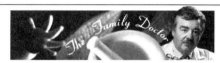

The Family Doctor

http://www.familydr.com/

The Family Doctor is divided into three main parts: (1) Ask the Doctor, (2) Doctor's Exam, and (3) Pharmacy. In Ask the Doctor, you may seek health information, which is categorized into 18 different sections. In Doctor's Exam, you may click on a body part, then seek a diagnosis, depending on a list of symptoms. In Pharmacy, you can find out what is in your new prescription via a search tool.

[About the Doctor] [Ask the Doctor] [Doctor's Exam] [Pharmacy]

Life has become so hectic that many of us can't find the time to explore important questions about our health. *The Family Doctor* website, based on the best-selling CD-ROM, can help make sense of your busy schedule by providing excellent, timely health information 24 hours a day. While you're here, browse through the thousands of questions and answers from the syndicated Family Doctor column. Got symptoms? Try the Doctor's Exam for a diagnosis of what might be the trouble. If you're wondering what's in your new prescription, search the Pharmacy for an answer. Relax – *The Family Doctor* is here to help.

Family Health

http://www.tcom.ohiou.edu/family-health.html

Family Health is Dr. Frank Myers' daily series of 2½-minute audio programs dealing with a wide variety of health-related topics. Program topics include attention deficit disorder, autologous blood donations, bee stings, and whiplash. To listen to these programs, download RealAudio, which can be accessed from this site.

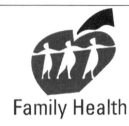

Family Health

A Production of the College of Osteopathic Medicine and the Telecommunications Center at Ohio University.

Welcome to *Family Health®* on the Net. Here you can find out more about the series and sample some of our programs.

Family Internet Health Clinic USA

http://www.familyinternet.com/healthclinicusa/

Family Internet offers Health Clinic USA where a consumer can browse or search for health information on diseases, injuries, poisons, medical tests, drugs, and diet.

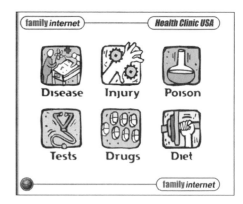

Family Medicine Online

http://www.aafp.org/family/

Family Medicine Online, provided by the American Academy of Family Physicians, contains health information for patients. The section on patients includes 200 health topics covering a variety of topics, a series of 60 patient education brochures from your family doctor, and a *Good Health Newsletter* with articles on preventive medicine.

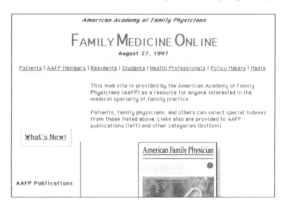

First Aid Book

http://www.medaccess.com/first_aid/FA_TOC.htm

First Aid Book is an online edition of the U.S. Department of Labor's book on first aid. This 11-chapter edition represents current recommended policies and procedures for handling emergencies requiring first aid.

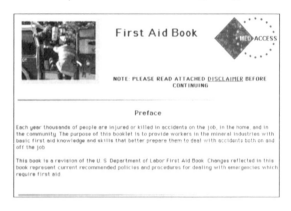

First Aid Online

http://www.prairienet.org/~autumn/firstaid/

First Aid Online presents remedies for small injuries and common medical problems such as blistering, burns, frostbite, poisoning, bites, and shock. The site includes a list of recommended first aid supplies.

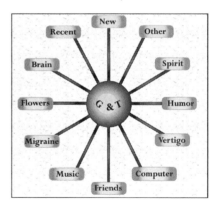

G & T

http://troost.rbdc.com/

The G & T home page provides consumer medical information on eye movements, migraines and other headaches, vertigo, dizziness, and hearing disorders.

Georgetown University Medical Center

http://dc.digitalcity.com/georgetownmed/

Georgetown University Medical Center provides a variety of health resources for consumers. To find a list of articles, click on **Health Information** and to find drug information on prescription or over-the-counter medications, click on **Medicine Chest.**

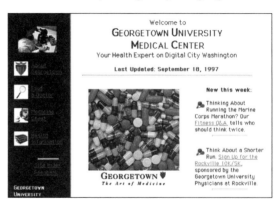

Good Health

http://www.goodhealth.com/

Good Health, from Seton, has online consumer information for wellness, fitness, disease prevention, and medical care. The site features an online searchable *Good Health* magazine and a reference page with sites for healthy living.

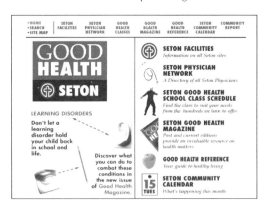

Gorden and Jacki's Home Page

http://www.supernet.net/~jackibar/

Gorden and Jacki Barineau's home page provides a wealth of information about the toxins in perfume, fabric softeners, dryer sheets, and air freshners.

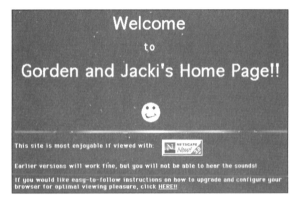

A Guide for Care of Your Back

http://www.halcyon.com/moonbeam/back/

A Guide for Care of Your Back has useful information from the doctors and therapists at the Virginia Mason Medical Center.

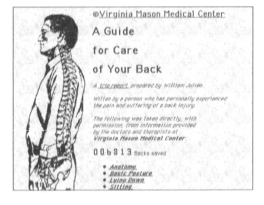

A Guide to Medical Information and Support on the Internet

http://www.geocities.com/HotSprings/1505/

A Guide to Medical Information and Support on the Internet contains medical chats, newsgroups, listservs, online doctors, Medline, and medical links.

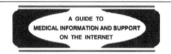

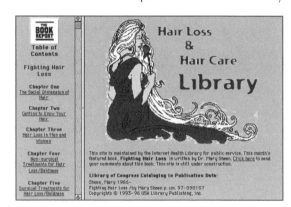

Hair Loss & Hair Care Library

http://members.aol.com/usalibrary

Hair Loss & Hair Care Library contains all eight chapters of a book entitled, *Fighting Hair Loss.* Among the chapter titles are "Nonsurgical Treatments for Hair Loss/Baldness," "Common Drugs That Cause Hair Loss," and "Secrets of Proper Hair Care." Two newspaper articles related to hair loss are also included.

Harvard University Health Services

http://www.uhs.harvard.edu/

Harvard University Health Services publishes *House Call,* an online quarterly magazine covering a variety of health-related topics. To find the articles, select **For HUGHP Members** and click on **House Call.** To find other health articles of interest to consumers, go to **Harvard Health & Fitness** and click on **HHF Presents** and go to **Clinician's Daily Journal.**

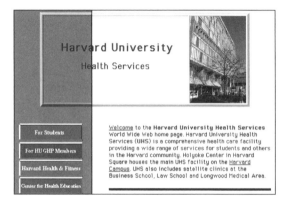

HazardNet

http://hoshi.cic.sfu.ca/~hazard/

HazardNet, from Simon Fraser University, provides information for people concerned with preventing and preparing for large-scale natural and technological emergencies. There is also alert and advisory information, hazard statistics, and emergency-response organizations. The site also includes extensive links to current information about droughts, severe storms, floods, and other perils to humans.

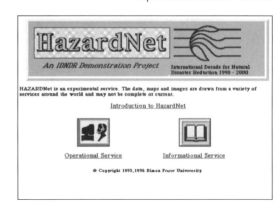

Headache Advice for Patients

http://www.bayer.com/Bayer2/EAuswahl.html

Headache Advice for Patients, provided by Bayer Aspirin, is an online questionnaire designed to differentiate between a tension-type headache and a migraine headache.

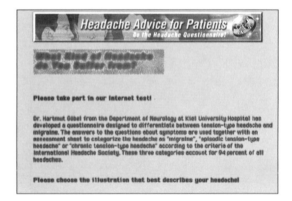

Headache Resource Center

http://www.womenslink.com/health/excedrin/

The Headache Resource Center, sponsored by Excedrin, provides advice on how to better manage headache pain.

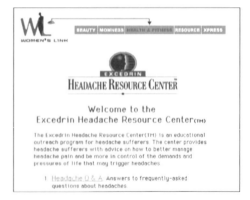

Health Care

http://www.med.upenn.edu/health/

Health Care, from the University of Pennsylvania Health System, contains a gold mine of health information for the consumer. Click on **Health Information** for news, online publications, tips, and quizzes to help you stay healthy. This site features a useful tip of the day such as "Hot liquids—even hot tapwater—can cause life-threatening burns."

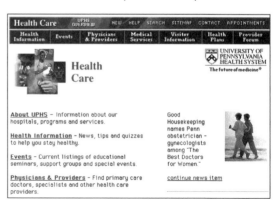

Health Education Page

http://www.nau.edu/~fronske/he.html

The Health Education Page, from the Fronske Health Center, provides an online brochure library with topics ranging from alcohol and other drugs to interactive health tests.

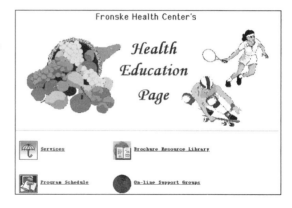

Health Explorer

http://www.healthexplorer.com/

Health Explorer features fast-search access to over 3000 health-related sites, descriptions, and reviews. Topics include aging, first aid, mortality, and men's health.

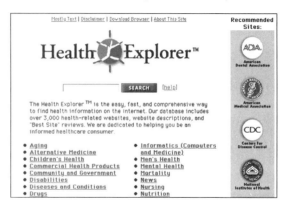

The Health Gazette

http://www.freenet.tlh.fl.us/HealthGazette/gazette.html

The Health Gazette, published by Dr. Karl Hempel, contains a list of consumer articles on various health topics, including acne, cancer, poison ivy, smoking, and stress.

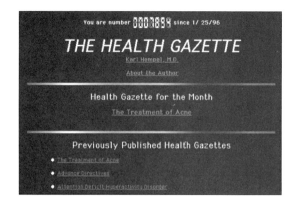

Health InfoNet

http://www.albert2.com/

Health InfoNet provides a wide selection of consumer health topics ranging from cataracts and colds and flu to family health and skin cancer. The site includes an excellent search engine.

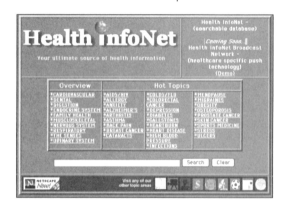

Health Information

http://www.ghc.org/health_info/contents.html

Health Information, from Group Health Cooperative, provides brief articles on the 30 medical conditions that account for 80% of all disease and death in the United States. In addition, there are topics on senior health, eyecare, health care for teenagers, safety, and injury prevention, as well as an excellent list of healthy Web sites.

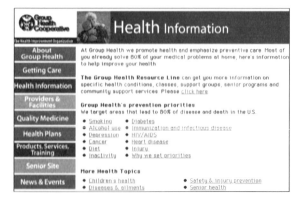

The Health Manual

http://www.columbia.net/consumer/

The Health Manual, Columbia/HCA Healthcare Corporation's online medical reference, provides the latest consumer health information for a variety of topics, including allergies and asthma, children's health, emergency care, orthopedics (muscles/bones), and many others.

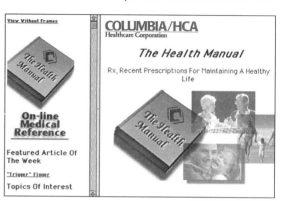

Health Net

http://www.healthnet.com/

Health Net includes a collection of monthly health themes in the Wellness section with extensive consumer information on topics such as cholesterol, taking care of yourself, nutrition, and children's health issues. The site also presents a new health tip after each reloading.

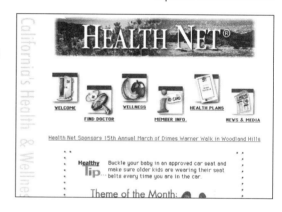

The-Health-Pages Directory

http://www.the-health-pages.com/directory.html

The-Health-Pages Directory contains a variety of topics with links to preventive care, education, medicine, emergency care, teenagers', men's, women's, and seniors' health, and much more.

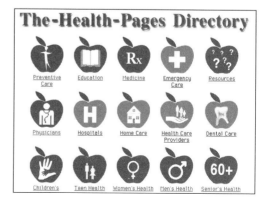

Health Status Questionnaire

http://www.mcw.edu/midas/health/

The Health Status Questionnaire is an online version of Rand's 36-question survey that evaluates your current state of physical and emotional health. You can learn how health status is assessed, see your own health status scores, and compare your scores with the general population. Just remember, no health questionaire should be considered perfectly reliable.

Your Health

Welcome to an **experiment** to test the feasibility of collecting health data via the Web. **We'd like your participation!** You can learn how health status is assessed, see your own health status scores, and compare your scores with the general population. We, meanwhile, are learning how to collect this information efficiently and reliably using the Web. More than 8000 users have already taken this survey and their e-mail says they enjoyed it. To participate, however, **you must understand the purpose and (minimal) risks of the experiment.**

The Test: 36 Questions

If you participate, we'll record your age, sex, and ethnicity, but we **will not record your identity.** You'll then take the **RAND 36-Item Health Survey**, which asks **multiple-choice questions** about your recent physical and emotional health. These are the same 36 questions that make up the **SF-36 "Short Form"** developed for the Medical Outcomes Study. The RAND version of the survey differs from the SF-36 only in its simpler scoring method. The survey takes less than 5 minutes on average. When you submit the completed form you'll immediately get your scores back. You may want to save your scores for future reference.

The Experiment

We are learning how to administer health surveys on the Web efficiently and reliably. To learn what works best, **some features of the survey you receive may be determined by random chance.**

Health Tips & Resource Guide

http://www.imgw.com/Insert.htm

Health Tips & Resource Guide, provided by GlaxoWellcome, is a compilation of facts, tips, self-tests, and resources on a variety of topics, including allergies, asthma, depression, heartburn, herpes, HIV and AIDS, and migraine headaches.

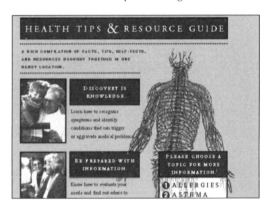

HealthAnswers

http://www.healthanswers.com/

HealthAnswers, from the American Academy of Pediatrics, provides a wealth of consumer health information, including **Get an Answer** where you can browse or search for tons of information on wellness, your body, and special medical groups. **Health Organizations** has information about the most common diseases and conditions, pediatric matters, and prescription and over-the-counter medications. **Health News** has the latest news from Reuters and the Orbis Broadcasting Group.

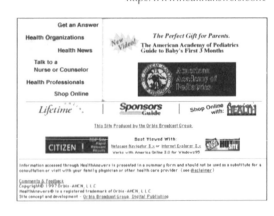

⌐HealthAtoZ Featured Articles

http://www.healthatoz.com/prev_month_news.htm#t1

HealthAtoZ provides a list of monthly featured articles covering topics such as osteoporosis, cholesterol, and colds and flu. Each featured article includes an interactive quiz to test your knowledge about that topic and offers related links for further information.

Featured Articles:

- Osteoporosis
- Heat Related Illnesses
- Vacation Safety and Travel Tips
- Men's Health
- Dealing with Allergies
- Planning a Healthy Pregnancy
- Healthy Parenting
- Diet And Fitness
- Colds And Flu
- Depression
- Breast Cancer
- Cholesterol
- Lyme Disease

[HealthAtoZ Home | Medline | HealthAtoz News | Message Board | Advertising | Register | Feedback | Add Site| About Us | Help]

⌐Healthcare Education Learning & Information Exchange

http://www.helix.com/

Healthcare Education Learning & Information Exchange, provided by GlaxoWellcome Healthcare Education, offers news and publications for health care professionals and patients. The **Consumer Health Info** section contains a **Consumer Education Information Catalog** where users can review and order health care resources at no charge from GlaxoWellcome and the **Medical Tribune** news service has synopses of up-to-date health-related articles on topics ranging from asking the doctor to preparing children for the dentist. In addition, the **Helibyte factoid of the day** features historical events in medicine.

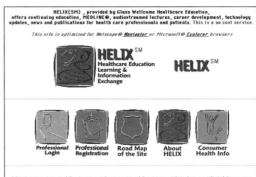

HELIX(SM) , provided by Glaxo Wellcome Healthcare Education, offers continuing education, MEDLINE®, audiostreamed lectures, career development, technology updates, news and publications for health care professionals and patients. This is a no cost service.

This site is optimized for Netscape® *Navigator* or Microsoft® *Explorer* browsers

HELIX SM
Healthcare Education Learning & Information Exchange

HELIX SM

Professional Login | Professional Registration | Road Map of the Site | About HELIX | Consumer Health Info

| Professional Login | Professional Registration | Road Map of Site | About HELIX | Consumer Health Info |

HealthCast

http://www.sb.com/health_news/

HealthCast, from SmithKline Beecham, provides health and science news and information intended for the general public. You can read featured articles on genetic testing and DNA research, download a video of the PBS special, "A Question of Genes: Inherited Risks," take the survey on DNA research issues, or review topical articles in the Index section.

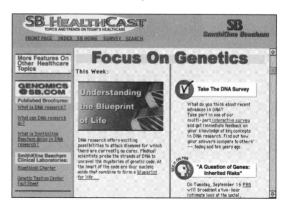

Healthfront.com

http://healthfront.com/

Healthfront.com, from Whitehall-Robins, provides answers to family health questions on a variety of topics, including treating asthma and preventing heatburn. There are also weekly articles on children's health, family health, and fitness and recreation.

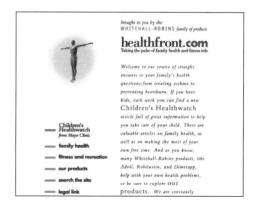

Healthline Publishing, Inc.

http://www.health-line.com/

Healthline Publishing, Inc. publishes topical online consumer magazines, *Healthline, Allergy & Asthma,* and *Skin Care Today,* written by health care professionals. Each magazine can be viewed by issue or articles can be searched in the extensive databases. The site also provides a collection of healthy recipes in the section **What's For Dinner.**

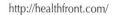
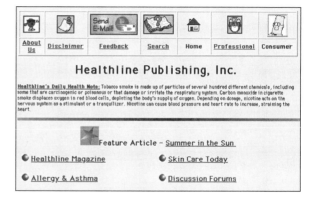

HealthLink

http://healthlink.stanford.edu/

HealthLink, a community outreach project of the Stanford University Medical Center News Bureau, provides a wealth of consumer health resources in its News, Health Tips, and Stanford Medicine sections. Each of these sections offers many topical and practical articles on a wide range of health and medical issues. The site features a daily health tip and includes a search tool.

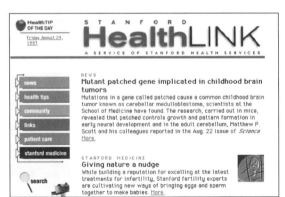

HealthLinks Health and Social Issue Resources

http://www.mcet.edu/healthlinks/health.html

HealthLinks Health and Social Issue Resources is a collection of health resources for sexuality education, conflict resolution, relationship violence, parenting skills, nutrition, and other topics.

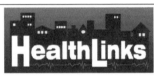

HealthSource

http://www.doctors-10tv.com/

HealthSource, from Doctors Hospital in Columbus, Ohio, contains a wide variety of consumer health information on heart health, occupational health, fitness, and other relevant topics.

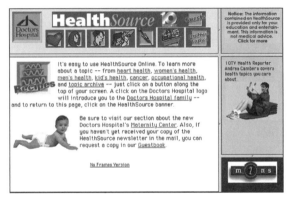

HealthTips

http://www-med.Stanford.EDU/center/communications/HealthTips/

HealthTips, from the Stanford University Medical Center News Bureau, is a series of monthly articles providing consumers with health information on a variety of topics from picking sunscreen to treating wounds.

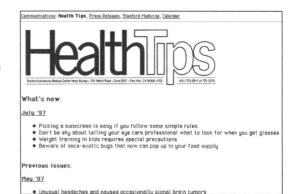

HealthWatch

http://www.newschannel9.com/healthwatch.html

HealthWatch, from NewsChannel 9 in Chattanooga, Tennessee, presents summaries of Maryellen Locher's reports on the latest health developments. For a collection of previous reports, scroll to bottom of the page and click on **Archives Index.**

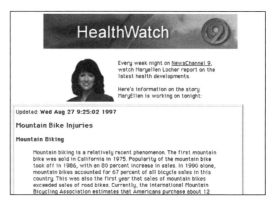

Healthwise

http://www.columbia.edu/cu/healthwise/

Healthwise features **Go Ask Alice,** an interactive question-and-answer service for teenagers and adults from Columbia University Health Service. You can ask Alice a personal health question anonymously or read her answers to your previous questions, which are categorized as follows: Sexuality, Sexual Health, Relationships, General Health, Fitness & Nutrition, Emotional Well-Being, and Alcohol & Other Drugs. Answers are posted weekly. In addition, the site provides articles from its online newsletter, *Healthwise Highlights,* presenting topics similiar to those in **Go Ask Alice.**

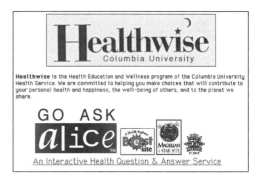

Healthy Devil Online

http://h-devil-www.mc.duke.edu/h-devil/

Healthy Devil Online provides consumer information on a variety of health-related topics for young adults. The topics include emotional health, men's and women's health, general health, drinking and smoking, and pregnancy.

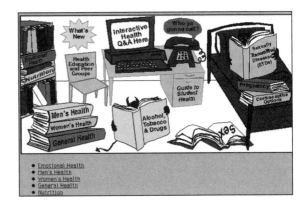

Healthy Living

http://www.healthgate.com/healthy/living/

Healthy Living, from HealthGate, is a collection of Web sites in the format of consumer magazines. The series includes health information for women, men, food choices, parenting, and sexuality. Each magazine covers the latest health news and timely feature articles to help you live a healthier life.

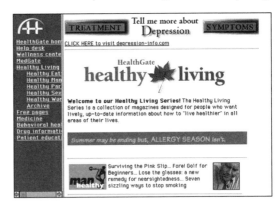

Highland Park Hospital

http://www.hphosp.org/

Highland Park Hospital, a member of Northwestern Healthcare Network, provides a variety of consumer health resources that include a physician finder service, osteoporosis prevention, parenting and pregnancy, and information about their nationally recognized fertility program. The site also contains a section entitled **Your Health I.Q.** with interactive online tests for diabetes, ovarian cancer, and heart attack and stroke.

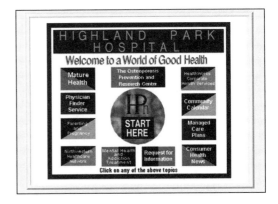

HomeArts Body & Soul

http://www.homearts.com/depts/health/00dphec1.htm

HomeArts Body & Soul provides a wide variety of consumer health resources that include sections on pregnancy and childbirth, health headlines, preventing or dealing with cancer, managing your weight, an ask the doctors feature, discussion forums, and special features such as the healthy traveler and managing menopause.

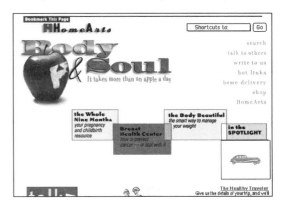

HomeArts Search Center

http://homearts.co-/waisform/find.htm

HomeArts provides a Search Center with hundreds of pages of health-related topics in its network. For example, enter the words "ask the doctors," "Dr. Joyce," or simply the word "health" in the **Search all of HomeArts** box to find 40 references for each of these searches. There are more health-related articles in either *Health, Good Housekeeping,* or *Redbook* under **Specialized Searches.** Try entering "exercise" in each of these specialized search tools.

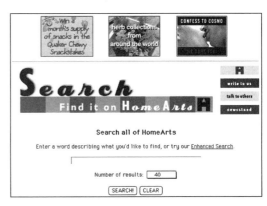

An Illustrated Guide to Muscles & Medical Massage Therapy

http://danke.com/Orthodoc/

An Illustrated Guide to Muscles & Medical Massage Therapy, presented by OrthoDoc, a pain and posture clinic, provides resources for pain relief and posture alignment in children, teenagers, and adults.

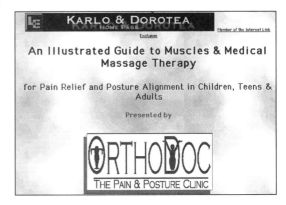

Info for Consumers

http://www.health.state.ny.us/nysdoh/consumer/consumer.htm

Info for Consumers, from the New York State Department of Health, provides consumer information on a variety of topics, including Alzheimer's disease and other dementias, communicable diseases, and environmental and occupational health.

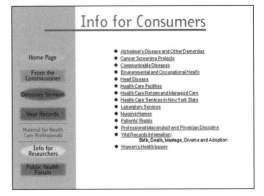

InfoPlex Medical Resources

http://www.ghsl.nwu.edu/nums/resource/mednews.html

InfoPlex Medical Resources, a part of the Medical UseNet newsgroups, is the place to listen in or participate in a lively discussion on a variety of issues and topics in medicine. There is a newsgroup for practically every issue.

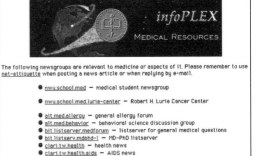

Information for Patients

http://www.aafp.org/patientinfo/

Information for Patients, developed by the American Academy of Family Physicians, contains a collection of handouts covering more than 200 health topics. The handout categories consist of the body, common conditions/diseases/disorders, treatments, and healthy living.

Injury Control Resource Information Network

http://www.injurycontrol.com/icrin/

The Injury Control Resource Information Network provides a comprehensive annotated list of links to sites for injury research and control. The site includes injury-specific resources related to fire and burns, various modes of transportation, poisonings, firearms, violence, falls, sports and recreation, occupations, consumer products, and others.

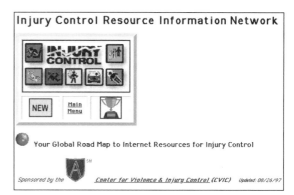

InteliHealth

http://www.intelihealth.com/

InteliHealth, home to Johns Hopkins Health Information, offers a treasure trove of health resources, including online quizzes, the top news headlines, fun interactive activities, and nearly one million pages of medical information. To have access to *all* the site's vast resources, you must register. It's free for the asking.

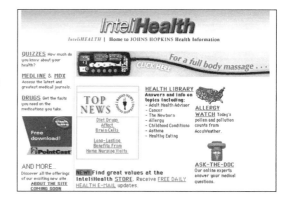

InteliHealth Health Library

http://www.intelihealth.com/ih/ihtHealthLibrary

InteliHealth Health Library is the one-stop Web site for answers to all your health concerns. From causes to cures, this site has the most accurate, practical, and up-to-date information on hundreds of ailments and conditions—in everyday language from some of the world's top medical authorities.

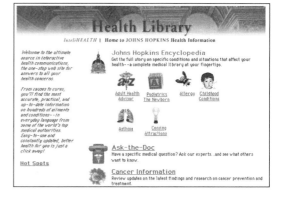

Intelligence Enterprises

http://opendoor.com/iehealth/IEHealthHomePage.html

Intelligence Enterprises health home page provides consumer information on a variety of health problems, including acne removal, weight loss, protecting your heart, protecting your unborn baby, and others.

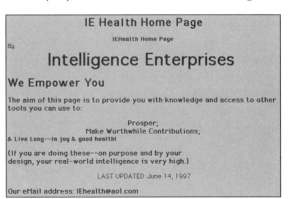

International Travelers Clinic

http://www.intmed.mcw.edu/travel.html

The International Travelers Clinic, from the Medical College of Wisconsin, provides comprehensive preventive health care resources for travelers planning trips abroad. The site includes information on pre-travel vaccinations and preventive medications, as well as links to related sites.

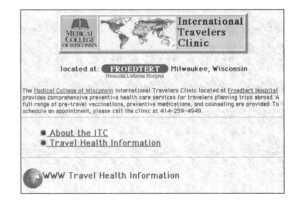

Jocularity

http://www.jocularity.com/toc.html

Jocularity, the humor magazine for nurses from the *Journal of Nursing,* contains over 45 articles and cartoons from past journal issues.

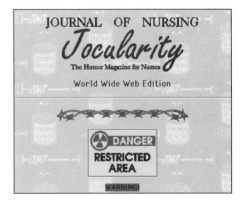

Johns Hopkins Bayview Medical Center

http://www.jhbmc.jhu.edu/cardiology/rehab/patientinfo.html

Johns Hopkins Bayview Medical Center provides cardiac rehabilitation and prevention patient information on nutrition, exercise, smoking, and stress. The site includes a list of related sites.

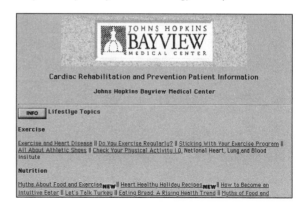

Kaiser Permanente Fremont Medical Center

http://slip-2.slip.net/~phend/

Kaiser Permanente Fremont Medical Center offers health tips and quizzes on a variety of topics from its resident doctors. To find this information, click on **Health Topics.**

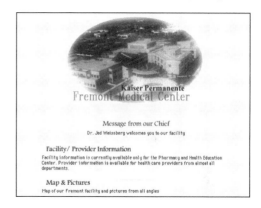

Kaiser Permanente Health Reference

http://www.scl.ncal.kaiperm.org/healthinfo/

Kaiser Permanente Health Reference, provided by the Santa Clara Medical Center, contains consumer health information on a variety of topics, including allergies, breast self-examination (BSE), exercises for the back and the heart, CPR, and others.

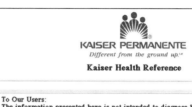

Lakes Region General Hospital

http://www.lrgh.org/healthfq.htm

Lakes Region General Hospital Community Affairs Department provides checkup facts for your health in the areas of breast cancer, skin cancer, hazards of smoking, tuberculosis, and other areas.

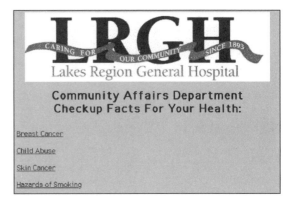

LARG*health

http://johns.largnet.uwo.ca/largh/healhome.html

LARG*health, a community health information network in southwestern Ontario, provides patient resources for AIDS, asthma and other respiratory disorders, general health, nutrition, transplants, and more.

The Longevity Game

http://www.northwesternmutual.com/games/
longevity/longevity-main.html

The Longevity Game is a means to calculate how long you can expect to live based on life insurance industry research. Each person starts with the average life expectancy of 73 years and adds or subtracts years from the score as he or she responds to a questionnaire.

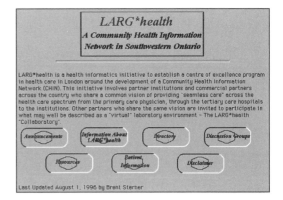

Maryland Poison Center

http://www.pharmacy.ab.umd.edu/~mpc/

The Maryland Poison Center supplies comprehensive emergency poison information, prevention, and educational resources for consumers. For online pamphlets on poisoning, bites, and safety, click on **Educational Info** and scroll to the bottom of the page.

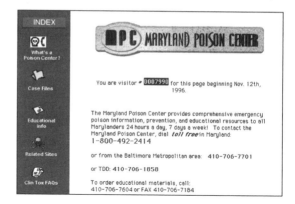

Mayo Health O@sis

http://www.mayohealth.org/

Mayo Health O@sis, sponsored by the Mayo Clinic and IVI Publishing, is an online service providing reliable, up-to-date health and wellness information on a wide variety of topics, including O@sis Library, Cancer Center, Diet & Nutrition, Heart Center, and Pregnancy & Children. Other features are Newsstand, with the most current breakthroughs and stories, and Ask Mayo, a place to talk with the experts. The site is updated daily.

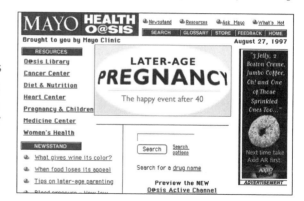

Mayo Health O@sis First Aid

http://www.mayohealth.org/mayo/library/htm/firstaid.htm

Mayo Health O@sis First Aid provides first aid information for a variety of topics ranging from bites and stings to trauma. The site also offers other references, including interactive quizzes and health tips.

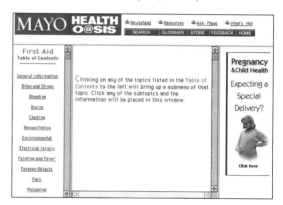

Mayo Health O@sis Library

http://www.mayohealth.org/mayo/common/htm/library.htm

Mayo Health O@sis Library is an immense collection of health information articles, reports, interactive quizzes, and other resources covering topics from eye disease to broken bones.

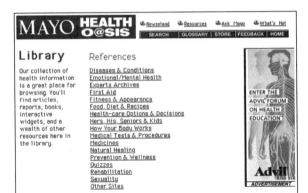

McKinley Health Center

http://www.uiuc.edu/departments/mckinley/mhc.html

McKinley Health Center, from Student Affairs at the University of Illinois at Urbana-Champaign, offers an **Easy-to-Use Index** with a comprehensive listing of health topics ranging from abnormal discharge to yellow fever.

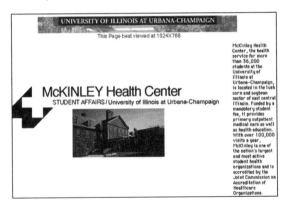

MedAccess On-Line

http://www.medaccess.com/

MedAccess On-Line provides a wide variety of health and wellness resources for the consumer. The **Better Information** section has thousands of pages of information on topics such as the healthy body, healthy mind, healthy children, just for seniors, you are what you eat, and others. Another section, **Health Quizzes,** checks your health IQ on diabetes and other subjects. The site also offers other sections, including health statistics and government agency addresses, environmental health, and a directory of hospitals.

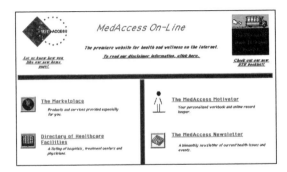

MedFacts.com

http://www.medfacts.com/

MedFacts.com, an interactive, learning discovery experience, features **SportsDoc** and **CardioDoc** simulations where you play the role of a rookie intern performing various (and often humorous) sports medicine injury-related and cardiology-related examinations.

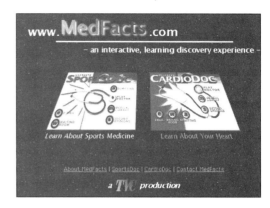

Medi Search

http://users.aol.com/mediinfo/medhome.htm

Medi Search, from Medical Information Research Services, has information on a variety of medical topics, including selecting a physician, and conditions such as asthma, breast lumps, AIDS and HIV and high blood pressure. To find these resources, scroll beyond **New Physicians Profiles Page.** In addition, you can ask Nurse Missy a general health question via e-mail.

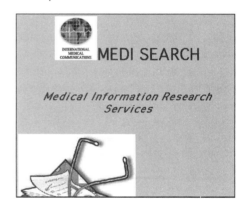

Medical Education Information Center

http://medic.med.uth.tmc.edu/

The Medical Education Information Center, provided by the University of Texas Houston Medical School, features **Health Explorer,** which contains consumer articles contibuted by their physicians. The site also includes a variety of health care resources in the section **MI-WAY Medical Information Super Highway.**

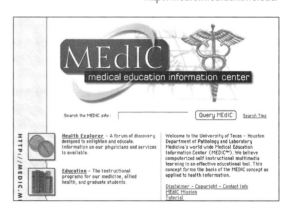

Medical Housecalls

http://www.familyinternet.com/peds/main.htm

Medical Housecalls is a searchable, online consumer medical encyclopedia with references for a wide variety of topics, including diseases, symptoms, drugs, nutrition, surgeries, general health, common injuries, and tests.

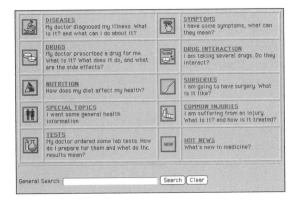

Medical Library

http://www.byu.edu/stlife/health/library/library.html

Medical Library, created by Brigham Young University, has consumer health information on a variety of topics ranging from acne to menstruation. The Library contains online books on common health concerns, mental health issues, nutrition, pediatrics, travel health, and women's health issues.

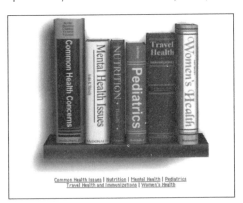

Medical Matrix
Patient Education
and Support

http://www.medmatrix.org/SPages/Patient_Education_and_Support.stm

Medical Matrix has a collection of patient education and support resources on the Internet.

Medical Quest

http://www.useekufind.com/medicin.htm

Medical Quest provides a rich variety of health resources, including medical information from A to Z, medical dictionaries and other references, Internet guides for dentists and chiropractors, health sites, and recipes and nutrition.

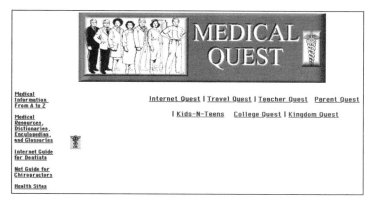

MedicineNet

http://www.medicinenet.com/

MedicineNet is an online comprehensive health reference written in plain language by board-certified physicians. Topics include diseases and treatments, drugs, health advice, what makes you tick, and health news. In addition, there is a medical dictionary. The site includes search tools and alphabetized indexes for different topics.

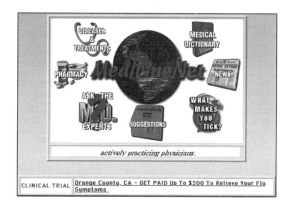

MedicineNet Ask The Experts

http://www.medicinenet.com/ate.asp?ag=Y&li=MNI&x=1

MedicineNet provides the Ask The Experts feature where consumers can ask all types of medical questions from the mundane to the technical. Consumers can submit questions to over 20 different specialty departments, including allergy, internal and family medicine, and cardiology, can view previous questions and answers in each specialty department, or can search the 1996 and 1997 databases.

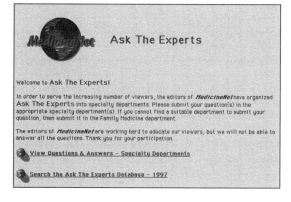

MedIQuiz

http://www.merck.com/quiz/

MedIQuiz is an interactive medical trivia quiz with four separate caregories. Questions change every month.

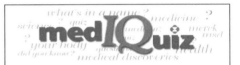

Our co-workers here at Merck may be taking their summer vacations, but our Quizmasters are still hard at work. We've got a whole new batch of questions for the August edition of **MedIQuiz**, and nothing -- not sun, not surf, not even relentless games of volleyball -- will distract us from our task. (Besides, all that sand really messes up our workstations.)

Don't be timid; you might know more than you think. Find out by taking our quiz, and you could **win a T-shirt!**

The multiple-choice quiz features five questions in each of four categories. Every month the first 10 winners who submit

MedWeb

http://www.gen.emory.edu/medweb/medweb.consumer.html

MedWeb, from Emory University Health Sciences Center Library, is an enormous consumer health index to a wide variety of medical information. Select from over 200 topics and then read specific data from a broad range of sources, including government agencies, hospitals, universities, support groups, invividuals, private firms, and research foundations.

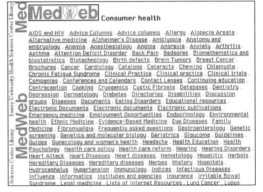

MedWorld

http://medworld.stanford.edu/medworld/

MedWorld, created by medical students from Stanford University, contains a variety of resources for everyone interested in health care. The site provides articles offering the latest health information, medical news, top-rated medical sites categorized by topic, a super search tool, MedBrot, for finding health and medical resources, and much more. To enter MedWorld, you must answer a random true/false medical question.

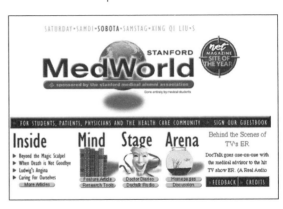

MetLife Online

http://www.metlife.com/

MetLife Online offers a Life Advice section containing a collection of online informative family brochures on health-related topics. Some of family/health brochures include "Being a Parent," "Caring for Aging Parents," "Choosing a Physician," "Coping with Major Illness," "Eating Right," and "Fitness and Exercise."

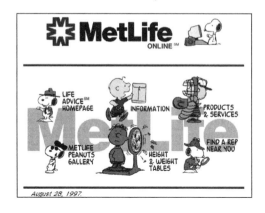

Myers Information Services

http://www.weight.com/

Myers Information Services, updated by Dr. Michael D. Myers, offers easy-to-read medical information on obesity, weight control, eating disorders, and other related medical conditions.

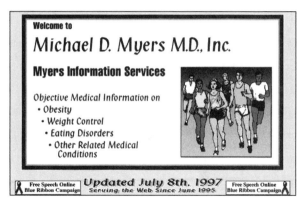

The Nashville Health Page

http://www.nashville.com/~Gsnace/

The Nashville Health Page, created by Dr. G. Stephen Nace, contains a compendium of consumer health resources. Click on **Health Information Topics** for today's health news, general health information sites, drug information, useful toll-free telephone numbers, and information on specific diseases.

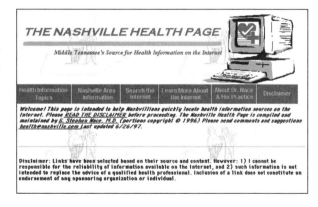

National Health Information Center

http://nhic-nt.health.org/

The National Health Information Center provides a directory of health resources and organizations just a free phone call away. This online list covers the gamut of medical ailments and disorders, as well as agencies dedicated to healthier living. Each link at the site contains toll-free numbers, mailing addresses, and a short abstract describing the organization's purpose and goals.

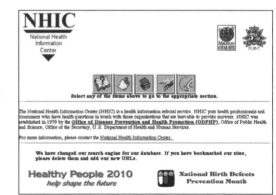

The National Heart, Lung, and Blood Institute

http://www.nhlbi.nih.gov/nhlbi/nhlbi.htm

The National Heart, Lung, and Blood Institute offers a collection of online articles about health information for cardiovascular, lung, blood, and sleep disorders. The articles cover topics ranging from obesity and cholesterol to high blood pressure.

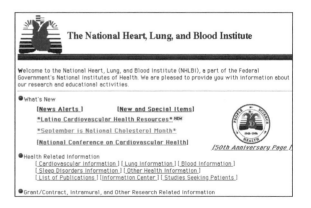

NetWellness

http://www.netwellness.org/

NetWellness is a Web-based consumer health information service developed by the University of Cincinnati Medical Center with many partners. The site contains a variety of topics, including diseases and conditions, your health and wellness, and general health. In addition, this service provides an electronic health library that is updated daily, a search tool, and ask an expert and in the news search features.

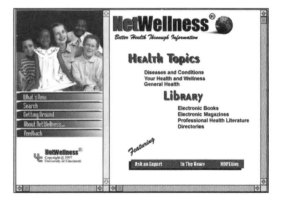

Oh, My Aching Back

http://www.achingback.com/

Oh, My Aching Back is an investigative guide to maintaining a healthy back. It is based on a CD-ROM and contains a wealth of helpful information on human anatomy, back problems, exercise, prevention techniques, lifestyle choices, and back-related links.

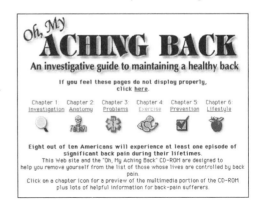

Olsten Health Services

http://www.okqchomehealth.com/

Olsten Health Services provides a wealth of information about home health services. The site includes additional health care resources.

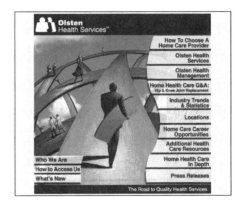

Onhealth

http://www.onhealth.com

Onhealth, from IVI Publishing, is a wonderful collection of health resources, including community health information, headline news, conditions from A to Z, an anatomy list, an online pharmacy with nearly 8000 different types of drugs, and much more.

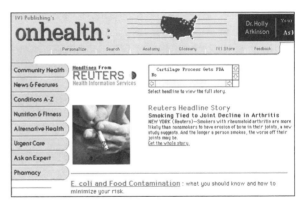

Openseason.com

http://openseason.com/

Openseason.com is an interactive site with information on health and health insurance. The site offers a variety of health resources for consumers in the **Healthy Living Area** section. The resources include food and nutrition articles and a library reading room with selected health articles ranging from early heart attack care to walking exercises. To learn about the different specialties, click on the **stethoscope** in the heading.

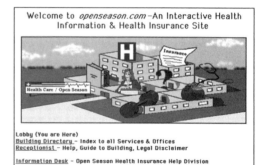

The Osteopathic Home Page

http://www.concentric.net/~Ericdo/

The main purpose of the Osteopathic Home Page is to further the public's understanding of osteopathic medicine. The site includes information about cranial osteopathy and a multitude of links to other osteopathic sites.

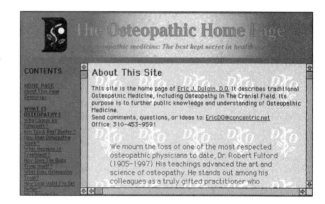

Patient Support Trust

http://www.patientsupport.org.uk/

Patient Support Trust provides a rich source of information and advice about a variety of illnesses and medical conditions. The Patient Support Centre section offers information about topics such as nicotine craving, migraine headaches, and impotence, while the Patient Advice on the Web addresses a great many topics, among them AIDS, allergies, child health, dental health, eye care, and mental health.

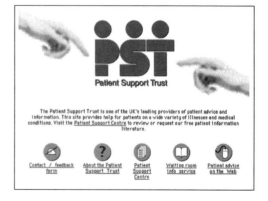

Physical Therapist Online

http://physicaltherapist.com/

Physical Therapist Online is a comprehensive physical therapist site that offers links to a number of physical therapy periodicals.

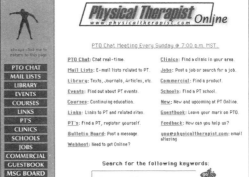

Physical Therapy

http://automailer.com/tws/

Physical Therapy, the Web space, lists links to other sites related not only to physical therapy but to health and medicine. Categories include Disease/Injury, Health/Medical, and Physical Therapy.

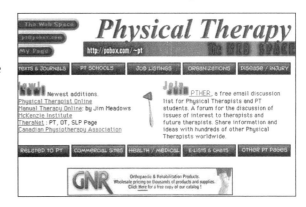

Princeton University Outdoor Action Program

http://www.princeton.edu/~oa/oa.html

The Princeton University Outdoor Action Program offers a wealth of resources about the outdoors, including online seasonal first aid guides. To find the *OA Guide to Heat* and the *OA Guide to Cold Weather,* scroll to Guide to the Outdoor Action Web Site and click on **First Aid & Safety Information.**

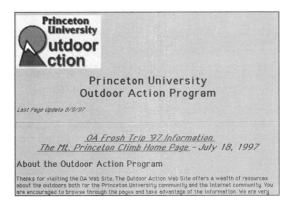

Reservoir

http://www.coolware.com/health/medical_reporter/health.html

Reservoir, a health information resource, has a wide variety of health and medical articles, including men's and women's health issues, stress, and sexuality topics. For a complete list of all the articles, click on **Table of Contents.**

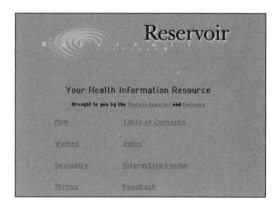

The Saturday Evening Post Medical Mailbox

http://www.satevepost.org/medical.html

The Saturday Evening Post Medical Mailbox is an online mailbox service where Dr. Cory SerVaas answers your questions on health and nutrition. You can either read about the latest medical research or use the keyword searchable database.

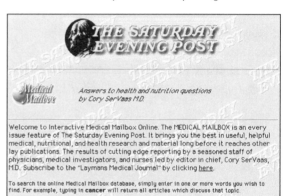

Selfcare Tips

http://www.aetnaaz.com/tips.html

Selfcare Tips, from Aetna Health Plans of Arizona, provides useful health information on a variety of topics, including allergies and asthma.

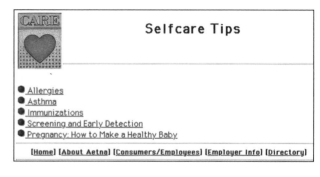

Stratospheric Ozone

http://www.epa.gov/ozone/

Stratospheric Ozone, from the U.S. Environmental Protection Agency, provides authoritative information about understanding ozone. The site includes public information and a national map of protection levels (see the **UV Index** link) so you can safely walk in the sun.

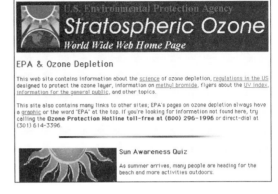

Timmy's Home Page

http://logic.csc.cuhk.edu.hk/~s965092/

Timmy's Home Page includes an interactive **life expectancy estimator** in which you enter personal data to determine your approximate life span.

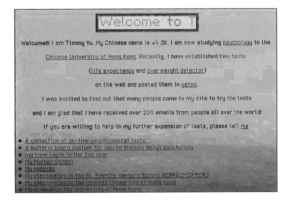

Trauma Home Page

http://rmstewart.uthscsa.edu/

The Trauma Home Page, from the University of Texas Health Science Center at San Antonio, focuses on issues dealing with injury, injury prevention, and surgical critical care.

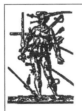

Travel Health Online

http://www.tripprep.com/

Travel Health Online, updated daily by Shoreland's, contains global health information and detailed health and safety information for over 225 countries, breaking news of health risks and vaccination requirements, current country maps showing regions of disease risk, and AIDS testing requirements in each country.

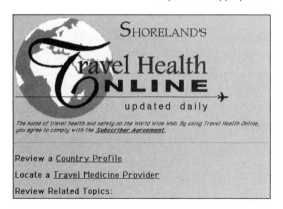

UCDavis Health System

http://www.ucdmc.ucdavis.edu/health/

UCDavis Health System has health information on a variety of topics of interest to consumers. The site includes the **Wellness Center** with information about childhood immunizations, healthy recipes, poison prevention, and much more. In addition, there are healthy recipes and health tips from *Pulse* and informative articles from *Health Journal,* the University of California Davis Health System's bimonthly publication for health care consumers.

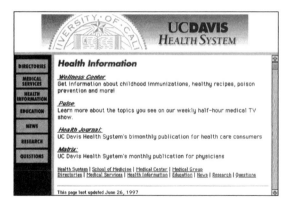

UCLA Student Health Service

http://www.saonet.ucla.edu/health.htm

UCLA Student Health Service contains a **Sexual Health and Wellness** section and an **Immunizations** section that provide health information and advice for college students. To find an A to Z index of health education handouts on such topics ranging from acne to yeast infection, click on **Health Education Outreach Services.**

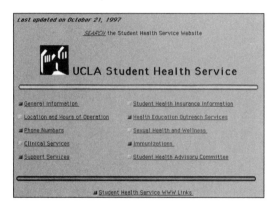

USA Today Health Index

http://web.usatoday.com/life/health/lhindex.htm

USA Today Health Index has a broad spectrum of articles on everything from AIDS to Women's Health. The *USA Today* articles are presented in synopsis form, as well as full length.

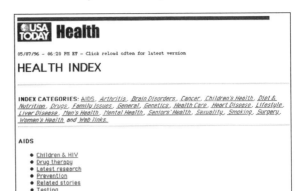

The Virtual Hospital
Iowa Health Book

http://www.vh.org/Patients/Patients.html

The Virtual Hospital presents the online *Iowa Health Book,* which contains a huge collection of patient educational materials for treating a wide variety of medical problems ranging from controlling pain to family safety. You can find patient information in the *Iowa Health Book* by searching for it or by browsing by department or by organ system. The site also provides an annotated list of these *Iowa Health Book* materials.

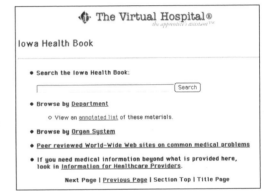

Warner-Lambert Products
and You

http://www.warner-lambert.com/conaffairs/

The Warner-Lambert Products and You Web site has product encyclopedias to find specific health information about a featured Warner-Lambert product. Each encyclopedia includes a symptom/product match service, an FAQs section, and interactive fun quizzes. Warner-Lambert offers health-related encyclopedias for allergy, cold cough and sinus relief, first aid, oral care, and others.

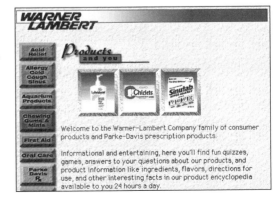

Weather-Health Link

http://www.inforamp.net/~eeyore/

Weather-Health Link, from the Canadian Medical Meteorology Network, features a wide range of articles on how the weather and the atmosphere affect various health aspects such as your skin, vision, asthma, diabetes, allergies, migraine headaches, and pollution.

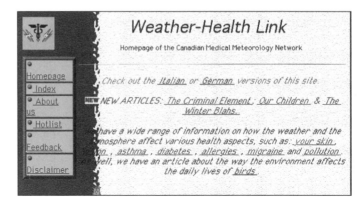

WebDoctor

http://www.gretmar.com/webdoctor/home.html

WebDoctor, the Internet navigator for physicians, provides a virtual library of up-to-date medical information. Resources are arranged by subject area and include information by disease, online journals, pharmacy resources, an online *WebDoctor Newsletter,* and late-breaking health news. Although the site is intended primarily for physicians, it can serve as an encyclopedia source for the interested consumer.

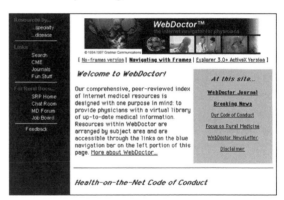

Wheaton Regional Library Health Information Center

http://www.mont.lib.md.us/hic.html

Wheaton Regional Library Health Information Center, in Silver Springs, Maryland, provides health information and consumer resources for a variety of topics, including health policy and issues, prescription and non-prescription drugs, wellness, HIV/AIDS, and environmental and occupational health.

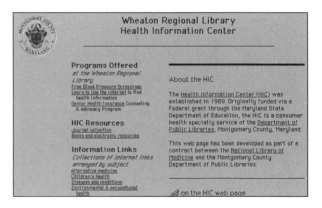

You First

http://www.youfirst.com/

You First provides a free, personalized, and confidential online health risk assessment report that includes recommendations to improve health and minimize potential future health problems. The site also includes summer health tips and health-related links on a variety of topics.

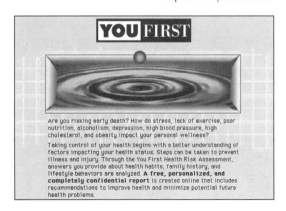

Your Health

http://www.cheshire-med.com/yourhealth1.html

Your Health, presented by The Cheshire Medical Center in New Hampshire, offers a wide variety of features, including monthly nutrition news, ask an ER nurse, prescription drug information, lung disease resource, and information for new moms.

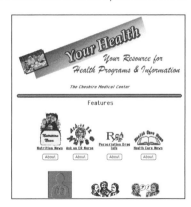

Your Personal Net Health

http://www.ypn.com/living/health/

Your Personal Net Health is a mega-site to gain access to descriptions of common ailments, trade information on the latest research, learn about alternative medicine, or tap into the database of the leading world health organizations. You can also download informational brochures, fitness regimens, and government reports on recently tested pharmaceuticals.

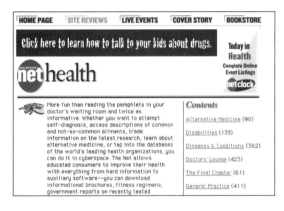

You and Your Children

CHAPTER 4

Aaron's Tracheostomy Page

http://members.aol.com/trachtube

Aaron's Tracheostomy Page is a guide to home care for a child with a tracheostomy. The site addresses problems such as eating and speech difficulties, equipment needs, changing the tube, and general precautions. There are links to other tracheostomy sites.

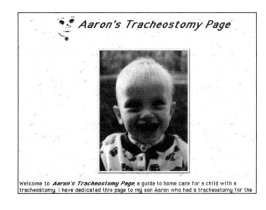

The ABCs of Safe and Healthy Child Care

http://www.cdc.gov/ncidod/hip/abc/abc.htm

The ABCs of Safe and Healthy Child Care, prepared by the Centers for Disease Control and Prevention (CDC), is an online handbook for child care providers, parents, or caregivers. The Handbook provides a whole alphabet of advice on keeping your child out of harm's way, including information on accident prevention, basic first aid, proper hygiene, common childhood diseases, and much more.

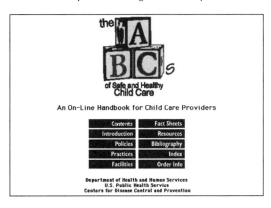

AIDS Now! for Teens

http://itec.sfsu.edu/aids/aids.html

AIDS Now! for Teens, designed for teenagers by Jeff Schwartz, provides an interactive multiple choice quiz on preventing AIDS.

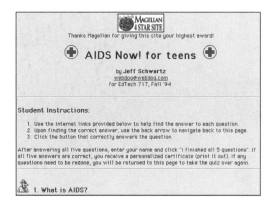

American Academy of Pediatrics

http://www.aap.org

The American Academy of Pediatrics site focuses on child and adolescent health. The site contains many articles published by nationally recognized magazines. The category entitled You and Your Family includes consumer-specific information such as "Air Bag Safety," "Caring for Your Adolescent," and "Reduce the Risk of Sudden Infant Death Syndrome."

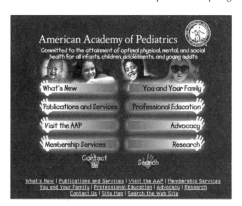

American Baby

http://www.enews.com/magazines/baby/

American Baby offers selected articles from current and back issues of the *American Baby* magazine. Articles focus on expectant parents and deal with such issues as diaper changing, discipline, the basics of baby care, and the health and medical concerns of pregnancy and infancy.

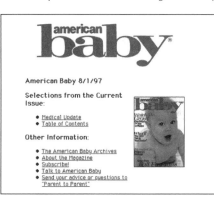

Attention Deficit Disorder

http://add.miningco.com/

Attention Deficit Disorder (ADD), part of the Mining Company Web site, contains a collection of articles and links to ADD sites.

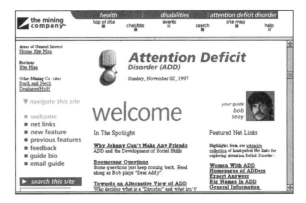

Attention Deficit Disorder and Related Issues

http://www.ns.net/users/BrandiV/

Attention Deficit Disorder and Related Issues, created by Brandi Valentine, offers a vast collection of online resources for ADD/ADHD.

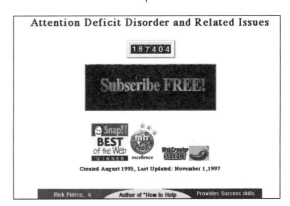

Attention Deficit Disorder WWW Archive

http://www.realtime.net/cyanosis/add/

Attention Deficit Disorder WWW Archive, started by Meng Meng Wong from the University of Pennsylvania, contains resources ranging from diagnostic criteria to tips for living with attention deficit disorder.

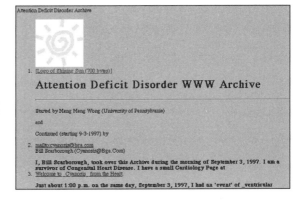

Baby Bag Online

http://www.babybag.com/

Baby Bag Online provides a wealth of resources for parents with children from prenatal stages to preschool. Among the topics are health and safety issues, pregnancy and childbirth information, parenting information, feeding and nutrition information, a cook's corner with recipes, an ask the professional section, and a variety of bulletin boards.

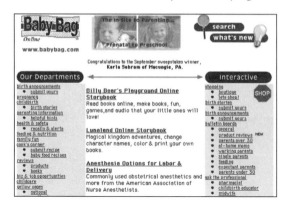

Canadian Parents Online

http://www.canadianparents.com/

Canadian Parents Online offers a variety of health-related topics and online activities of interest to parents. You can enter into a discussion forum, read parenting articles from the library, and get healthy recipes from the Canada Cooks section. In addition, you can get help from a team of parenting experts in Ask an Expert. The experts include family and teenage counselors and health care professionals.

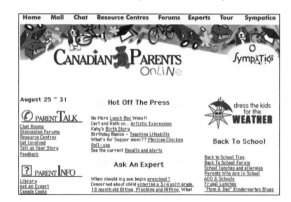

Careguide

http://www.careguide.net/

Careguide is a comprehensive searchable, national reference guide with thousands of listings of child care and elder care facilities. The site also provides online bulletin boards where ideas and experiences can be exchanged.

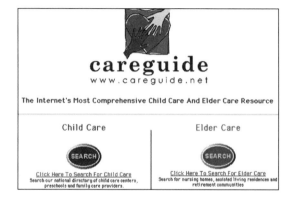

CAT HIV/AIDS Info

http://www.qcfurball.com/cat/aids.html

CAT HIV/AIDS Info, from Children's Animated Television (CAT), has many informative documents regarding AIDS prevention, AIDS testing, condom usage, food safety advice for people with AIDS, caring for people with AIDS, AIDS hotline numbers, an Ask Dr. Rick feature, exercise and HIV, women and AIDS, and needle exchange. The site also includes a list of other AIDS links.

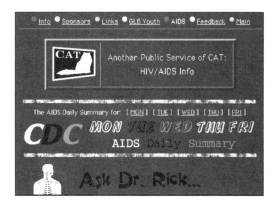

Child & Family Canada

http://www.cfc-efc.ca/

Child & Family Canada, a bilingual site developed through the cooperation of more than 30 Canadian non-profit health and family organizations, provides a variety of well-written articles indexed under 14 categories on the **Information by Theme** page. Examples include allergies in children from the health theme, working with families and children from the the parenting theme, suicide from the adolescent theme.

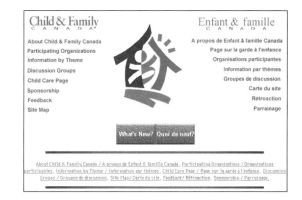

Child Secure

http://www.childsecure.com/

Child Secure has more than 400 online pages of timely information on children's health and safety. The site contains health archives, safety archives, related links, an ask the doctor feature, and much more.

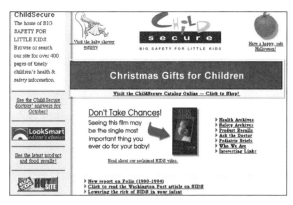

Child-Neuro Home Page

http://waisman.wisc.edu/child-neuro/

The Child-Neuro home page is a collection of child neurology sites. Links to other sites include categories such as Academy sites, disease information, clinical service information, two search tools, e-mail and Internet resources, and the latest in research.

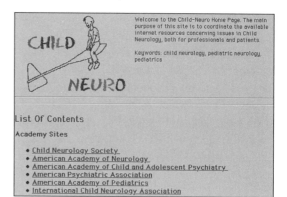

Childhood Infections

http://kidshealth.org/parent/common/

Childhood Infections, from the Nemours Foundation site, KidsHealth.org, provides information about a variety of childhood diseases.

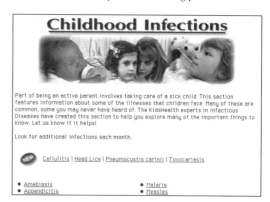

Children Now

http://www.childrennow.org

Children Now offers many articles, reports, and links to other sites, all of which deal with the health and welfare of children, both nationally and in California. The topic entitled Children's Health provides a link called **Internet Resources** on children's health. This link lists hundreds of resources covering a broad range of issues related to the health of children.

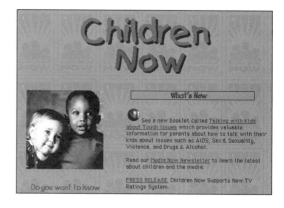

Children with Diabetes

http://www.castleweb.com/diabetes

Children with Diabetes tells you everything you might want to know about diabetes, whether in children or in adults, briefly, concisely, and in language that is easy to understand. Naturally, many articles discuss diet, but other offerings include diet camps, a diabetes dictionary, related Web sites, and a search tool.

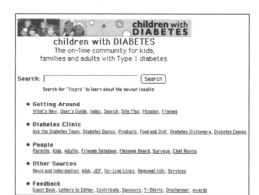

Children with Milk, Egg and other Food Allergies

http://users.aol.com/katherinez/kath2.htm

The Children with Milk, Egg, and other Food Allergies site provides information about food allergies in children, especially allergies to eggs and dairy products. A mother of two children with food allergies reports her experiences and research. Of particular interest may be the brand names of specific products that claim to be "dairy free" according to federal guidelines but which, according to the author, contain dairy products or by-products.

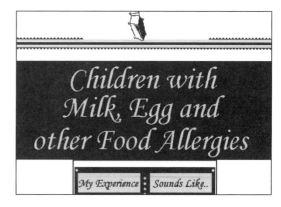

Children with Spina Bifida

http://www.waisman.wisc.edu/~rowley/sb_kids.htmlx

Children with Spina Bifida is a comprehensive resource for information about spina bifida and includes topics such as other spina bifida sites, spina bifida organizations, mailing lists, newsgroups and chat rooms, and links to research sites.

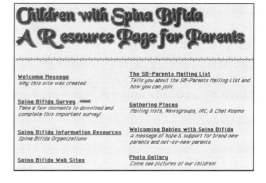

The Children's Health Page

http://www.best.com/~gazissax/chealth.html

The Children's Health Page, by Lynn Gazis-Sax, is a collection of FAQs and links to Internet resources related to children's health. The FAQs are divided into four general areas: (1) diseases and vaccinations, (2) prenatal tests, (3) allergies, and (4) safety and childproofing.

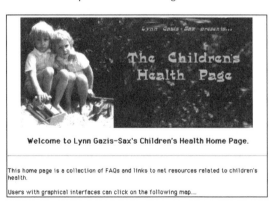

Chronic Cough in Children

http://www.bcm.tmc.edu/cme/courses/oto_01/

Chronic Cough in Children is an online course from Baylor Medical School on chronic cough in children. The topics include etiology of cough, a diagnostic protocol, pulmonary function testing, and many others, all with accompanying illustrations.

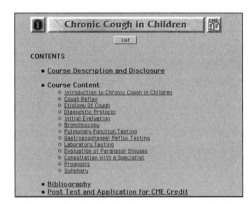

CNN Interactive Parenting

http://cnnplus.cnn.com/consumer/parenting/

CNN Interactive Parenting provides information on immunization schedules, physical examinations, common childhood ailments, sudden infant death syndrome (SIDS), and much more. In addition, the site offers Internet guidelines for parents.

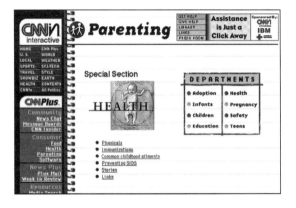

Combined Internal Medicine & Pediatrics

http://ourworld.compuserve.com/homepages/anduril/medicine.htm

Combined Internal Medicine & Pediatrics is an extensive directory of internal medicine and pediatric sites on the Internet. Categories include general information, medical links, specific pediatric sites, medical associations, doctors' home pages, and others.

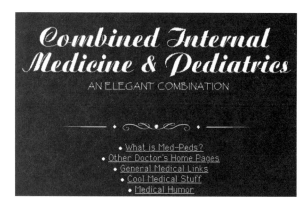

Congenital Heart Disease Information and Resources

http://www.tchin.org/

Congenital Heart Disease Information and Resources, from the Children's Health Information Network, provides information and resources to families of children with congenital and acquired heart disease, adults with congenital heart disease, and the professionals who work with them.

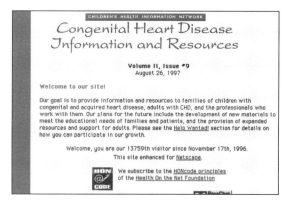

The Congenital Heart Disease Resource Page

http://www.csun.edu/~hcmth011/heart/

The Congenital Heart Disease Resource Page provides parents of children with congenital heart disease a place to find information about specific diseases and other support resources. The site includes personal pages, support information, and a list of newsgroups and other heart-related sites.

A Consumer's Guide to Bicycle Helmets

http://www.bhsi.org/webdocs/guide.htm

A Consumer's Guide to Bicycle Helmets, prepared by the Bicycle Helmet Safety Institute (BHSI), is a "must-read" for all cyclists, especially children. The Guide is an extensive online pamphlet describing everything you need to know about choosing and using a bike helmet.

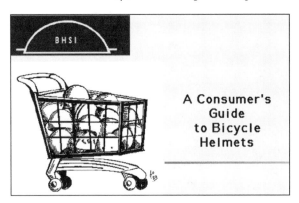

Doctor Paula's Web Site

http://www.drpaula.com/

Doctor Paula's Web Site has daily free online pediatric advice and information on what to keep in the medicine cabinet. There are answers to questions about children and teenagers with topics ranging from abdominal pain to the wheeze. The site also includes a wealth of related pediatric links.

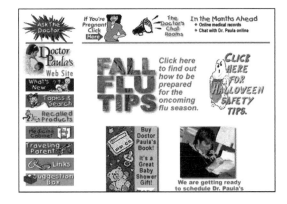

Dr. Greene's HouseCalls

http://www.drgreene.com/

Dr. Greene's HouseCalls provides a multitude of health resources. The site features a search tool and articles divided into seven categories: prenatal, newborns, infants, toddlers, pre-schoolers, school age, and adolescents. Articles are also subdivided into 13 areas by content. Links to other sites are available.

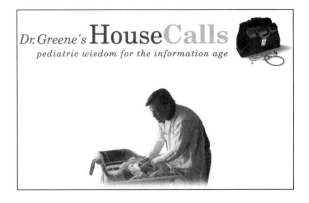

The Dr. Judy Column

http://www.parentsplace.com/readroom/doctor/drjudy.html

The Dr. Judy Column contains some 30 articles about children's health, arranged in four general categories: (1) sports and recreation (sample title: "Baby, It's Cold Outside"), (2) at home (sample title: "Pick Your Poison"), (3) medical issues (sample title: "Go for the Throat"), and (4) other issues (sample title: "If the Shoe Fits").

ParentsPlace.com | Health Reading Room | Children's Literature, A Newsletter for Adults.

The Dr. Judy Column
Pediatric Advice for Parents

Dr. Judy Rowen is a pediatrician at Baylor College of Medicine, Houston, Texas. Her column here is reprinted with permission from *Children's Literature, A Newsletter for Adults*. Please feel free to browse several of the selections below.

Sport and Recreation

- Baby It's Cold Outside Cold Weather and Frostbite *NEW*
- Is your child "suiting up" for a sport that is suitable?
- Be Hardheaded About Helmets!
- Playground Safety
- Sun Protection for Tender Tots
- I've Got You Under My Skin Tick Bites
- Something's Afoot Athlete's Foot
- Ankle Sprains

At Home

- Clean Up Your Act Handwashing *NEW*
- Pick Your Poison: Surprising Household Hazards
- Pet Peeves Contracting Illnesses from Pets

Dr. Warren's Web Page

http://www.mindspring.com/~drwarren/DrWarren.html

Dr. Warren's Web Page offers an informative newsletter in a question-and-answer format. Dr. Warren addresses a wide variety of topics from "My newborn Looks Like a Cone Head" to "How Can I Tell if My Girlfriend is Really Pregnant?" The site also includes sugar-free dessert recipes for diabetics. Other articles by Dr. Warren can be found in the **Pediatrics at the Mining Company** link.

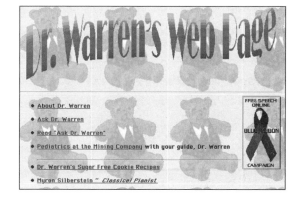

- About Dr. Warren
- Ask Dr. Warren
- Read "Ask Dr. Warren"
- Pediatrics at the Mining Company with your guide, Dr. Warren
- Dr. Warren's Sugar Free Cookie Recipes
- Myron Silberstein – *Classical Pianist*

Dyslexia

http://www.dyslexiaonline.com/

Dyslexia, maintained by Dr. Harold Levinson, presents information about the misconceptions of dyslexia and related attention deficit and anxiety disorders.

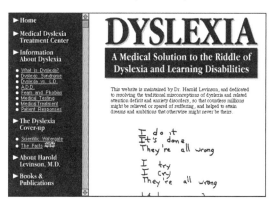

Dyslexia The Gift

http://www.dyslexia.com/

Dyslexia The Gift, based on the Ron Davis book, provides a forum for sharing information about dyslexia and other learning difficulties. The site contains information and articles on materials and methods for overcoming academic dyslexic problems.

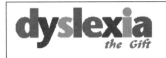

Epilepsy in Young Children

http://www.geocities.com/HotSprings/1000/

Epilepsy in Young Children features a list of children diagnosed with epilepsy. The site includes each parent's e-mail address, which helps to create a large support network of parents of children with epilepsy.

FactLine

http://www.drugs.indiana.edu/publications/iprc/factline/ritalin.html

FactLine, from the Indiana Prevention Resource Center at Indiana University, includes a reprint of William J. Bailey's article on the non-medical use of Ritalin. The article presents information on patterns of non-medical use, health consequences, and legal issues.

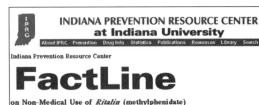

Get It Straight! The Facts About Drugs

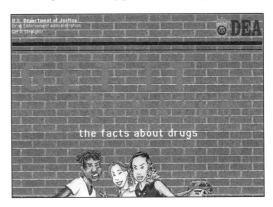

http://www.usdoj.gov/dea/pubs/straight/cover.htm

Get It Straight! The Facts About Drugs is an online book for teenagers presented by the U.S. Department of Justice Drug Enforcement Administration (DEA).

Girl Power!

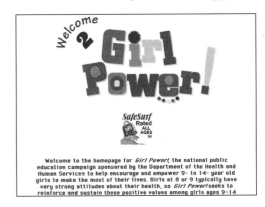

http://www.health.org/gpower/

Girl Power!, presented by the U.S. Department of Health and Human Services, seeks to turn things around for girls ages 9 to 14 with tips for healthy living.

HeadLice.org

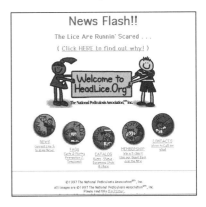

http://www.headlice.org

HeadLice.org presents the latest news on headlice and scabies, answers to FAQs, and a catalog listing related products.

Health Ink

http://www.healthink.com/

Health Ink, a publisher of consumer health books and magazines, provides reliable, up-to-date, and entertaining information on a variety of health topics of interest to parents and children. The topics include the **Fresh Air Cafe,** a smoke-free cool zone; **Doctors Tell All,** why they do their stuff; **Starting Out Healthy,** kids' health advice; **Teen Truth,** teen counseling online; and **Dr. Brian McDonough,** a real TV Doc who fields questions. In addition, the site offers crossword health puzzles, nutrition quizzes, and an informative report on the leading health care businesses on the Net.

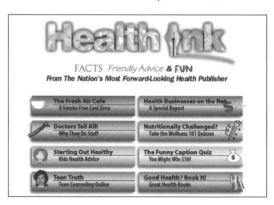

Health-Net

http://www.parentzone.com/health/

Health-Net, from the Parent Zone, provides a collection of health topics with articles written by medical professionals. Topics range from arthritis to wellness, and the Ask the Doctor feature contains a list of the readers' questions answered by the experts.

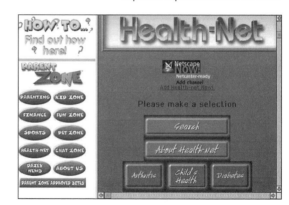

Healthy Living with Sunshine

http://www.mb.ec.gc.ca/ENGLISH/AIR/HLWS/mmenu.html

Healthy Living with Sunshine, part of the Environment Canada Web site, provides useful health information to protect children from skin cancer. The site also explains, in terms understandable to kids, "What's happening to the ozone layer?"

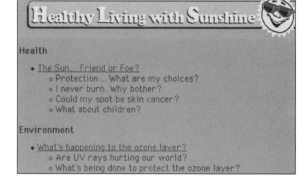

Infectious Diseases in Children

http://www.slackinc.com/child/idc/idchome.htm

Infectious Diseases in Children, an online version of the monthly Slack periodical, *Diseases in Children,* includes new drugs and procedures for diagnosing and testing pediatric infectious diseases. The site features key articles from current and past issues, breaking news bulletins, a searchable directory, and a comprehensive pediatric Internet directory.

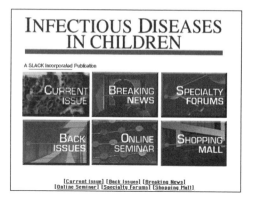

Info for Kids

http://ach.uams.edu/kids/

Info for Kids, from Arkansas Children's Hospital, is jam-packed with useful information for parents of newborns to young adults age 21. The site is divided into the following sections: My Visit to the Hospital, Kid's Health and Safety Tips, Cool Stuff for Kids, and Teens and Young Adults.

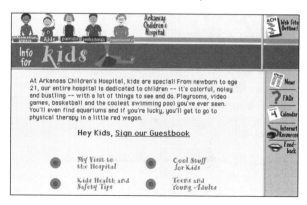

Information for Patients

http://ww2.med.jhu.edu/cancerctr/peds/pedinfo.htm

Information for Patients, from Johns Hopkins Oncology Center, provides useful patient information about a variety of children's cancer diseases. You can read about prevention, symptoms, treatment, clinical trials, and support groups by clicking on **Search for Information by Cancer Type.**

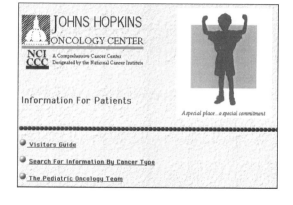

Juvenile Diabetes Foundation International

http://www.jdfcure.com/

The Juvenile Diabetes Foundation International, a non-profit health agency, supports and funds diabetes research. The site contains a mail-order pharmacy, information and online publications about diabetes, and related sites.

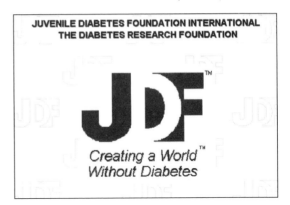

Kid Safety on the Internet

http://www.uoknor.edu/oupd/kidsafe/start.htm

Kid Safety on the Internet, provided by the University of Oklahoma Department of Public Safety, features a fun and colorful "slide-show" presentation on 27 important safety topics. The topics include strangers, drugs and alcohol, finding needles, getting lost, home emergencies, and even Internet safety.

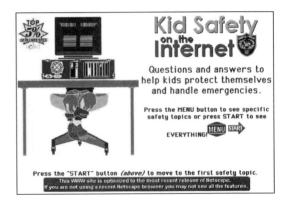

Kid's Health at the AMA

http://www.ama-assn.org/insight/h_focus/nemours

Kid's Health at the AMA covers a range of topics, including childhood infections, emergencies and first aid, safety and accident prevention, and child development.

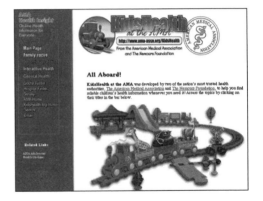

Kids Campaigns

http://www.kidscampaigns.org

Kids Campaigns, a project of the Coalition for America's Children, is an invaluable social and health resource for parents and community leaders. For an overview of the site, click on **Contents At A Glance** and scroll to the Features section to find health information about Teens, Drugs, and Parenting.

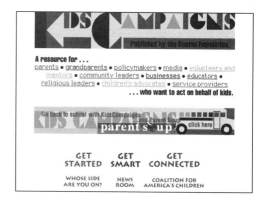

KidsDoctor

http://www.kidsdoctor.com/

KidsDoctor contains a search tool to look up information on topics such as poison oak, fever, earache, and many others. Click on **list** to find an alphabetical listing of articles, everything from bubble baths to bug bites.

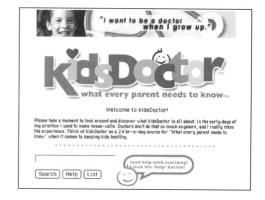

KidsHealth.org

http://kidshealth.org/

KidsHealth.org, a premiere site for kids and parents created by the Nemours Foundation, provides a comprehensive collection of resources and accurate up-to-date information about growth, food and fitness, childhood infections, immunizations, laboratory tests, medical and surgical conditions, and the most recent treatments.

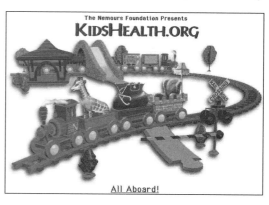

KidSource OnLine

http://www.kidsource.com/

KidSource OnLine provides a wealth of health care resources for newborns, toddlers, preschoolers, school-age children from K to grade 12, and parenting. Each section on the bottom of the page includes online forums, related Web sites, and age-appropriate health-related articles that are rated. In addition, the comprehensive health section contains articles on topics such as childhood diseases and illnesses, general health and medicine, and preventive care and nutrition.

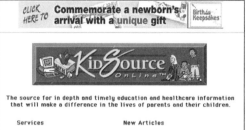

KidsVision

http://www.children-special-needs.org

KidsVision provides parents with comprehensive information on children's vision care and eye health. The site also includes a directory of vision care providers.

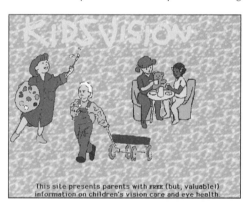

Managing Your Health

http://www.warrencl.com/health.html

Managing Your Health, prepared by the Warren Clinic at Saint Francis Children's Hospital in Tulsa, Oklahoma, contains a variety of health topics of interest to parents. Topics include choosing a physician, the benefits of physical activity and fitness, looking at food labels, facts about osteoporosis, the flu, and childhood immunizations.

Mi Pediatra

http://eureka.tamnet.com.mx/~rmurguia/

The Mi Pediatra home page, written in Spanish, contains general pediatric information, including information on vaccinations and Spanish medical periodicals.

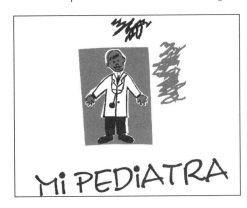

Multimedia Tutorials for Children and Parents

http://galen.med.virginia.edu/~smb4v/tutorial.html

Multimedia Tutorials for Children and Parents presents general information about several medical conditions that might strike children: (1) gastroesophageal reflux in infants, (2) cerebral palsy, (3) asthma, and (4) chronic constipation. Several links to searchable databases are available. Click on one of the general categories. The potential for additional information is almost unlimited.

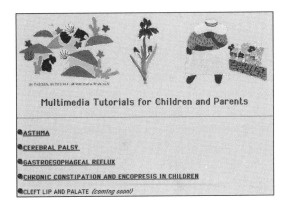

National Immunization Program

http://www.cdc.gov/nip/

The National Immunization Program, from The Centers for Disease Control and Prevention (CDC), offers recommendations to protect the nation's children and adults from vaccine-preventable diseases. To find consumer immunization information for a variety of diseases, select **Frequently Asked Questions** and click on **General Q & A.**

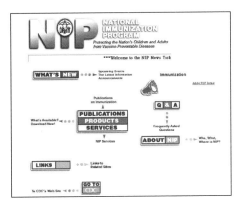

National Information Center for Children and Youth with Disabilities

http://www.kidsource.com/NICHCY/

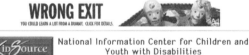

The National Information Center for Children and Youth with Disabilities, part of KidSource Online, contains a collection of articles, fact sheets, and information for parenting children with a range of disabilities and developmental disorders.

National Parent Information Network

http://ericps.ed.uiuc.edu/npin/npinhome.html

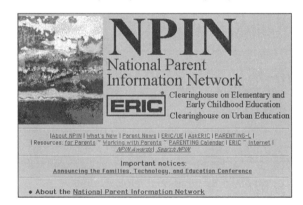

National Parent Information Network provides information to parents and those who work with parents. The site includes an online monthly newsletter, *Parent News,* with health-related articles, parenting resources with electronic versions of childhood development pamphlets and guides. The site also includes a search tool for your inquiries.

Not Me, Not Now

http://www.notmenotnow.org/

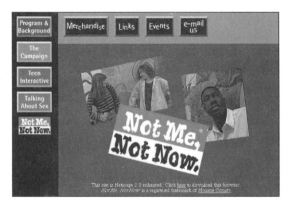

Not Me, Not Now provides information for parents and teenagers interested in learning more about premarital sex. The site offers a listing of educational journal articles, facts about teenage pregnancy, and sample conversations about how to talk with your child about sensitive issues. Teens should check out the online quizzes, testing one's resilience against peer pressure and judgment when dealing with sticky situations.

OncoLink Pediatric Leukemias

http://cancer.med.upenn.edu/disease/leukemia/

OncoLink Pediatric Leukemias, from the University of Pennsylvania Cancer Center, contains an index to hundreds of articles about cancer and leukemias in children. The site also includes other cancer-related sites.

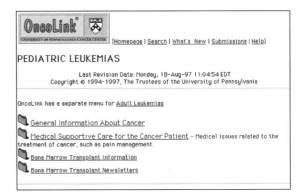

One A.D.D. Place

http://www.greatconnect.com/oneaddplace/

One A.D.D. Place has a wealth of information about attention deficit disorder/attention deficit hyperactivity disorder (ADD/ADHD), including an adult checklist, famous people with ADD, an online library with newsletters, articles, and references, and related links to ADD/ADHD sites.

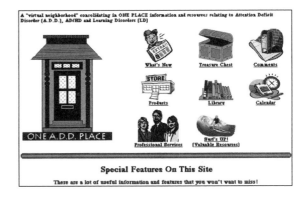

Our-Kids

http://rdz.stjohns.edu/library/support/our-kids/

Our-Kids is an excellent source of information for parents and caregivers of children with various disabilities. The site also contains links to disability-related sites and listservs.

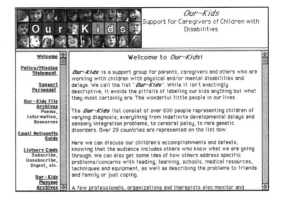

Paediatrics on the Internet

http://www.healey.com.au/users/nghmc/paedlinks.html

Paediatrics on the Internet is a huge index to other pediatric Web sites with thousands of articles dealing with children's health.

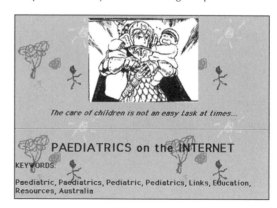

ParenthoodWeb

http://www.parenthoodweb.com/

ParenthoodWeb offers a team of 19 health experts who will answer your questions each week. The experts include a child psychologist, an obstetrician/gynecologist, a midwife, a pediatrician, and others. Each expert area contains an archive of previous questions and answers. You can also use a topics pull-down menu or a search engine to find health-related articles on a variety of topics ranging from allergies to vaccinations.

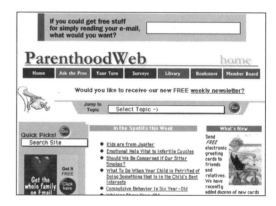

Parenting Library

http://www.parentsoup.com/library/

Parenting Library, from Parent Soup, contains a plethora of useful articles on everything from health and safety tips to complications in childbirth. Click on **Browse** to find categories that include baby and toddlers, pregnancy and birth, relationships, and much more. The site includes a search tool.

Parents' Page

http://members.aol.com/AllianceMD/parents.html

Parents' Page contains selected excerpts from Dr. Lewis Wasserman's e-mail publication, *Parents' Letter,* offering medical advice and helpful hints. The site also includes The Baby Booklet, a new parents' brochure, information about attention deficit/hyperactivity disorder, and related parent sites. For an overview of the site, click on **Tour.**

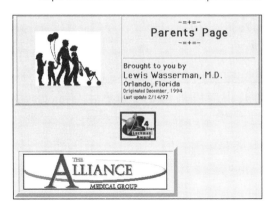

ParentsPlace.com

http://www.parentsplace.com/genobject.cgi/readroom/dr_answers.html

ParentsPlace.com contains a Children's Health Center reading room with hundreds of articles on a wide variety of health-related topics ranging from childhood illnesses to nutrition. To find other reading rooms, click on **Articles.** The site also features in-depth articles on many health topics, a search engine, and over 250 parenting bulletin boards, including one on kid's health and ages and stages dialog groups.

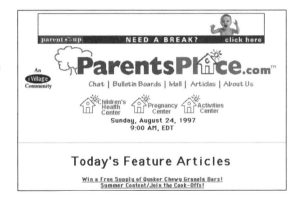

ParentTime

http://www.pathfinder.com/ParentTime/

ParentTime contains resources related to the health of children in the category Health Matters. There are articles from a comprehensive guide to childhood illnesses, first-aid techniques, prevention strategies, and other topics. The site also includes an Ask Dr. Bill & Martha Sears and a Home Talk feature for health and safety information.

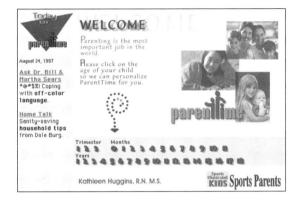

Pediatric Critical Care Medicine

http://PedsCCM.wustl.edu/

Pediatric Critical Care Medicine contains an immense amount of pediatric information and related Web sites for both health professionals and parents.

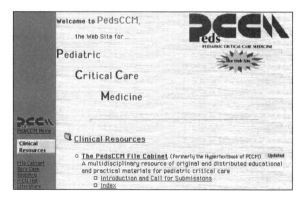

Pediatric Database (PEDBASE) Homepage

http://www.icondata.com/health/pedbase/

The Pediatric Database (PEDBASE) Homepage, designed by Dr. Alan Gandy, contains an alphabetical listing and descriptions of over 500 childhood illnesses.

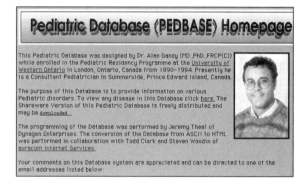

Pediatric Neurosurgery

http://cait.cpmc.columbia.edu/dept/nsg/PNS/

The Pediatric Neurosurgery home page, from Columbia-Presbyterian Medical Center, provides information about many aspects of pediatric neurosurgery. Ten general areas are discussed, all in "plain English." Several links to related sites are offered.

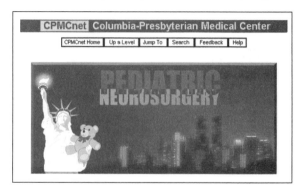

Pediatric Points of Interest

http://www.med.jhu.edu/peds/neonatology/

Pediatric Points of Interest, from Johns Hopkins University School of Medicine, contains 20 broad categories of pediatric information. Among the 20 general categories are parenting resources, e-mail discussion lists, and electronic consultations.

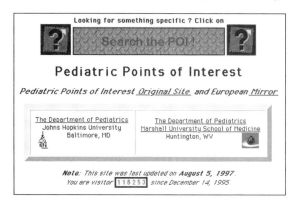

Pediatrics LinkExchange

http://www.med.auth.gr/medsurf/Pediatrics.html

Pediatrics LinkExchange is a supermarket for pediatric Web sites.

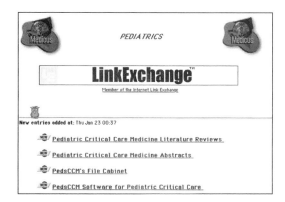

PEDINFO: An Index of the Pediatric Internet

http://www.uab.edu/pedinfo/

PEDINFO: An Index of the Pediatric Internet is a pediatrics Webserver of the University of Alabama at Birmingham disseminating online information for pediatricians and others interested in child health. The site offers pediatric forums, information on childhood diseases, a mailing list, and many other resources.

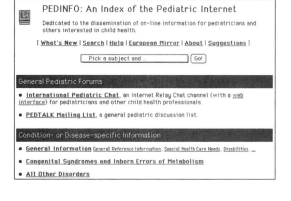

PediWeb

http://solar.rtd.utk.edu/~esmith/pedi.html

PediWeb is a pediatric pharmacy Web site with drug information and related sites.

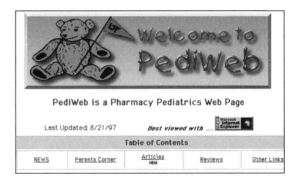

Puberty 101

http://www.jgeoff.com/puberty101/

Puberty 101, maintained by adolescent therapist J. Geoff Malta, is an interactive forum for teenagers. The **Q&A Archives** has a large collection of topics ranging from breast size to masturbation. The site also offers links to related counseling sites.

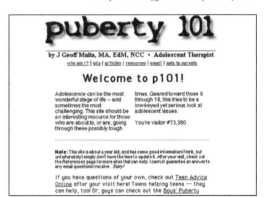

The SaferSex Page

http://www.safersex.org/

The SaferSex Page, written for teenage girls, contains important information on safer sex. For an overview of the site, click on site **index.**

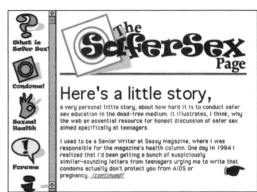

Self-Help Resources

http://www.dal.ca/~pedpain/selfhp.html
Dalhousie University

Self-Help Resources, from Dalhousie Medical School, contains online booklets to help parents understand pain and teach children how to deal with pain from cancer. The site also provides links to related sites.

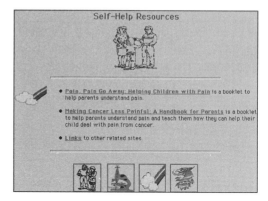

Should Ritalin Be Used to Treat ADD?

http://pubweb.nwu.edu/~cah682/ritalin/

Should Ritalin Be Used to Treat ADD? is the title of an article that presents clear information in everyday terms on Ritalin and ADD.

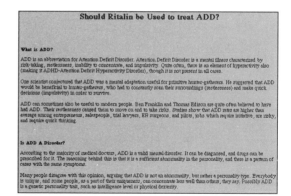

SpeciaLove

http://minuteman.com/specialove/

SpeciaLove offers year-round programs to children with cancer so they have a chance to enjoy normal activities. SpeciaLove also offers cancer families a network of support made up of other patients and families.

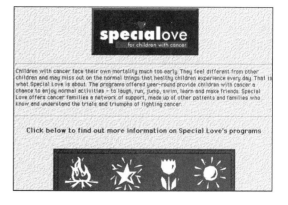

STD Home Page

http://med-www.bu.edu/people/sycamore/std/std.htm

The STD Home Page, prepared for the teenagers of East Boston, is an online guide to sexually transmitted diseases (STDs), including a glossary and images. The site contains information about AIDS, chlamydia, gonorrhea, lice, syphilis, warts, chancroid, scabies, and other STDs.

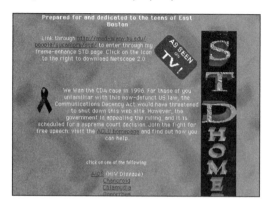

Sudden Infant Death Syndrome (SIDS) Sibling Information Web Site

http://sids-network.org/sibtocsids.htm

The Sudden Infant Death Syndrome (SIDS) Sibling Information Web Site, created by Eagle Scout Jay Alan Mihalko, contains basic SIDS information, brochures, support groups, FAQs contributed by parents and experts, and other SIDS and health-related resources worldwide.

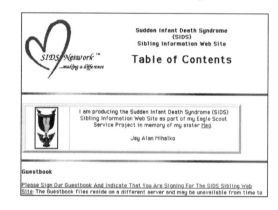

Sun Protection for Children

http://tray.dermatology.uiowa.edu/PIPs/ABCsFunSun.html

Sun Protection for Children, from the American Academy of Dermatology, presents a parents' online guide with specific details on how, when, and why to cover up from the sun. The Guide also includes information for treating and preventing sunburn.

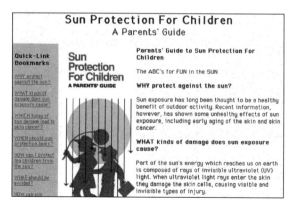

Teen Health Home Page

http://chebucto.ns.ca/Health/TeenHealth/

The Teen Health home page contains a growing series of well-written and informative articles targeted to teenagers and young adults about sexual and reproductive health. The articles are arranged by category and listed in an alphabetical index. Content is based on input from teens and written by Dalhousie University medical students under the supervision of medical and faculty staff.

Teen Health Home Page

On this page are some links to subjects which have been identified in meetings with teens as health concerns. Through these links, the Teen Health Project hopes to provide some basic information about these concerns, and to suggest where to go to find more information.

Table of Contents
- Healthy Sexuality
- Sexual Orientation
- Sexually Transmitted Diseases
- Pregnancy
- Women's Health
- Men's Health
- Sexual Assault

Teen Health Alphabetic Index
Search Teen Health Web Site

Feedback

Let us know what you think of these pages. Fill out the Teen Health Web Site Survey.

Total Baby Care

http://www.pampers.com/

Total Baby Care, sponsored by the Pampers Parenting Institute, features child development information from Dr. T. Berry Brazelton. The **Well Baby** section is a comprehensive encyclopedia of child care information and the **Skin Care Clinic** examines common skin ailments and remedies. The site also offers information on diapering for new parents. The site can be searched by key word or topic.

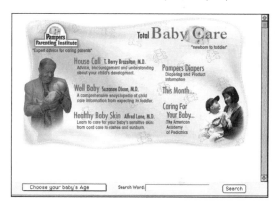

Touchstone Support Network

http://www-med.stanford.edu/touchstone/

Touchstone Support Network is a non-profit, non-sectarian, completely autonomous volunteer organization that provides emotional and practical support services for children with chronic or life-threatening illnesses. The site also provides pediatric e-mail discussion groups.

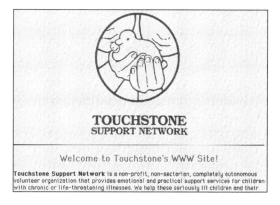

TOUCHSTONE
SUPPORT NETWORK

Welcome to Touchstone's WWW Site!

Touchstone Support Network is a non-profit, non-sectarian, completely autonomous volunteer organization that provides emotional and practical support services for children with chronic or life-threatening illnesses. We help these seriously ill children and their

The Virtual Pediatrician

http://www.geocities.com/HotSprings/1364/vphome.html

The Virtual Pediatrician provides links to pediatric sites for parents, kids, professionals, and anyone involved in the care of children.

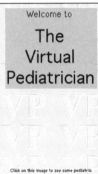

Welcome to **The Virtual Pediatrician**

A web site for parents and others involved in the care of children, devoted to providing information about children's health and maintained by Dr. Joel Selanikio, MD, a practicing pediatrician and public health researcher.

Now, in association with **Amazon.com**, the world's largest bookstore, the Virtual Pediatrician is proud to feature **direct-ordering** of a wide selection of pediatric and parenting books.

Let me see the books!

Click on this image to see some pediatric images from the National Library of Medicine

Read any good pediatric or parenting books lately? Is there a children's book your kids really love? Want to share your thoughts?

Wee Willie Wheezie Asthma Education Web Site

http://enterprise.newcomm.net/ies/

The Wee Willie Wheezie Asthma Education Web Site provides a Parent Zone with a list of asthma sites and kids' activities featuring a demo computer game and an online coloring book.

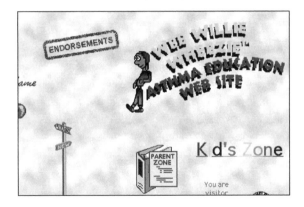

YPWCNet's Info Source

http://www.ypwcnet.org/resource/

YPWCNet's Info Source contains information about childhood diseases, including chronic fatigue syndrome. The site also offers toll-free numbers in the **Charitable Organizations** section and a rich variety of pediatric sites in the **Children's Health** section.

YPWCNET'S INFO SOURCE

The main idea of our site revolves around sick kids with Chronic Fatigue Syndrome, but that does not mean that we are blind to all the other diseases. The truth is, CFS has many things in common with other diseases, and some of these on the list below are not related at all. But because of the tie that is that we share, no matter what the reason for that is, our site is like a "sister site" to other sick kids sites.

This page has what we hope to be a very complete list of sites all over the net on all different diseases, places for more information, newsgroups, mailing lists etc. If you have something to contribute, please contact us, we are trying to build a comprehensive list, but it is going to take some time, and we could use all the help we can get.

Charitable Organizations - Toll Free Number Listing

Children's Health - List of Pediatric Sites

- AIDS and HIV
- Attention Deficit Disorder (ADD)
- Cancer
- Chronic Fatigue and Immune Dysfunction Syndrome (CFIDS/CFS/ME)
- Epilepsy

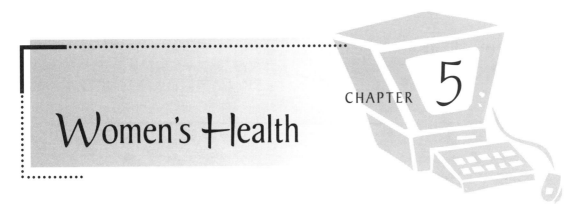

CHAPTER 5

Women's Health

General Health Issues
Breast and Ovarian Cancer
Pregnancy and Childbirth
Menopause

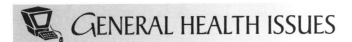

GENERAL HEALTH ISSUES

Always a Woman

http://www.always.com/

Always a Woman features a special topic monthly where women worldwide can voice their concerns and share information online. The current topic is breast cancer awareness but other topics can be found in the **Last Month's Topic** section. The site also contains a wealth of women's health information and issues in the **Straight Talk** section and plain and simple facts for teenagers about their bodies in the **Growing** section.

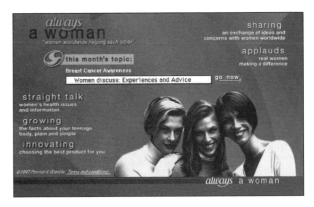

The American College of Obstetricians and Gynecologists

http://www.acog.com/

The American College of Obstetricians and Gynecologists is the nation's leading group of professionals providing health care for women. The site offers women's health information in the **Publications** section with weekly columns from the *Woman's Health* magazine, excerpts from patient education pamphlets, and news releases.

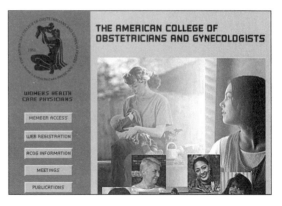

The American Surrogacy Center, Inc.

http://www.surrogacy.com/

The American Surrogacy Center, Inc. contains the most complete source of surrogacy information on the Web. The site provides a wide variety of surrogacy articles and stories on legal, medical, psychological, and personal issues and includes a list of agencies, directories of surrogacy providers, message boards, and classified ads. In addition, there is information from surrogate mothers, intended parents, egg donors, and leading experts in the field.

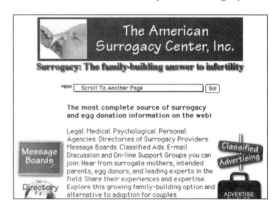

Ask a Woman Doctor

http://www.womenshealth.org/ask.htm

Ask a Woman Doctor, sponsored by GenneX Corporation, offers a comprehensive database of answered questions on women's health topics. Topics are arranged in categories by reproductive system, other medical issues, social and psychological issues, and wellness issues. In addition, personal questions will be answered by a woman medical doctor.

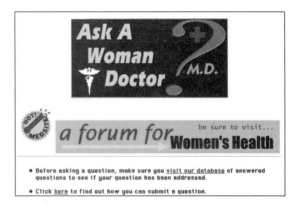

Atlanta Reproductive Health Centre WWW

http://www.ivf.com

The Atlanta Reproductive Health Centre WWW Web site, maintained by Dr. Mark Perloe, provides comprehensive online resources on many aspects of women's health such as reproduction, endometriosis, breast cancer, gynecological cancer, infertility, medical tests, and procedures. In addition, Dr. Perloe invites you to submit your own medical questions.

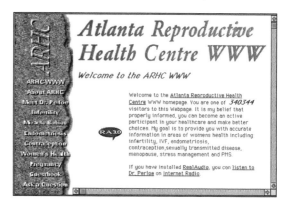

Because You're A Woman

http://www.saintfrancis.com/because.html

Because You're A Woman, from Saint Francis Hospital in Tulsa, Oklahoma, contains information on women's health issues, including numerous resources and online links. The section **Topics in Women's Health** highlights a variety of health topics ranging from osteoporosis to sexually transmitted diseases. The **Women's Perspective on Heart Disease and Cancer** section includes risk factors associated with heart disease and an in-depth look at breast cancer. Some of the other major sections are **The Status of Women's Health, Help Yourself: Living Healthy,** and **Having Your Baby.**

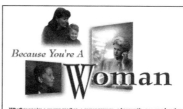

The Canadian Women's Health Network

http://www.cwhn.ca/

The Canadian Women's Health Network provides access to health information, resources, and research on women's health issues. The contents include **Women's Health Resources,** a comprehensive listing of Internet resources, and **CWHN's Network,** a timely newsletter from the Canadian Women's Health Network.

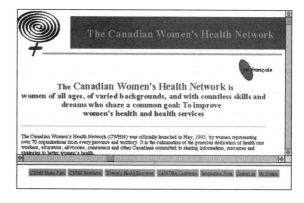

CBS News Up to the Minute

http://uttm.com/rx_women/

The Rx: Women Weekly Report, from the CBS News weekly spot on women's health, provides a wealth of information and expert opinions on a wide variety of women's health issues. You can read the current topic online or review a large selection of past reports. You can also listen to the reports with RealAudio 3.0.

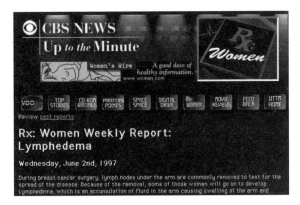

Chatelaine Connects Women to Women

http://www.canoe.ca/Chatelaine/

Chatelaine Connects Women to Women is an online version of the Canadian Women's Health Network magazine, *Chatelaine.* The site contains a **Sources** section with libraries ranging from family to food and recipes. A search engine provides quick access to information on various health topics. In addition, the site has a huge health resource guide with descriptions and phone numbers of different health-related agencies and organizations.

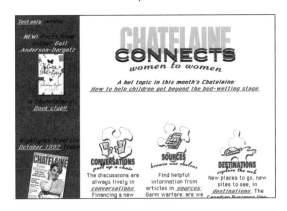

The Chronic Candidiasis Syndrome

http://members.aol.com/docdarren/med/candida.html

The Chronic Candidiasis Syndrome (yeast infection) page is a well-organized index that includes the symptoms, diagnosis, treatment, a doctor referral list, what to do after treatment, and related links.

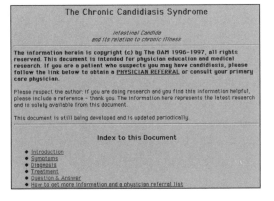

Endometriosis Care Center

http://www.dunwoodymed.com/endo/

Endometriosis Care Center diagnoses, treats, and educates women with endometriosis. To learn more about this troubling disease that affects millions of women worldwide, scroll to table of contents and click on **basic q and a** for Dr. Robert B. Albee's clear explanation of endometriosis.

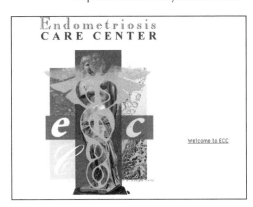

Femina

http://femina.cybergrrl.com/femina/HealthandWellness/

Femina provides a collection of women's health and wellness sites categorized by topic. Topics range from AIDS/HIV to weight. The site also includes links to other women's health resources.

Feminist.com

http://www.feminist.com/health.htm

Feminist.com provides a vast collection of links on women's health issues. Topics include general women's health, breast cancer, reproductive health, and women and AIDS.

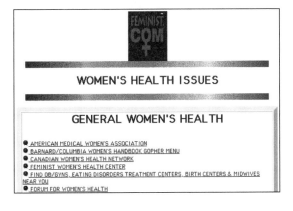

A Forum for Women's Health

A Forum for Women's Health, sponsored by GenneX Corporation, contains a collection of facts, information, advice, and suggestions to help women deal with their health concerns. The pages were written and developed by women physicians along with other women's health professionals. You can ask a woman doctor a question, learn about the life cycle, and find out the latest on birth control, pregnancy, reproduction, menopause, sexuality, and much more.

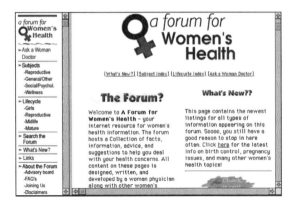

Gyn 101

Gyn 101, sponsored by Pfizer, provides accurate information about visiting a gynecologist. The site helps you find a doctor, do your homework, tells you what to expect during an examination, and lets you test yourself.

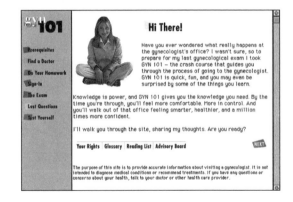

Healthy Ideas

Healthy Ideas, an online version of the women's magazine, *Prevention,* contains information on eating healthy, natural remedies, common vitamins, and losing weight. The site also offers the services, **Ask Mom MD** and **Doctor Oncall,** where doctors answer your questions.

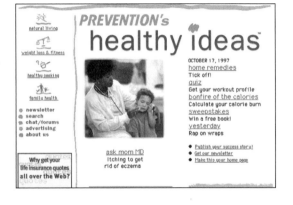

HomeArts Winning @ Losing

http://homearts.com/depts/health/0dietf1.htm

Winning @ Losing, from HomeArts, is a realistic way for women to manage their weight no matter how active or sedentary they are. The first three weeks of the plan focus on getting the pounds off; the last week helps you keep them off for good. The plan includes an online **Kitchen Counter,** which keeps track of what you eat, and an interactive **Burn Barometer,** which shows how many calories you have worked off doing anything from aerobics to yoga.

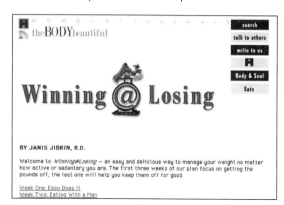

Leading Ladies.com

http://www.leadingladies.com/

Leading Ladies.com, presented by Women's Wire, *Reader's Digest,* and the National Alliance of Breast Cancer Organizations, gives you a health quiz geared to your age level, lets you post messages to a forum, sends a postcard to remind a friend about a mammogram, and gives a checklist of things to do to prevent breast cancer.

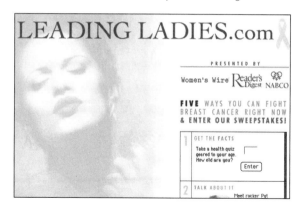

Lifetime Online

http://www.lifetimetv.com/healthtimes/

Lifetime Online provides a wealth of health resources for women, including breast cancer information, healthy recipes, women's wellness, and nutritional information.

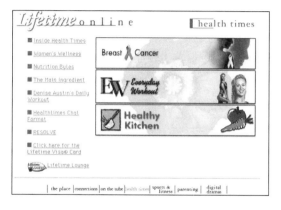

Mediconsult.com

http://www.mediconsult.com/frames/women/

Mediconsult.com features a library of medical and women's health articles from leading medical journals, medical institutions, government agencies, and non-profit organizations. Medical topics include breast cancer, fitness/prevention, osteoporosis, and pregnancy complications. The site also includes a variety of support groups where questions can be posted to a message board about a specific disease.

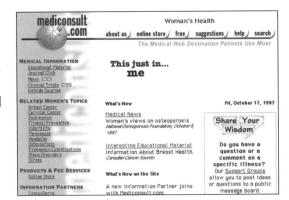

Melpomene Institute

http://www.melpomene.org/

Melpomene Institute is a non-profit research organization dedicated to women's health and physical activity. The site contains a brief discussion and related links on topics such as eating disorders, aging well, osteoporosis, menopause, body image, and exercise and pregnancy.

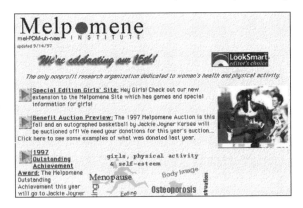

Museum of Menstruation & Women's Health

http://www.mum.org/

The Museum of Menstruation & Women's Health is devoted to menstruation and selected topics on women's health. For an overview of this site, click on **Directory.**

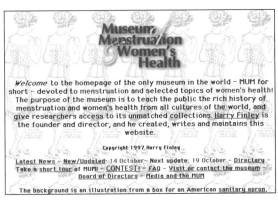

National Women's Health Resource Center

http://www.healthywomen.org/

The National Women's Health Resource Center is the national clearinghouse for women's health information. The site contains women's resources, including the *National Women's Health Report* newsletter and The Bod Squad. In addition, there are questions and answers to women's health concerns from the newsletter and a huge collection of links organized by topic.

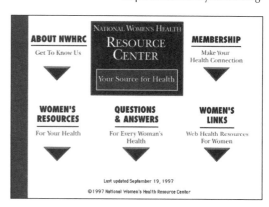

National Women's Resource Center

http://www.nwrc.org/

The National Women's Resource Center provides information on the prevention and treatment of alcohol, tobacco, and other drug abuse, as well as mental illness. The site has a **searchable bibliography database** on substance abuse and mental illness in women, an extensive **virtual library** for women's organizations, and other Web resources related to women's health and environment. The **document** section has reports and bibliographies on fetal alcohol syndrome (FAS), violence against women, gender-specific substance abuse treatment, and related subjects.

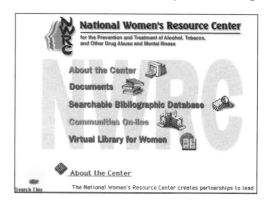

The New York Times Women's Health

http://www.nytimes.com/specials/women/whome/

The New York Times provides a comprehensive guide to women's health issues. From a topic index, you can choose an issue from a range of topics such as aging, explore the special edition with information on a wide variety of women's health concerns, or go to resources to browse an annotated list of over 100 women's health sites. The site also provides a search engine.

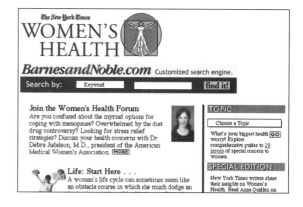

ObGyn.net Women and Patients

http://www.obgyn.net/women/women.htm

ObGyn.net Women and Patients, designed by obstetricians and gynecologists, provides reliable and comprehensive women's health resources. The site includes a women's health section with a tremendous collection of links divided into categories, including health topics, discussion forums, ObGyn.net doctors, archives, and resources. The category on health contains topics such as medical procedures, conditions, menopause, and pregnancy and birth, and the archives category offers special features, a medicine chest, news, and articles.

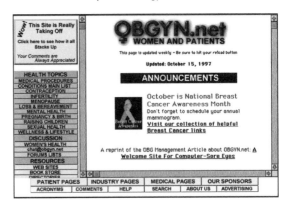

Phys Nutrition for Normal People

http://www.phys.com/

Phys Nutrition for Normal People, an online interactive magazine for health-conscious women in their twenties, thirties, and forties, has articles and information from a number of sources, including the U.S. Department of Agriculture. The site includes measuring tools for self-analysis, daily fat-fighting tips, an encyclopedia of nutrients and additives, and discussion boards. The site's personal nutritionist will also provide a customized diet plan and a sample menu.

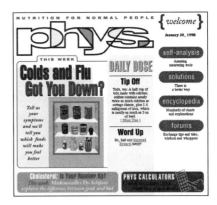

S.P.O.T.

http://critpath.org/~tracy/spot.html

S.P.O.T., the tampon health Website, provides health information about tampons. For other women's health resources, click on **Information** to find The Yeast Infection home page.

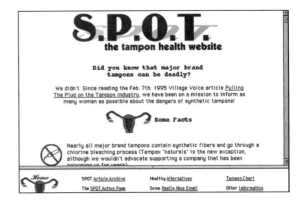

Saint Francis Osteoporosis Center at Warren Clinic

http://www.warrencl.com/ocosteo.html

Saint Francis Osteoporosis Center at Warren Clinic provides a variety of osteoporosis resources for women. Scroll to the bottom of the page for an online osteoporosis risk questionnaire and information about calcium and vitamin D, exercise and osteoporosis, osteoporosis therapy, and home safety.

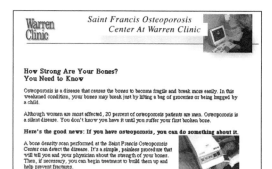

The Singapore Obstetrics & Gynecology Web

http://vhp.nus.sg/kkh/

The Singapore Obstetrics & Gynecology Web provides obstetric and gynecologic health information for female consumers. Click on **Patient & Public Information** to find online patient education pamphlets among the site's rich resources.

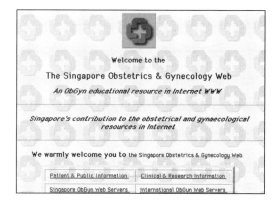
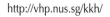

Voices of Women

http://www.voiceofwomen.com/

The Voices of Women, a journal and resource guide, contains articles on a variety of topics of interest to women. For articles on women's health issues, click on **Article Index.** The site also includes links to other women's resources, including reproductive health.

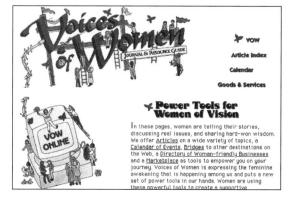

Web by Women for Women

http://www.io.com/~wwwomen/

Web by Women for Women contains a wealth of
information on pregnancy, contraception, abortion,
censorship, sexuality, and menstruation. To find
these topics scroll to **What You'll Find** near the
bottom of the page.

A Woman's Perspective

http://www.uvol.com/woman/

A Woman's Perspective is an online monthly
newsletter by Becky Ward. The newsletter provides women's health information on topics
such as health, fitness, nutrition, emotions,
relationships, menopause, child rearing,
and diseases.

Women and Health

http://www.wellweb.com/women/women.htm

Women and Health, from the WellnessWeb, provides a variety of women and health topics, including
medical tests for women, women's illnesses, menopause and hormone therapy, women's health
pages, and violence against women.

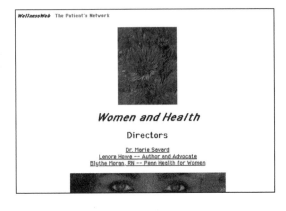

Women Care

http://www.womencare.com

Women Care, Karen Lee's virtual clinic, offers general information about cervical cancer, breast examination, ovarian cancer, menopause, and other topics specific to women's health.

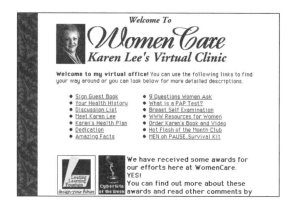

Women Know

http://tampax.com/

Women Know, sponsored by the Tampax company's corporate headquarters, provides general information about menstruation and the use of tampons. The site also includes information about toxic shock syndrome.

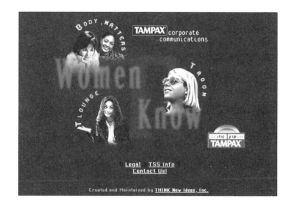

Women's Health

http://info.pitt.edu/HOME/GHNet/GHNet.html

Women's Health, from the Global Health Network at the University of Pittsburgh, features an index of women's health sites organized by category. Categories include aging, cancer, domestic violence, heart disease, infectious diseases, mental health, and nutrition and fitness.

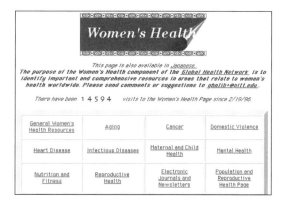

Women's Health 2000 Links Page

http://www.itvisus.com/hwlinks.htm

Women's Health 2000 Links Page, from the Information Television Network, contains a wide variety of health and medical resources of interest to women.

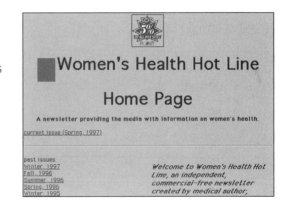

Women's Health Hot Line

http://www.soft-design.com/softinfo/womens-health.html

Women's Health Hot Line, created by medical journalist Charlotte Libov, is a quarterly newsletter dating back to 1994. The online newsletter provides women's health information on topics ranging from aspirin as a heart attack preventive to smoking kills.

Women's Health Interactive

http://www.womens-health.com/

Women's Health Interactive provides health resources for women that emphasize learning and doing, not simply gathering information. The featured topics are the **Gynecologic Health** and the **Infertility** Centers. Click on **Topics** to find other centers, including the Heart Disease Health Center and the Nutrition Health Center. The site also offers information on cancer, diabetes, osteoporosis, and other topics.

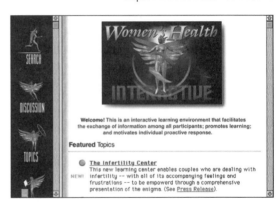

Women's Health Place

http://women.shn.net/

Women's Health Place, from Sapient Health Network, offers the latest women's medical information on a variety of topics, including uterine fibroids, endometriosis, and pelvic pain.

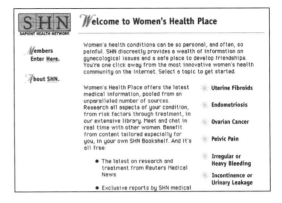

Women's Health Platform

http://www.whp.com/

Women's Health Platform, sponsored by Bristol-Myers Squibb Company, provides information on women's health care issues and includes health sites of interest to women.

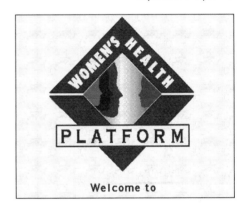

Women's Health Weekly

http://www.newsfile.com/1w.htm

Women's Health Weekly contains summaries of women's disease-related articles from CW Henderson weekly publications. The site also includes full-text articles of the top news stories.

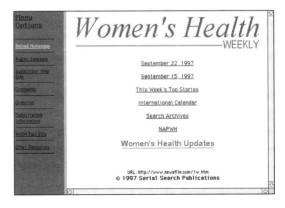

The Women's Heart Disease and Stroke Quiz

http://www.hsf.ca/test/4quiz.htm

The Women's Heart Disease and Stroke Quiz, from the Heart and Stroke Foundation of Canada, is designed to test and increase women's knowledge of their risk for heart disease and stroke. Links at the end of the quiz provide more information about risk factors you can control (e.g., cholesterol, high blood pressure, smoking, stress), as well as three broad questions women should ask their doctors to help identify and lower risk for these diseases.

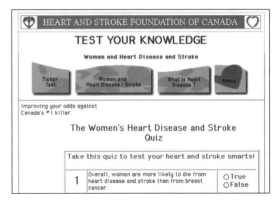

Women's Medical Health Page

http://www.best.com/~sirlou/wmhp.html

The Women's Medical Health Page provides summaries of scholarly articles from medical journals. It is written primarily for health professionals, but anyone with an interest in women's health will find the articles useful.

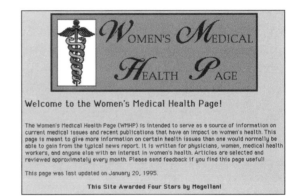

Women's Wire

http://www.women.com/body/

The Women's Wire offers personal health information and frank talk for women. The topics covered are breast health, parenting, sex health, health news, plus health quizzes and more. In addition, the site provides an interactive nutritionist.

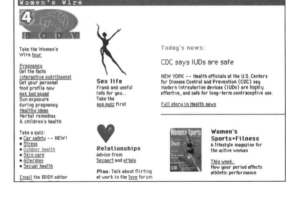

BREAST AND OVARIAN CANCER

American Cancer Society

http://www.cancer.org/

The American Cancer Society provides a variety of cancer resources for prevention, detection, and treatment. The **Cancer Info** section has a wealth of information for specific cancers, patients and families, statistics, guidelines, and tobacco information. The site also contains the latest research progress, news, and extensive links to other cancer sites in the **WWW Directory** section. Furthermore, you can jump directly to a site category using a pull-down menu to find a link to a local ACS chapter.

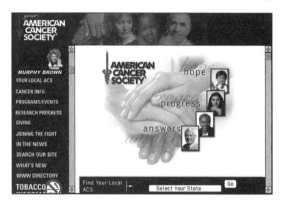

Best Web Sites on Breast Cancer

http://darkwing.uoregon.edu/~jbonine/bc_sources.html

The Best Web Sites on Breast Cancer, compiled by John E. Bonine, contains a collection of the best breast cancer resources.

Breast Cancer

http://www.ca.cancer.org/services/breast/

Breast Cancer, from the American Cancer Society, California Division, provides online resources for the early detection, treatment, and support of breast cancer. The site offers more information on breast cancer, including the network resources, FAQs, breast cancer risk factors, and other topics.

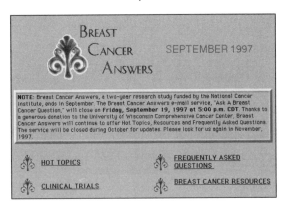

Breast Cancer Answers

http://www.biostat.wisc.edu/bca/

Breast Cancer Answers provides a variety of cancer online resources. Topics include hot topics, the latest developments in diagnosis and treatment, clinical trials, questions you should ask your doctor, FAQs, and breast cancer resources. In addition, you many call the Cancer Information Service using the toll-free number 1-800-4-CANCER (1-800-422-6237).

Breast Cancer Awareness

http://www.harvardpilgrim.org/html/frontpage/
breast_cancer/breast_cancer.htm

Breast Cancer Awareness, from the Harvard Pilgrim HMO, offers a variety of breast cancer resources, including breast self-examination, mammography information, a breast cancer screening guide, and survival stories.

Breast Cancer Awareness Crusade

http://avon.com/showpage.asp?thepage=crusade

Breast Cancer Awareness Crusade, from Avon, provides a variety of online breast cancer resources in the **library** section. Topics include a breast cancer glossary, common questions about mammograms, ten common questions about breast cancer, and support groups. Avon also offers a bulletin board where you can join others in open and supportive dialogues about the many aspects of breast cancer.

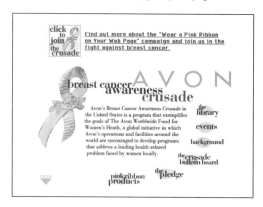

Breast Cancer Information Center

http://www.feminist.org/other/bc/bchome.html

The Breast Cancer Information Center offers a compendium of breast cancer resources. Categories include What You Need to Know, Mammography Information, and breast cancer Internet resources. The site also provides a list of toll-free numbers in the **Hotline** section.

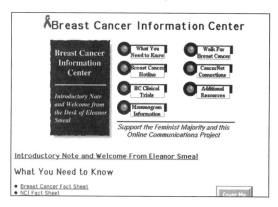

Breast Cancer Information Clearinghouse

http://nysernet.org/bcic/

The Breast Cancer Information Clearinghouse, maintained by the New York State Education and Research Network, provides a wealth of breast cancer resources for patients and their families. The site contains information ranging from instructions on breast self-examination to a comprehensive, nation-wide listing of breast cancer support groups. For a list of updates dating back to 1994, click on **What's New in the BCIC?** and for an overview of the site, click on **Subject Oriented Index.** BCIC includes a searchable database.

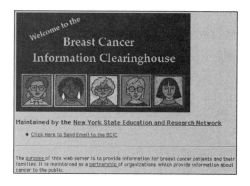

Breast Cancer Network

http://www.cancer.org/bcn/bcn.html

The Breast Cancer Network, part of the American Cancer Society home page, provides reliable information on breast cancer and breast reconstruction and includes the latest breast cancer news and an easy-to-understand glossary.

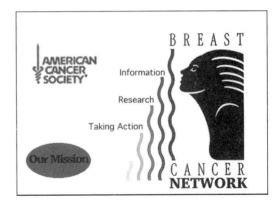

The Breast Cancer Roundtable

http://www.seas.gwu.edu/student/tlooms/MGT243/bcr.html

The Breast Cancer Roundtable contains information about breast cancer and breast health with an emphasis on myths, facts, and early detection guidelines. The site includes information about mammograms, specific directions for doing a breast self-examination, FAQs about breast cancer, a non-technical glossary to cancer terms, and links to other breast cancer sites.

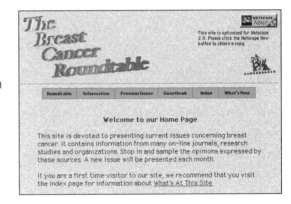

Breast Reconstruction

http://www2.centerplasticsurgery.com/cps/
breastreconstruction/breastreconstruction.html

Breast Reconstruction, from the Center of Plastic Surgery, provides information on a variety of topics related to breast reconstruction, including reconstruction candidates, types of mastectomies, radiation and chemotherapy, reconstruction techniques, nipple-areolar reconstruction, and more.

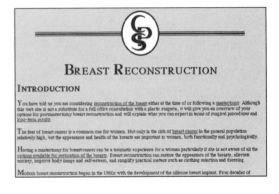

Breast Tutorial

http://www.biostat.wisc.edu/surgery/wolberg/breast.html

Breast Tutorial, written by Dr. William H. Wolberg, presents information and illustrations on breast problems for the layperson. Among the topics are breast anatomy, physiology, and examination, differential diagnosis and cancer types, role and type of definitive surgery, and self-help questions.

BREAST TUTORIAL

William H. Wolberg, M.D.

If you are a lay person desiring information on breast problems click here.

If you want information about Dr. Wolberg and what he does click here)

NOTE: The abstracted references are available by clicking on the reference. Pathology examples and links leading to a more detailed discussions are accessed by clicking on the highlighted word or term.

Table of Contents

Breast Anatomy, Physiology and Examination

Differential Diagnosis & Cancer Types

Screening & Risk

Postmenopausal Hormonal Replacement

Genetic Considerations

Diagnosis and Prognosis

Role and Type of Definitive Surgery

BreastCancer.net

http://www.breastcancer.net/

BreastCancer.net is a "linked list" of Internet-based resources on the prevention, detection, and treatment of breast cancer. The site is updated daily, monitors every major news source for breast cancer-related topics, offers a free e-mail newsletter, and has an extensive list of related sites.

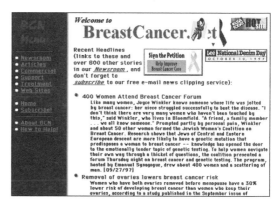

BreastNet

http://www.bci.org.au

BreastNet, from the New South Wales Breast Cancer Institute in Australia, provides a **Best Practice** section with helpful online breast cancer guides. The site includes a list of related cancer links.

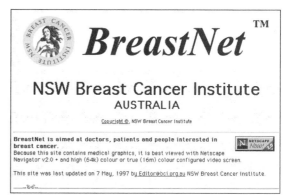

The Community Breast Health Project

http://www-med.Stanford.EDU/CBHP/

The Community Breast Health Project is a grassroots, patient-driven project whose mission is to improve the lives of people touched by breast cancer by acting as a clearinghouse for information and support.

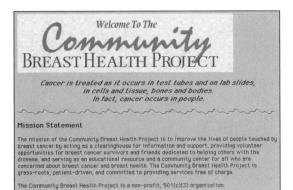

A Consumer's Guide: Early Breast Cancer

http://www.nbcc.org.au/pages/clincon/content.htm

A Consumer's Guide: Early Breast Cancer, from the Australian National Breast Cancer Centre, provides an online guide of breast cancer articles. Some of the topics include the impact of breast cancer, dealing with breast cancer, tests, options for treatment, alternative therapies, and women with special needs.

EduCare Inc.

http://www.cancerhelp.com/ed

EduCare, Inc., a network for breast health and breast cancer, offers patient resources for breast cancer, including breast lumps and diagnosis guides, a guide for support partner's questions, a glossary of breast cancer terms, and links to related sites.

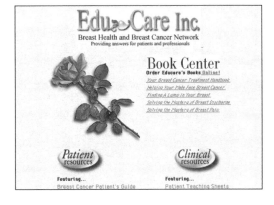

Emory University School of Medicine Department of Surgery

The Division of Plastic, Reconstructive, and Maxillofacial Surgery, from the Department of Surgery at Emory University School of Medicine, provides comprehensive services in reconstructive and aesthetic surgery. For inquiries, call the director, Dr. John Bostwick III, at 1-404-778-5761.

http://www.emory.edu/WHSC/MED/SURGERY/plastic/

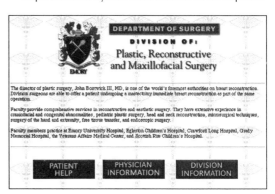

HomeArts Breast Health Center

HomeArts Breast Health Center has topics such as the latest news, breast health, and breast cancer. The site also includes authoritative related links and lets you talk to others on a multitude of topics and ask doctors health questions.

http://homearts.com/depts/health/00breaf1.htm

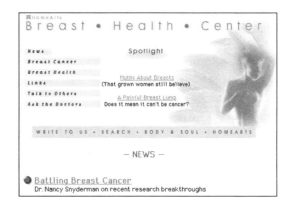

Komen.org

Komen.org, the home page of the Susan G. Komen Breast Cancer Foundation, provides comprehensive news and information on breast cancer research, programs, support, and "talk back" sessions where survivors can share their experiences. In addition, the site includes a toll-free number 1-800-I'M AWARE (1-800-462-9273) and a link to **Race for the Cure.**

http://www.komen.org/

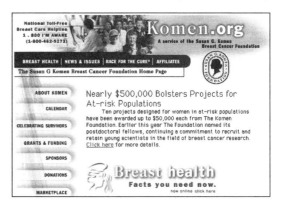

Mammograms

http://rex.nci.nih.gov/MAMMOG_WEB/MAMMOG_DOC.html

Mammograms, from the National Cancer Institute, offers women a resource on mammograms. Topics range from background information to an index of printable materials.

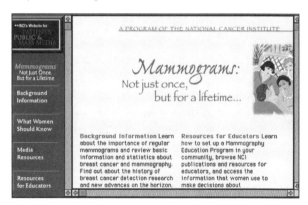

Mind2Body Ovarian Cancer Links

http://www.ovarian.org/m2b/m2b.shtml

Mind2body Ovarian Cancer Links, created by an ovarian cancer victim, offers a comprehensive collection of sites for women with ovarian cancer and their support providers. Categories of information include Ovarian Cancer, Your Medical Team, Support, Chemotherapy and Medications, Tests and Procedures, Alternative Therapies, and others.

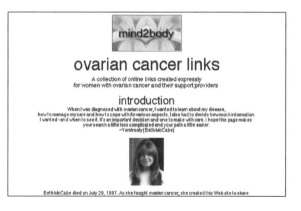

The National Alliance of Breast Cancer Organizations

http://www.nabco.org/

The National Alliance of Breast Cancer Organizations is a rich breast cancer resource. The site contains fact sheets ranging from breast cancer in the United States to managing lymphedema, related links, and addresses and phone numbers of support groups nationwide. You can also get answers to your questions about breast cancer via e-mail.

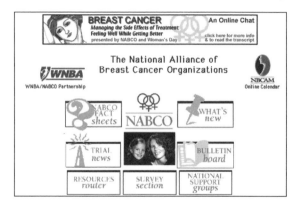

National Ovarian Cancer Coalition

http://www.ovarian.org/

The National Ovarian Cancer Coalition is the national clearinghouse providing information on the detection, prevention, risks, symptoms, and treatment of ovarian cancer.

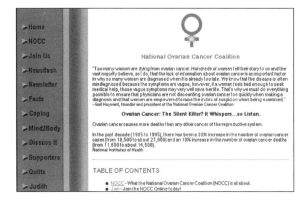

OncoLink NCI/PDQ Patient Statement Breast Cancer

http://oncolink.upenn.edu/pdq_html/2/engl/200013.html

OncoLink NCI/PDQ Patient Statements, from the University of Pennsylvania Cancer Center, provides up-to-date summary information for the treatment of breast cancer. Click on the **Table of Contents** for the complete list of information.

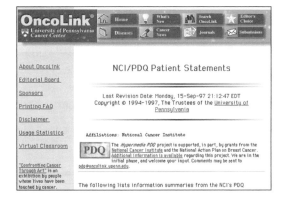

OncoLink Ovarian Cancer

http://www.oncolink.upenn.edu/specialty/gyn_onc/ovarian/

OncoLink Ovarian Cancer, from the University of Pennsylvania Cancer Center, provides a list of online resources for ovarian cancer. The site also accesses resources for information about cancer and hormones and cancer.

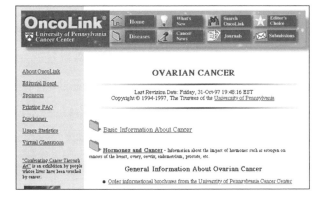

Patient's Guide to Breast Cancer

http://www.bimc.edu/netscape2/breastcancer/bctoc.html

The Patient's Guide to Breast Cancer, developed by
the Beth Israel Medical Center in New York, contains
detailed information and illustrations on breast cancer.
Categories include Making a Diagnosis, Understanding
Breast Cancer, Breast Reconstruction, and Follow-Up
Care. The site also provides a glossary of breast cancer
medical terms.

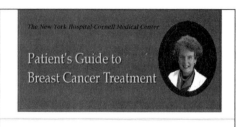

Patient's Guide to Breast Cancer Treatment

http://nysernet.org/bcic/patients/mooretitle.html

The Patient's Guide to Breast Cancer Treatment,
from the New York Hospital-Cornell Medical Center,
provides an invaluable online guide for women on the
treatment of breast cancer. Click on **Contents** to access
this information.

Plastic Surgery Information Service

http://www.plasticsurgery.org/surgery/brstrec.htm

The Plastic Surgery Information Service presents
an illustrated guide to breast reconstruction
prepared by the American Society of Plastic and
Reconstructive Surgeons (ASPRS).

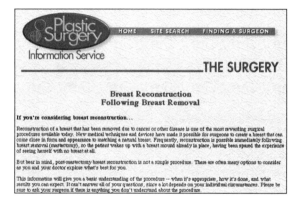

Self Magazine's Breast Cancer Handbook

http://nysernet.org/bcic/self

Self Magazine's Breast Cancer Handbook includes its 1994 handbook and selected articles from its 1993 handbook.

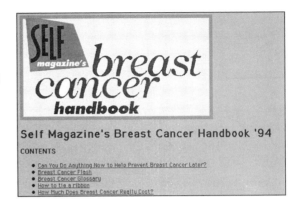

Y-Me National Breast Cancer Organization

http://www.y-me.org/

Y-Me National Breast Cancer Organization, founded in 1978 by two breast cancer survivors, provides information and support to anyone who is touched by cancer. Topics include breast health, general information about breast cancer, and related cancer links. There is also a search engine and a 24-hour toll-free hotline number 1-800-221-2141. In General Information about Cancer, click on **Facts About Breast Cancer** or **Frequently Asked Questions** to negate your misconceptions about breast cancer.

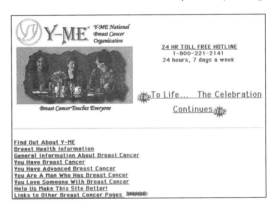

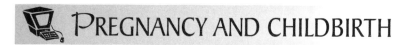 PREGNANCY AND CHILDBIRTH

Ask NOAH About: Pregnancy

http://www.noah.cuny.edu/pregnancy/pregnancy/.html

The New York Online Access to Health (NOAH) is the combined effort of the New York Public Library and other educational institutions. Ask NOAH About: Pregnancy is an extensive guide to the issues dealing with pregnancy. Among them are teen pregnancy, family planning, contraception, sexual lifesyles, problems and risks, prenatal care, and postnatal care. Other pregnancy resources are offered through links to related sites.

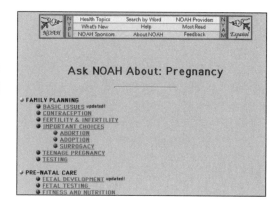

Ask the Professional

http://www.babybag.com/askpro/

Ask the Professional, from Baby Bag Online, is a source for advice from a childbirth educator, a pharmacist, a home-based employment specialist, or from a midwife. The site includes previous questions and answers.

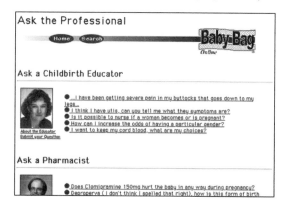

Baby123

http://www.meadjohnson.com/baby123/

Baby123, from MeadJohnson, answers your questions about feeding your baby. The site also includes **Mom & Baby** links on everything from prenatal care and breastfeeding to daycare and preschool readiness.

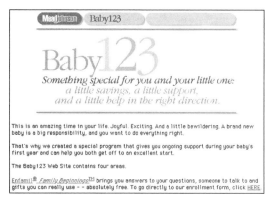

BabyCenter

http://www.babycenter.com/

BabyCenter provides a comprehensive collection of news and articles for expectant mothers and parents in the **Resource Section.** The entire list of articles can be viewed using the A to Z index or by categories. Categories include Pregnancy, Baby Care, Mother Care, Family Life, and Working Parents. In addition, there is a glossary of terms, breaking news, buying tips, and interactive calculators.

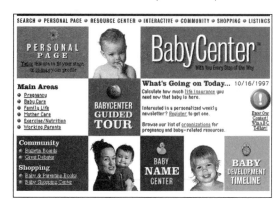

The Billings Ovulation Method of Natural Family Planning

http://www.billings-centre.ab.ca

The Billings Ovulation Method of Natural Family Planning provides basic information about female sexuality in simple medical terms and probably far more thoroughly than your mother ever explained it to you.

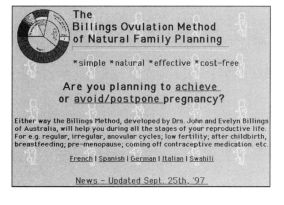

Breastfeeding and Parenting Resources on the Internet

http://www.prairienet.org/laleche/other.html

Breastfeeding and Parenting Resources on the Internet, from the La Leche League of Champaign-Urbana, Illinois, is a collection of Web pages featuring breastfeeding, lactation, and parenting techniques.

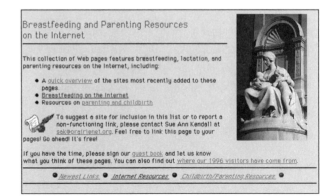

The Breastfeeding Page

http://www.islandnet.com/~bedford/brstfeed.html

The Breastfeeding Page provides a variety of resources on breastfeeding. Topics include how to breastfeed, benefits, problems associated with breastfeeding, three newsgroups, related sites, and breastfeeding organizations.

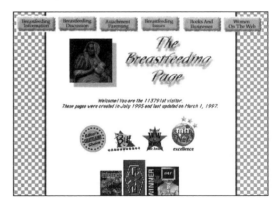

Childbirth.org

http://www.childbirth.org/

Childbirth.org has a vast collection of childbirth-related sites. Topics include infertility, postpartum care, feeding, cesarean delivery, pregnancy, FAQs, and reproductive health.

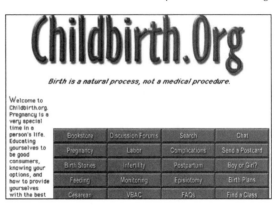

Creative Consultants, Inc.

http://members.aol.com/creaconinc/

Creative Consultants, Inc. contains useful information about pregnancy, fetal alcohol syndrome, and related sites.

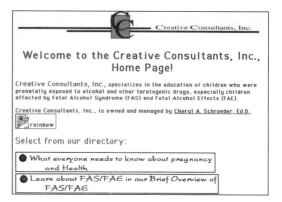

Directory of Resources

http://birthandbeyond.simplenet.com/

The Directory of Resources is an A to Z index on women's health. Categories include breastfeeding and human milk banking, childbirth and related associations, drugs in pregnancy and breast-feeding, midwifery, infertility, vaccines, and women's health issues.

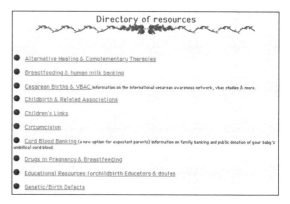

Group B Streptococcus Infections

http://www.geocities.com/HotSprings/3017/

Group B Streptococcus Infections, the number one cause of life-threatening infections in newborn babies, are more common than other illnesses for which pregnant women are screened, such as Down's syndrome, rubella, and spina bifida. The site, also in a Spanish version, contains invaluable GBS information from the news sources and Medline and includes a list of related links.

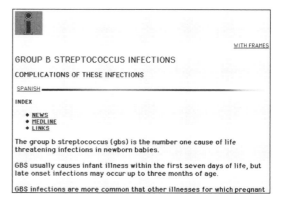

HomeArts The Whole Nine Months

http://homearts.com/depts/health/00ninec1.htm

The Whole Nine Months, from HomeArts and Parent Soup, provides a bevy of online resources and interactive activities for expectant mothers. **Preparing for Pregnancy** features an ovulation calculator, a fetal development calendar, and a checklist with sound medical advice and information, while the **Baby's Bottom Line** provides a calculator for estimating your baby's cost as a new little tax deduction. In addition, **How Your Baby Grows,** a month-to-month guide, lets you pick a month and see how your baby will change and what you can do to have the healthiest baby.

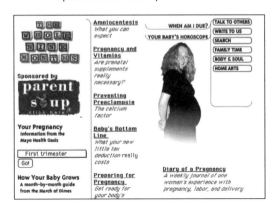

Jane's Breastfeeding & Childbirth Resources

http://webzone1.co.uk/www/cathus/janelink.htm

Jane's Breastfeeding & Childbirth Resources home page contains over 600 sites for breastfeeding and childbirth.

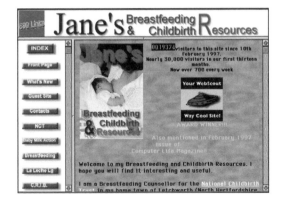

La Leche League International

http://www.lalecheleague.org/

The La Leche League International site provides a rich variety of breastfeeding information for women. The **Breastfeeding Information from LLLI Periodicals** section has articles on weaning, breastfeeding adopted babies, breastfeeding in public, breastfeeding premature infants, and breastfeeding with implants. In addition, the site includes related links, a help forum, FAQs, La Leche League local offices, and a search tool.

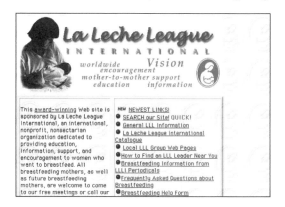

Mother Stuff

http://www.teramonger.com/dwan/mother.htm

Mother Stuff is a meta-index of mother knowledge. Topics include birth, health, midwifery, and pregnancy and each topic features articles and related links. The site includes a complete table of contents and a search tool.

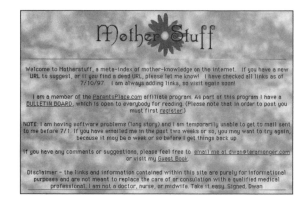

Olen Interactive Pregnancy Calendar

http://www.olen.com/baby/

Olen Interactive Pregnancy Calendar provides a month-by-month customized calendar for the expectant mother. Enter the date of conception and the expected due date appears. Enter any month of the gestation period and a calendar appears that includes dos and don'ts and helpful advice. The site also includes scheduled chat rooms.

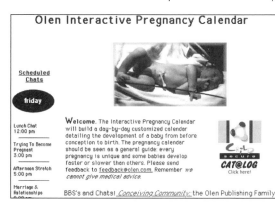

Online Birth Center

http://www.efn.org/~djz/birth/birthindex.html

Online Birth Center has information on midwifery, pregnancy, birth, and breastfeeding. The topics include women's resources, high-risk situations and complications, a parent's page, and the midwifery page for both practicing and aspiring midwives.

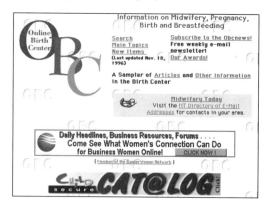

ParentsPlace.com

http://www.parentsplace.com/readroom/pregnant.html

ParentsPlace.com features a Pregnancy and Birth Center with a variety of parenting resources. The **Ask the Midwife** section contains over 500 online pregnancy parents'questions answered by midwife Peg Plumbo. The **Family Care** section contains hundreds of relationship questions answered by family and marriage therapist Dr. Gayle Peterson. ParentsPlace.com lets you ask Dr. Gayle advice on your own family problem. The site also includes a collection of birth and adoption stories and various bulletin boards.

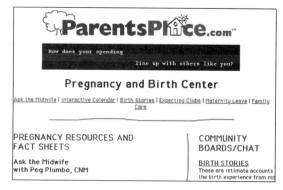

The Pregnancy Place

http://www.familyinternet.com/fisites/pregcom/

The Pregnancy Place offers articles about pregnancy in the following categories: Planning for a Family, Fertility and Infertility, The Three Trimesters of Pregnancy, Planning for Baby (Birth Planning), Labor and Delivery, and Products for Moms, Dads, and Babies.

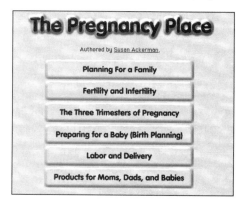

Redbook The Exercise Tricks That Really Take Off Pounds

http://homearts.com/rb/health/11tricf1.htm

The Exercise Tricks That Really Take Off Pounds, from a *Redbook* magazine article, provides exercise tips to help moms lose weight.

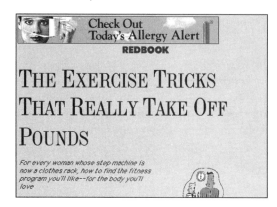

Running on Full

http://lifematters.com/rofintro.html

Running on Full, from Lifematters, contains practical information on pregnancy and exercising, healthy eating, and breastfeeding.

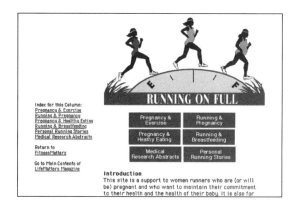

Toni's Angel Pages

http://www.geocities.com/heartland/8242/

Toni's Angel Pages reaches out to women interested in pregnancy, infertility, pregnancy loss, and related topics.

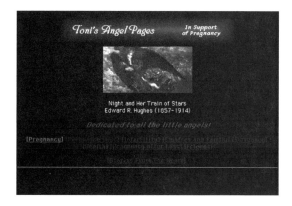

Ultrasound and Other Prenatal Diagnostic Tests

http://www-leland.stanford.edu/~holbrook

Ultrasound and Other Prenatal Diagnostic Tests, by Dr. R. Harold Holbrook, Jr., contains articles on topics such as ultrasound, genetic amniocentesis, and Rh disease. A link to the **Centers for Disease Control and Prevention** (CDC) provides information about the prevention of prenatal Group B streptococcus infections.

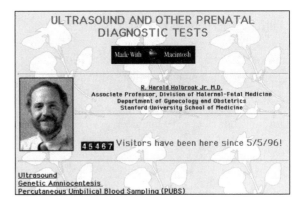

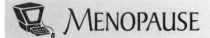 MENOPAUSE

Doctor's Guide to Menopause Information & Resources

http://www.pslgroup.com/MENOPAUSE.HTM

The Doctor's Guide to Menopause Information & Resources presents the latest medical news and online resources for patients or friends and parents of patients with menopause and menopause-related disorders. Categories include Medical News and Alerts, Menopause Information, Stay Abreast (mailing list), Discussion Groups and Newsgroups, and Other Related Sites.

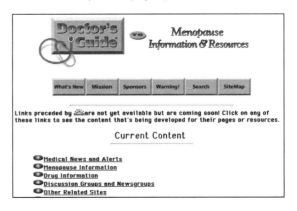

Menopause

http://www1.medaccess.com/physical/menop/meno_toc.htm

Menopause, from Med Access, provides information that can help you better understand menopause as well as put you in touch with organizations that offer additional information and assistance.

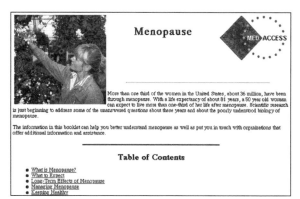

Menopause—Another Change in Life

http://www.ppfa.org/ppfa/menopub.html

Menopause—Another Change in Life is an online resource from the Planned Parenthood Federation of America that includes information on signs and indications, osteoporosis, and traditional and alternative therapies.

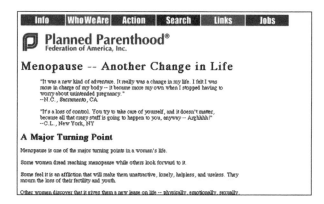

The Menopause Link

http://www.progest.com/

The Menopause Link contains online holistic medicine resources for women in menopause. Women can read humorous stories about their menopause experiences, sample articles in the newsletter, *Natural Solutions,* or review previously answered menopause questions. Women can also e-mail their own stories with the possibility of publication, and even get answers to a menopause question from a homeopathic doctor.

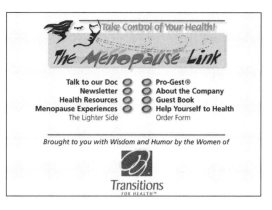

Menopause Online

http://www.menopause-online.com/

Menopause Online provides women with up-to-date, easy-to-use information about the natural changes from reproductive life to midlife. Topics are menopause updates with late-breaking news and scientific studies, health problems associated with menopause, therapies and treatments for menopausal women, and health resources, including bibliographies and Web sites.

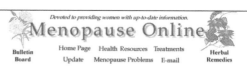

The North American Menopause Society

http://www.menopause.org/

The North American Menopause Society offers information, advice, and more for women in menopause.

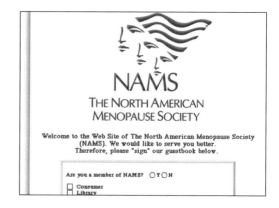

Power Surge

http://members.aol.com/dearest/

Power Surge is an online network for women in menopause. The site offers twice weekly live chats, an active database monitored by physicians, monthly newsletters, and related health links.

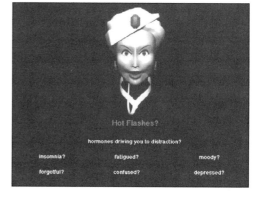

Men's Health

CHAPTER 6

A Man's Life

http://www.manslife.com/

A Man's Life, a magazine published by Real Life Publishing, provides an online edition with complete instructions for health and wealth. The **Health** section features Dr. Bob Arnot's weekly updates for active healthy living and Dr. George Fleming's e-mail service for answering your medical questions and giving free medical advice in his health forum. The **Fitness** section offers the Big Sweat, an interactive personal trainer, where you can click on a part of the body for exercise tips and a fitness forum for exchanging workout notes. For an overview of the entire site, click on **Contents.**

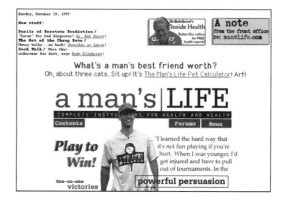

Circumcision Facts On-Line

http://www.gepps.com/circ.htm

Circumcision Facts On-Line is a comprehensive resource that deals with many of the issues related to circumcision. The site presents actual pictures of circumcisions performed, as well as pictures of complications of circumcisions both in infants and adults. In addition, the site provides forum feedback from expectant parents and others.

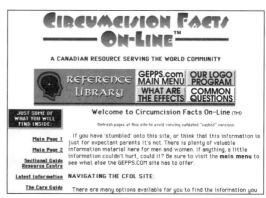

175

Circumcision Information and Resource Pages

http://www.cirp.org/CIRP/

The Circumcision Information and Resource Pages provides information on all aspects of the genital surgery known as circumcision. The site is divided into two parts: (1) the **Circumcision Reference Library** containing technical material, medical and historical articles, and statistics, and (2) the **Circumcision Information Pages** containing readable collections of information for consumers.

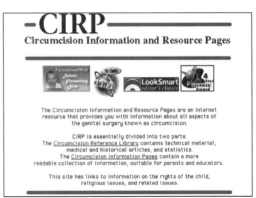

Circumcision Online News

http://www.geocities.com/hotsprings/2754

Circumcision Online News has the latest information on the benefits of male circumcision from doctors, medical establishments, and researchers. Circumcision is practiced throughout the world because of the potential benefits, parental preference, religious beliefs, traditions, and customs.

The Diagnostic Center for Men

http://www.for-men.com/

The Diagnostic Center for Men provides help and information on impotence and premature ejaculation.

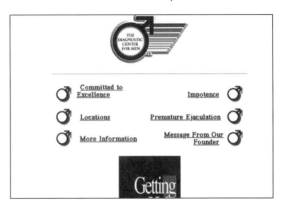

Fun With Urology

http://users.alphainfo.com/wlynes/

Fun With Urology, created by Dr. William Lynes, features a variety of genitourinary topics, including prostate cancer, cystitis, interstitial cystitis, urine infection, Peyronie's disease, and many others. The site also includes a section for female topics and a collection of related links.

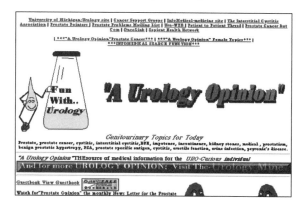

Impotence Resource Center

http://www.impotence.org/

The Impotence Resource Center, from the Geddings Osbon, Sr. Foundation, provides information about the causes, treatments, and facts about impotence. Impotence is often called "the most common untreated treatable medical disorder in the United States."

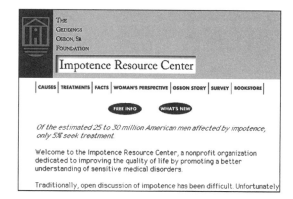

Kidney & Urologic Health

http://www.healthtouch.com/level1/leaflets/106107/106107.htm

Kidney & Urologic Health, from Healthtouch Online, provides a variety of resources on urologic disorders such as urinary tract infections and bladder control, benign prostatic hyperplasia (BPH), penis disorders, and other topics.

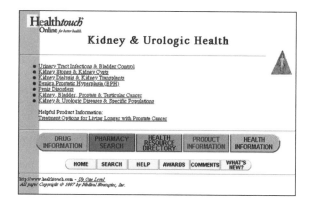

Men: Test Your Knowledge of Women's Health

http://www.coolware.com/health/medical_reporter/quiz.html

Men: Test Your Knowledge of Women's Health, created by the Rose Men's Health Resource in Denver, is an interactive quiz for men about women's health issues.

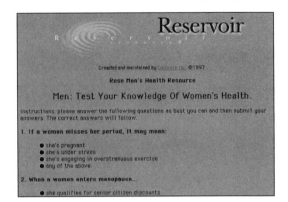

Men's Health

http://www.menshealth.com/

Men's Health, an online version of *Men's Health* magazine, invites you to check out "tons of useful stuff," including a new health angle on pushups and an ask the sex doc feature that lets you post questions about relationships.

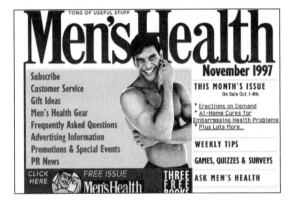

Men's Health Issues

http://medic.med.uth.tmc.edu/ptnt/00000391.htm

Men's Health Issues, from the University of Texas at Houston Medical School, provides men's health information on exercise, fat and cholesterol, prostatic cancer screening, and benign prostatic hyperplasia (BPH).

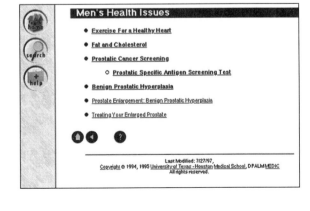

Men's Health Topics

http://www.uro.com/mhealth.htm

Men's Health Topics, provided by the Virginia Urology Center, contains information on prostate cancer, impotence, kidney stones, vasectomy, and other topics.

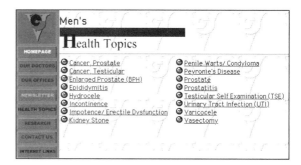

Not For Men Only

http://www.malehealthcenter.com/

Not For Men Only, the Male Health Center Internet Education Site from Dallas, Texas, covers a broad range of special medical problems of men ranging from impotence to how to live "as long as women." Scroll to **Site Map** to find a list of men's health topics, including all about male health, symptoms, self-care, sex, and others. "His Health" is an encyclopedia on male health featuring Dr. Goldberg's syndicated columns.

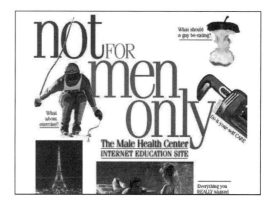

Prostate Cancer

http://www.ca.cancer.org/services/prostate/

Prostate Cancer, from the American Cancer Society, California Division, provides online resources for the early detection and treatment of prostate cancer. The site also includes a link to **California Facts and Figures about Cancer** at the bottom of the page.

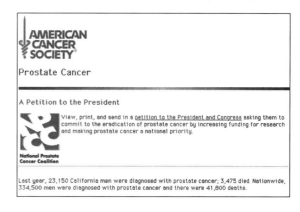

Prostate Cancer

http://wellweb.com/prostate/prostate.htm

Prostate Cancer, from the WellnessWeb, provides a variety of prostate resources, including new patient information, available treatments, and an Ask the Expert feature with selected questions answered by WellnessWeb doctors.

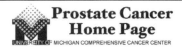

WellnessWeb The Patient's Network

Prostate Cancer

Effective New Drug For Prostate Cancer

Join the NPCC National Prostate Cancer Petition Drive.
New Patient Information
Available Treatments
Impotence
Incontinence
What's New
Prostate Pointers -- Gary Huckaby's Site
Ask The Expert
The Screening Controversy
Reliability of Single PSA Readings
My Story
Get a Second Opinion
Look-It-Up -- Glossary
Resources
Complementary, Experimental, and Unconventional

Send email to: CaP@wellweb.com

Reliability of Single PSA Readings

Prostate Cancer Home Page

http://www.cancer.med.umich.edu/prostcan/prostcan.html

The Prostate Cancer Home Page, from the University of Michigan Comprehensive Cancer Center, contains a wealth of resources about prostate cancer, including information on the various stages of prostate cancer, treatment options, medical journal articles, and related links.

Prostate Cancer Home Page

UNIVERSITY OF MICHIGAN COMPREHENSIVE CANCER CENTER

Kenneth J. Pienta, M.D.

A resource for prostate cancer related information pertaining to diagnosis, staging, treatment options, specialists, investigational studies and current research. It is intended for health professionals and patients, alike.

Articles on Prostate Cancer
A collection of scientific and general articles.

Prostate Cancer Clinical Trials
A listing of clinical trials being conducted.

The Prostate Cancer InfoLink

http://www.comed.com/Prostate/

The Prostate Cancer InfoLink, from the CoMed Communications Internet Health Forum, provides information and resources for patients with prostate cancer, their families, and the professionals who are involved in the diagnosis and treatment of the most common male cancer in the United States.

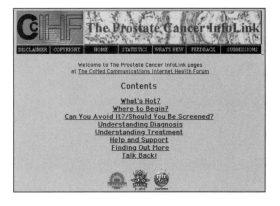

The Prostate Cancer InfoLink

DISCLAIMER | COPYRIGHT | HOME | STATISTICS | WHATS NEW | FEEDBACK | SUBMISSIONS

Welcome to The Prostate Cancer InfoLink pages
at The CoMed Communications Internet Health Forum

Contents

What's Hot?
Where to Begin?
Can You Avoid It?/Should You Be Screened?
Understanding Diagnosis
Understanding Treatment
Help and Support
Finding Out More
Talk Back!

Prostate Enlargement: Benign Prostatic Hyperplasia

http://www.niddk.nih.gov/ProstateEnlargement/
ProstateEnlargement.html

Prostate Enlargement: Benign Prostatic Hyperplasia, from the National Institute of Diabetes and Digestive and Kidney Diseases, provides a comprehensive online brochure about the prostate gland and prostate enlargement or hyperplasia (BPH), featuring symptoms, diagnosis, and treatment. The site includes illustrations and numerous links to medical definitions.

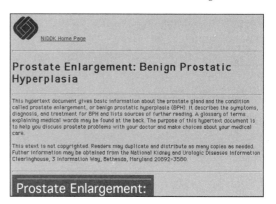

Prostate Health

http://www.prostatehealth.com/

Prostate Health, an official site of the Prostate Health Council of the American Foundation for Urologic Disease, Inc., is a comprehensive, interactive resource where men and their families can learn about current prostate health topics, including anatomy and physiology, symptoms and treatment, articles and reports, an American Urologic Association's survey for determining the severity of your urinating problems, and related links.

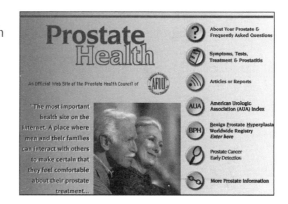

Prostate Pointers

http://rattler.cameron.edu/prostate/

Prostate Pointers, maintained by prostate cancer survivors, provides a collection of prostate cancer resources and information about general problems of the prostate.

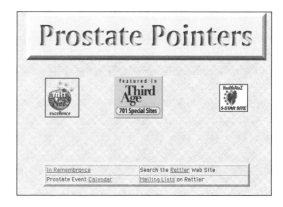

Prostatitis

http://www.prostate.org/

The Prostatitis home page has a wide variety of online resources on urinary tract diseases and prostate problems. The site includes an annotated alphabetical index and an extensive list of related sites.

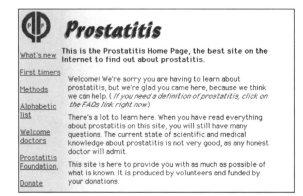

Successfully Treating Impotence

http://www.impotent.com/

Successfully Treating Impotence, prepared by Pharmacia and Upjohn, provides an online guide for the causes and cures to impotence.

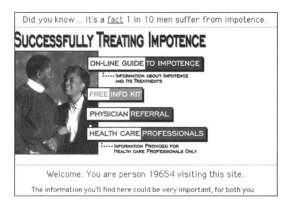

Testicular Cancer and TSE

http://raven.jmu.edu/~taylorbw/

Testicular Cancer and TSE, contributed by the Department of Health Science at James Madison University, provides information on testicular cancer and how to conduct a testicular self-examination (TSE). Graphics also help the reader (men 15 years and over) understand the specific instructions.

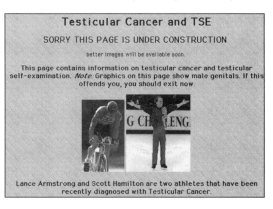

The Testicular Cancer Resource Center

http://www.acor.org/diseases/TC/

The Testicular Cancer Resource Center provides must-know information about the most common cancer among young men. The site includes a primer on testicular cancer, a testicular self-examination, a dictionary, information on treating testicular cancer, and over 590 related links.

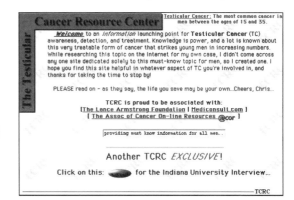

The Testosterone Source

http://www.testosteronesource.com/

The Testosterone Source provides you with intelligent, factual information on testosterone and testosterone deficiency—a problem that affects more than 5 million men in the United States.

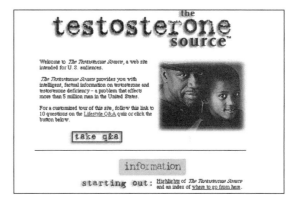

Urologic and Male Genital Diseases

http://www.mic.ki.se/Diseases/c12.html

Urologic and Male Genital Diseases, prepared by the Karolinska Institute Library and Information Center in Stockholm for its Medical Information Center, contains a comprehensive collection of links to infectious and noninfectious urologic and male genital diseases.

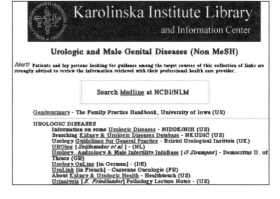

Urology Page

http://www.urolog.nl/uropage/uroeng.htm

The Urology Page provides patient information about urologic health problems of the kidneys, urinary bladder, urethra, prostate, penis, and testicles.

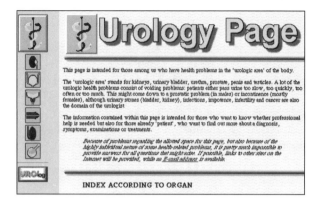

Virgil's Prostate On-line

http://www.prostate-online.com/

Virgil's Prostate On-line is a guide to and personal story of fighting prostate cancer with help from related online resources.

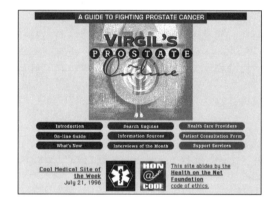

Human Sexuality and Fertility

CHAPTER 7

Alt.sex

http://www.halcyon.com/elf/altsex/

Alt.sex is a newsgroup site containing discussions on the subject of human sexuality. The FAQs include explicit information but are not erotic.

alt.sex

Alt.sex is a newsgroup dealing in human sexuality. Discussions on alt.sex are often frank and honest, and the language used on alt.sex is reflected in this FAQ. People who feel they are likely to be offended by educational materials dealing with human sexuality should not delve any farther into this archive.

This FAQ uses sexually explicit words, phrases, and even images as part of its educational mission. This material is for information purposes only. **No material of an explicit erotic nature is intended in this FAQ.**

"You know, talking. That other thing you do with your mouth to make sex more enjoyable." - MegaZone

A FAQ (Frequently Answered Questions) sheet is intended, according to news.answers, to reduce the amount of traffic on a typical newsgroup by answering the most common questions that would be asked of someone conversant in that newsgroup's topic.

Alt.sex is not a typical newsgroup. It receives significantly more traffic than the average newsgroup, for one thing. If the statistics are to be believed, alt.sex is the singlemost widely read newsgroup of Usenet-- a significant statement when one-quarter of all machines receiving Usenet do not include alt.sex as part of their feed.

Ann Rose's Ultimate Birth Control Links Page

http://gynpages.com/ultimate/

Ann Rose's Ultimate Birth Control Links Page provides numerous resources for information on birth control, sexuality, and fertility.

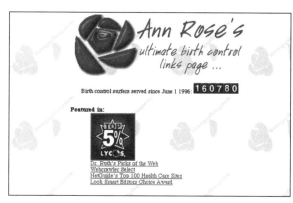

Ann Rose's ultimate birth control links page ...

Birth control surfers served since June 1 1996: 160780

Featured in:

TOP 5% LYCOS

Dr. Ruth's Picks of the Web
Webcrawler Select
NetGuide's Top 100 Health Care Sites
Look Smart Editors Choice Award

Ask a Sex Therapist

http:/www.mindspring.com/~debfox/

Ask a Sex Therapist is a fee-based e-mail question-and-answer forum to get answers from sex therapist Deborah J. Fox.

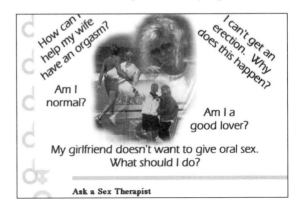

Ask Eve . . . Anything!

http://www.evesplace.com/sensuous/askeve.html

Ask Eve . . . Anything!, dating from 1995, contains archives with questions and answers about sex. The site discusses sexuality topics appropriate only for those 21 years and older.

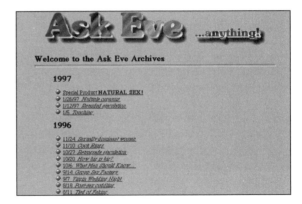

Coalition for Positive Sexuality

http://www.positive.org/

The Coalition for Positive Sexuality promotes positive attitudes about sexuality and encourages safe sex among teens.

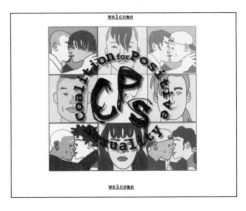

The Diagnostic Center for Men

http://www.for-men.com/

The Diagnostic Center for Men provides help and information on impotence and premature ejaculation.

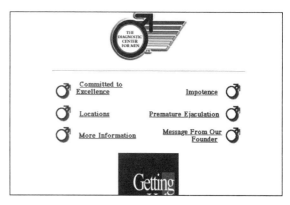

Dr. Derman's Infertility Home Page

http://members.aol.com/fertilmd

Dr. Derman's Infertility Home Page, created by Dr. Seth G. Derman, a reproductive endocrinologist, provides infertility information and resources for the diagnosis and treatment of infertility. The site also includes other infertility links.

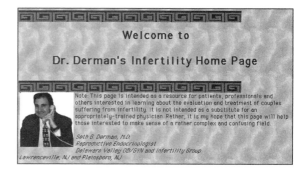

Dr. Ruth Online

http://www.drruth.com/

Dr. Ruth, a famous talk show host, provides information on sex and sex therapy. You can ask Dr. Ruth questions, read previous FAQs and answers, access her top mental health sites, and get sex tips.

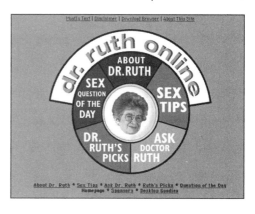

Fertilitext

http://www.fertilitext.org/

Fertilitext provides information about fertility and reproductive problems to those who need it. In addition, it offers a telephone hotline service with specific recorded information on fertility problems, as well as the names and locations of physicians.

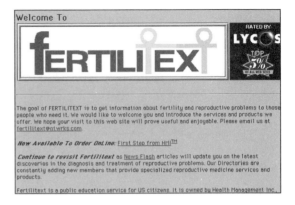

Fertility

http://www.fertilityuk.org

The Fertility home page is a comprehensive introduction to fertility awareness and natural family planning. This site includes an overview, description of the physiology of the male and female fertility cycle, information on recording and interpreting the indicators of fertility, a quiz to test your knowledge of fertility, and a glossary of fertility terms.

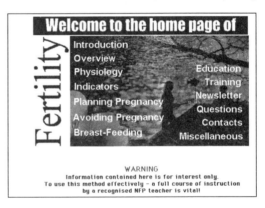

The Kinsey Institute

http://www.indiana.edu/~kinsey/

The Kinsey Institute site supports interdisciplinary research and the study of human sexuality. This venerable 50-year-old Institute was founded by Dr. Alfred Kinsey (1894-1956).

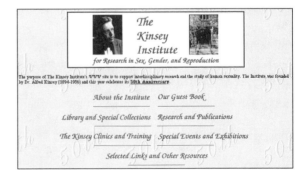

Not Me, Not Now

http://www.notmenotnow.org/

Not Me, Not Now provides information for parents and teenagers interested in learning more about premarital sex. The site offers a listing of educational journal articles, facts about teenage pregnancy, and sample conversations about how to talk with your child about sensitive issues. Teens should check out the online quizzes, testing one's resilience against peer pressure and judgment when dealing with sticky situations.

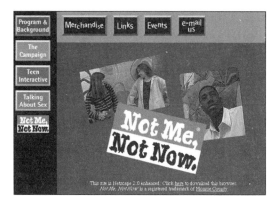

Reproductive Health and Rights Center

http://www.choice.org/

Reproductive Health and Rights Center, sponsored by the CARAL Pro-Choice Education Fund, features breaking news on reproductive rights and health and an activist center with information on how you can have an effect on your local officials and your government. The Resources section contains numerous links to other sites and topics ranging from medical information and sexuality education to legal issues concerning reproductive rights.

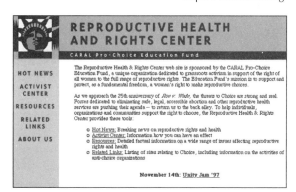

Sexual & Reproductive Health

http://www.ppfa.org/ppfa/lev2-hlt.html

Sexual & Reproductive Health, from the Planned Parenthood Federation of America, provides sexual and reproductive health information on a variety of topics, including AIDS and HIV, herpes, pregnancy and prenatal health, a man's and a woman's guide to sexuality, and commonly asked questions about vaginitis. The site also offers breast cancer and adolescent information, excerpts from *The Planned Parenthood Women's Health Encyclopedia,* and current fact sheets on sexual and reproductive health.

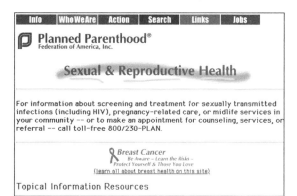

The Sexuality Forum

http://www.askisadora.com

The Sexuality Forum, hosted by Isadora Alman, a syndicated sex and relationship columnist, is an advanced birds-and-bees forum offering mature discussion of sexuality and relationships.

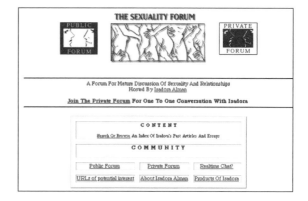

Society for Human Sexuality

http://weber.u.washington.edu/~humsex/

The Society for Human Sexuality, at the University of Washington, is an all-volunteer social and educational organization devoted to the understanding and enjoyment of all safe and consensual forms of sexual and sensual expression.

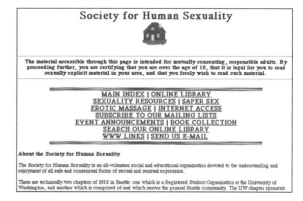

Topics on Sexuality and Relationships

http://www.campuslife.utoronto.ca/services/sec/infotops.html

Topics on Sexuality and Relationships, from the University of Toronto Sexual Education & Peer Counselling Centre, contains a list of topics in sexuality and relationships for young adults. Among the topics are sexually transmitted diseases (STDs), birth control, basic anatomy and human reproduction, and safer sex.

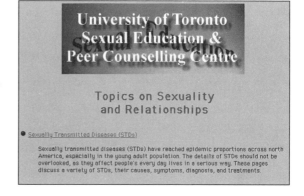

Unspeakable The Naked Truth About STDs

http://www.unspeakable.com/

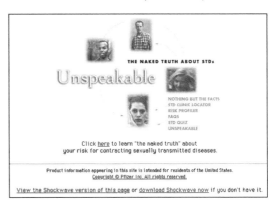

Unspeakable The Naked Truth About STDs, sponsored by Pfizer, provides a variety of online resources for the prevention and treatment of sexually transmitted diseases (STDs). The site presents an interactive questionnaire, which enables the user to construct a risk profile for contracting an STD, offers a search tool for locating an STD clinic in your geographical area, and makes suggestions for more comfortably discussing the risk of STDs with your partner.

Virginia Johnson Masters Learning Center

http://www.vjmlc.com/home.htm

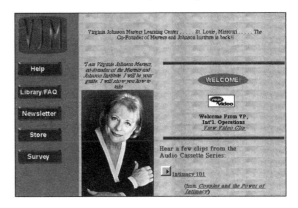

Virginia Johnson Masters Learning Center provides information about relationships based on 40 years of research in the field of human sexuality. To participate in a weekly survey on sex, love, and relationships, click on **Survey.**

The Virtual Hospital
What You Need to Know About Sexually Transmitted Diseases, HIV Disease, and AIDS

What You Need to Know About Sexually Transmitted Diseases, HIV Disease, and AIDS provides topical information on the most common sexually transmitted diseases (STDs): how you get one, how it's transmitted, what it looks like and what the symptoms are, how you get tested, and what will happen to you if you don't get treatment. The site also includes articles on the proper use of a condom and HIV disease.

http://www.vh.org/Patients/IHB/IntMed/Infectious/
STDs/STDAIDS.html

The Virtual Hospital®
the apprentice's assistant™

Iowa Health Book: Infectious Diseases

What You Need to Know About Sexually Transmitted Diseases, HIV Disease, and AIDS

Burroughs Wellcome Co.
Peer Review Status: Externally reviewed by Burroughs Wellcome Co.

Distributed at The American Medical Association Conference on Sexually Transmitted Diseases: Risk Assessment, Diagnosis, and Treatment

About STDs

"STDs" (sexually transmitted diseases) is a broad term that refers to as many as 20 different sicknesses, all of them transmitted by sex – usually through the exchange of body fluids such as semen, vaginal fluid, and blood. STDs can also be given by mothers to their babies. You can get some STDs, such as herpes, by kissing and caressing or close contact with infected areas – not just intercourse. Some STDs just make you feel uncomfortable. Some are more dangerous – if left untreated, they can cause permanent damage that leaves you blind, brain-damaged, or unable to have children. One, HIV (human immunodeficiency virus) disease, often leads to AIDS (acquired

CHAPTER 8

Mental Health

The A-Z Index

http://www.xs4all.nl/~kyjoshi/

The A-Z Index is an alphabetical, self-help directory of various links with information on medical and psychological disorders and related sites.

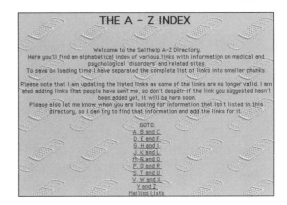

THE A - Z INDEX

Welcome to the Selfhelp A-Z Directory.
Here you'll find an alphabetical index of various links with information on medical and psychological 'disorders' and related sites.
To save on loading time I have separated the complete list of links into smaller chunks.

Please note that I am updating the listed links as some of the links are no longer valid. I am also adding links that people have sent me, so don't despair if the link you suggested hasn't been added yet, it will be here soon.
Please also let me know when you are looking for information that isn't listed in this directory, so I can try to find that information and add the links for it.

GOTO:
A, B and C
D, E and F
G, H and I
J, K and L
M, N and O
P, Q and R
S, T and U
V, W and X
Y and Z
Mailing Lists

Abuse Survivors' Resources

http://www.tezcat.com/~tina/psych.shtml

Abuse Survivors' Resources is an immense site providing survival resources for anyone who has suffered sexual, emotional, or physical abuse. In addition to FAQs, newsgroups, and innumerable links, the site includes psychology- and psychiatry-related links.

Topical Pages
Resource Lists
Newsgroups & FAQs
Publications
Miscellany
SANCTUARY
Search me!
Feedback

Hate frames? Reload this page via this link and you can browse without them.

Blue Ribbon Campaign
Free Speech Online

This page supports EFF's blue ribbon campaign. Some of the content on the pages linked to maybe be disturbing to those of a sensitive nature, and may be unsuitable for minors.

Abuse Survivors' Resources

Welcome to Discord's Abuse Survivor's Resources pages. Although this page is primarily aimed at abuse survivors, friends and family of survivors, victims still in their abusive situation, and other interested parties will find most of these links useful as well. Most of the links on these pages are either about abuse (whether it is sexual, physical, emotional, or ritual) or its effects (which vary widely but can include such things as depression, anxiety disorders, and dissociation). The pages here are split by type of resource, and then on each page are split by topic.

Please do not e-mail me asking me for further help or information. If it's not up on the page, I almost certainly don't have access to it. It's just frustrating when people ask me stuff I can't answer. Thanks.

Try the search program -- now updated slightly.

American Academy of Child & Adolescent Psychiatry

http://www.aacap.org/web/aacap/

The American Academy of Child & Adolescent Psychiatry provides a variety of resources about child and adolescent psychiatry. The site contains a collection of online family fact sheets in English, Spanish, and French ranging from the "The Adopted Child" to "When Children Have Children." In addition, the site has the latest breaking news, information on clinical practice, managed care, and health care, and related links.

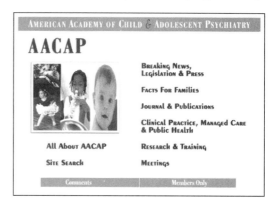

American Psychological Association

http://www.apa.org/

The American Psychological Association home page offers a wealth of psychology resources in the **PsychNET** section. It includes a **Help Center,** which provides information on modern life problems, as well as a **Public Information** area, which features online brochures ranging from "Sexual Harassment: Myths and Realities" to "Controlling Anger Before It Controls You." For an overview of resources, click on the **Site Map.**

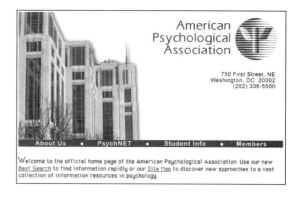

Andrew's Depression Page

http://www.blarg.net/~charlatn/Depression.html

Andrew's Depression Page contains a multitude of resources on mental depression ranging from treatment to mood scales. The site includes a large collection of related links.

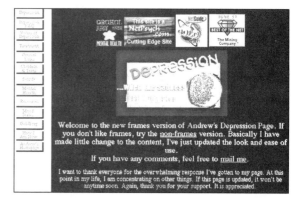

Anxiety and Phobia Clinic of White Plains Hospital

http://www.phobia-anxiety.com/

The Anxiety and Phobia Clinic of White Plains Hospital is one of three founding groups of the Phobia Society of America, now known as the Anxiety Disorders Association of America. The site includes an **Ask the Doctors** section to answer your questions about anxiety and phobias.

Last updated: Monday, August 18, 1997

Welcome to the

Anxiety and Phobia Clinic of White Plains Hospital

Davis Ave. at East Post Rd White
Plains, NY 10601

Phone: (914) 681-1038 Facsimile:
(914) 681-2284

➤ Celebrating our 26th year helping people overcome their fears, phobias and anxieties.

➤ The Anxiety and Phobia Clinic is one of three founding groups of the Phobia Society of America, now known as the Anxiety Disorders Association of America.

Director Emeritus	Manual D. Zane, M.D., author of Your Phobia: Understanding Your Fears Through Contextual Therapy
Director	Fredric Neuman, M.D., author of Fighting Fear: An Eight Week Guide to Treating Your Own Phobias Published by Macmillian and Pinpoint Press. Caring: Home Treatment for the Emotionally Disturbed
Coordinator	Judy Lake Chessa

Anxiety Disorders Association of America

http://www.adaa.org

The headquarters of the Anxiety Disorders Association of America provides a wealth of information about anxiety disorders such as panic disorder phobias, obsessive-compulsive disorder, post-traumatic stress disorder, and generalized anxiety disorder. Each topic in the **Information about Anxiety Disorders** section includes an online self-test. The site also offers an anxiety disorder glossary, a table of contents, and related links.

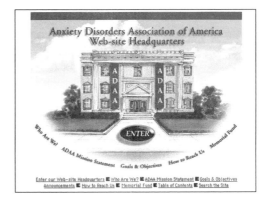

The Anxiety-Panic Internet Resource

http://www.algy.com/anxiety/

The Anxiety-Panic Internet Resource involves thousands of people interested in anxiety disorders such as panic attacks, phobias, shyness, generalized anxiety, obsessive-compulsive behavior, and post-traumatic stress. It is a self-help network dedicated to overcoming and curing overwhelming anxiety. Click on The **A-Z Index** to find an encyclopedia of anxiety and self-help information.

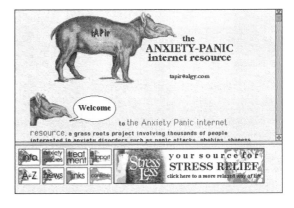

APA Online

http://www.psych.org/

APA Online, from the American Psychiatric Association, is a rich resource covering a variety of topics with related links. Click on **Public Information Section** to find the Let's Talk Facts pamphlet series, a collection of articles on everything from anxiety disorders to teenage suicides. In addition, you can choose a psychiatrist, find out about mental illness coverage issues, and psychiatric medications. For an overview of the site, click on **Index.**

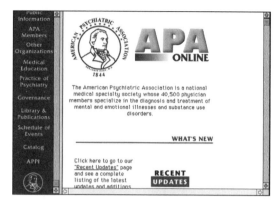

Arnot Ogden Medical Center

http://www.aomc.org/HOD2/general/stress.html

The Arnot Ogden Medical Center features a collection of articles on every aspect of stress management. There are articles dealing with family stress levels, chronic fatigue, coping with anxiety, helping children through a crisis, and dealing with anger.

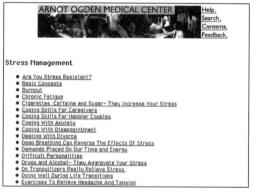

Behavior OnLine

http://www.behavior.net/

Behavior OnLine houses online discussion forums on topics ranging from arts therapy to anxiety disorders. It includes pages from related behavioral institutes and interviews with Jungian and Adlerian therapists. The site also offers mind games and puzzles, as well as links to institutes and organizations.

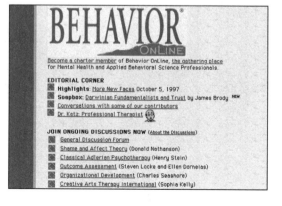

Buros Institute of Mental Measurements

http://www.unl.edu/buros/

The Buros Institute of Mental Measurements, renowned in the field of measurement, provides online reviews of tests ranging from vocational interest inventories to personality and mental tests. Select the **ERIC/AE Test Locator** and then click on **ETS/ERIC Test** file. At the search query, type in your test and click on **Search.** To get a more in-depth discussion of this test, click on the **magnifying glass.**

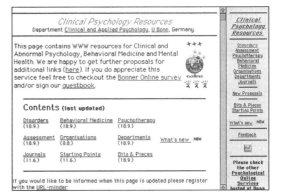

Clinical Psychology Resources

http://www.psychologie.uni-bonn.de/kap/links_20.htm

Clinical Psychology Resources, prepared by the Clinical and Applied Psychology Department at the University of Bonn, Germany, contains a collection of sites for clinical and abnormal psychology, behavioral medicine, and mental health. Categories include Disorders, Psychotherapy, Assessment, and Journals. For a list of general mental health sites, click on **Starting Points.**

Counseling Center Self-Help Home Page

http://ub-counseling.buffalo.edu/

The Counseling Center Self-Help Home Page, from the State University of New York at Buffalo, offers a wide selection of articles, Internet resources, referrals, and reading lists to help college students with day-to-day stresses and difficult periods in their lives.

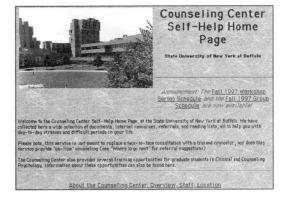

Cyber-Psych

http://www.webweaver.net/psych/

Cyber-Psych provides a variety of mental health resources that discuss addictions and eating and mood disorders, present sex information, and provide lists of psychology journals, national psychological organizations, and self-help and support groups. There are also fun psychology-related sites in the **Other Neat Stuff** section.

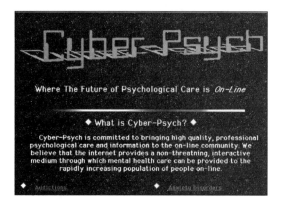

David Baldwin's Trauma Info Pages

http://www.teleport.com~dvb/trauma.htm

David Baldwin's Trauma Info Pages provides a variety of traumatic stress resources, including disaster handouts, research-related trauma information, and general support information about trauma and mental health, in addition to related links.

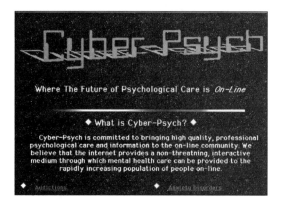

Dear Abby

http://www.uexpress.com/ups/abby/

Dear Abby provides sample letters from her column with advice on snoring, homosexuality, marriage, and other earthy topics. You may browse previously answered questions or post your own question in the **Forum** section.

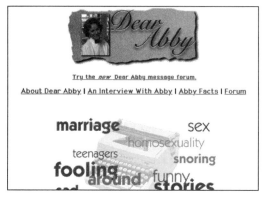

Depression

http://www.ns.net/users/adhd/depress.htm

Depression, by Brandi Valentine, provides information on depression, a message board, and related links.

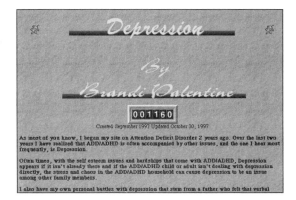

Doctor's Guide to Schizophrenia Information & Resources

http://www.pslgroup.com/SCHIZOPHR.HTM

The Doctor's Guide to Schizophrenia Information & Resources presents the latest medical news and online resources for patients or friends or parents of patients diagnosed with schizophrenia and schizophrenia-related disorders. Categories include Medical News and Alerts, Schizophrenia Information, Discussion Groups and Newsgroups, Stay Abreast of Schizophrenia Development (a mailing list), and Other Related Sites.

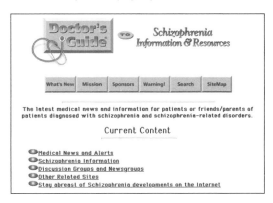

Dr. Bob's Mental Health Links

http://uhs.bsd.uchicago.edu/~bhsiung/mental.html

Dr. Bob's Mental Health Links presents a plethora of mental health resources. Among them are psychopharmacology tips, an Rx Qx section with information on psychiatric medications and conditions, a virtual pamphlets section for university students, and links to other psychology and psychiatry sites.

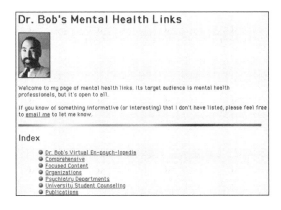

Dr. Bob's Psychopharmacology Tips

http://uhs.bsd.uchicago.edu/dr-bob/tips/tips.html

Dr. Bob's Psychopharmacology Tips provides information on drugs designed to assist in coping with mental health problems. A searchable database, as well as many links to other mental health sites, is offered.

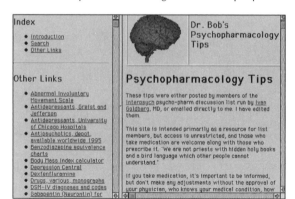

Dr. Ivan's Depression Central

http://www.psycom.net/depression.central.html

Dr. Ivan's Depression Central, created by Dr. Ivan Goldberg, is a clearinghouse for information on all types of depressive disorders and effective treatments for individuals suffering from major depression illnesses.

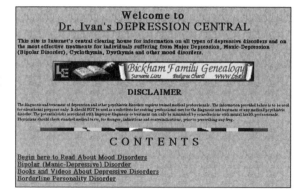

Eating Disorders Awareness and Prevention, Inc.

http://members.aol.com/edapinc/home.html

Eating Disorders Awareness and Prevention, Inc. presents a variety of eating disorder resources, including basic facts, prevention, how parents and friends can help, and much more.

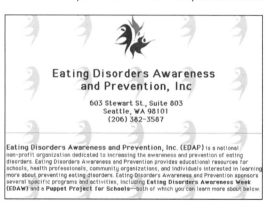

Eating Disorders Shared Awareness

http://www.mirror-mirror.org/eatdis.htm

Eating Disorders Shared Awareness provides a collection of articles offering information about eating disorders. The articles are arranged in more than 25 categories, including college students, older women, men, athletes, self-injury, addictions, and society. The site also presents an eating behavior test to help you determine if you have an eating disorder.

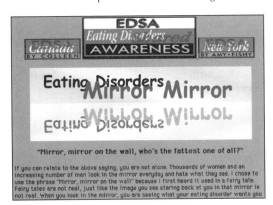

Good Housekeeping Your Questions Answered

http://www.homearts.com/gh/advice/97brotf1.htm

The *Good Houskeeping* magazine contains an online feature in which Dr. Joyce Brothers answers your questions and offers advice about mental health problems. Some of the topics include Father's Broken Promise and Four Things You Should Never Say in Anger.

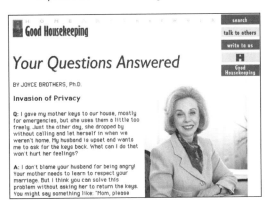

Guide to Psychotherapy

http://www.shef.ac.uk/~psysc/psychotherapy/

Guide to Psychotherapy, from the Centre for Psychotherapeutic Studies at the University of Sheffield, England, features an **Online Dictionary of Mental Health** with thousands of alphabetical and searchable links to mental health resources. In addition, the site provides a library with innumerable reference resources for further inquiry.

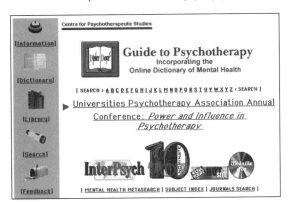

InStream PsychLink

http://www.psychlink.com/

InStream PsychLink presents the latest mental health news daily from a variety of media sources, an index of medical databases, forums, and discussion groups, and a humor page.

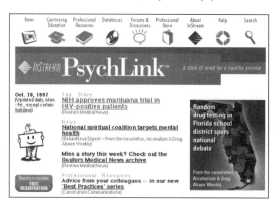

Interlude

http://www.teleport.com/~interlud/

Interlude is a universal retreat for anyone seeking peace of mind and a shelter away from the cares of the world. The site contains thoughts, meditations, prayers, relaxation techniques, a bibliography, inspirational e-mails, and related links.

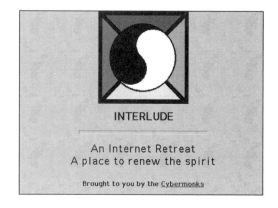

Internet Mental Health

http://www.mentalhealth.com/

Internet Mental Health is an encyclopedia of mental health information, including disorders, diagnosis, medications, magazines, and related links. Click on the **Index** to quickly access the site's resources.

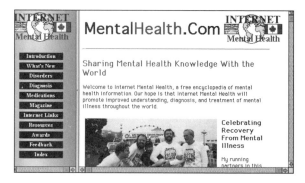

Internet Mental Health Resources

Internet Mental Health Resources, maintained by Herbert D. Stockley, contains an index of mental health topics, including bipolar disorders, cults, suicide, and Tourette's syndrome.

http://ub-counseling.buffalo.edu/Internet/herbs.html

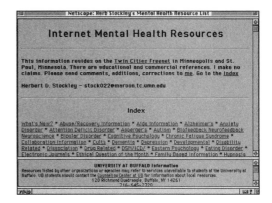

A Layperson's Short Classification of Psychotherapeutic Drugs

A Layperson's Short Classification of Psychotherapeutic Drugs, by Judith Michelsen, is a comprehensive guide to common medications prescribed for mental health disorders and their side effects.

http://onlinepsych.com/treat/drugs.htm

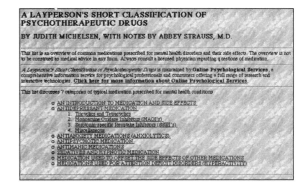

A Look at Sleep Disorders

A Look at Sleep Disorders, from the Saint Francis Hospital Sleep Disorders Center in Tulsa, Oklahoma, has information about sleep disorders and their treatments. Among the topics are the various sleep disorders, good sleeping habits, a sleeping disorder test, FAQs, and related links.

http://www.saintfrancis.com/sleepintro.html

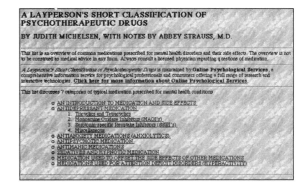

Magic Stream Journal

http://fly.hiwaay.net/~garson/

The Magic Stream Journal offers a holistic and emotional wellness approach providing extensive self-help and mental health references for professionals, consumers, family members, and individuals seeking professional advice. Among the site's resources is **WebDex,** which contains a wealth of information on addictions, eating disorders, recovery, child abuse, fitness, nutrition, and depression. The site also includes a self-help discussion group, articles and poetry, and an online or telephone counseling service available 24 hours a day.

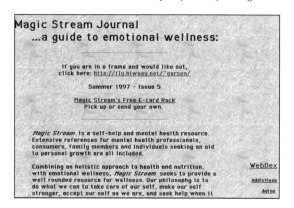

The Medical Basis of Stress, Depression, Anxiety, Sleep Problems, and Drug Use

http://www.teachhealth.com/

The Medical Basis of Stress, Depression, Anxiety, Sleep Problems, and Drug Use is the online version of *How to Survive Unbearable Stress* by Steve Burns, M.D., and Kimberley Burns. The site contains chapters on topics such as recognizing stress, stress tolerance, patterns of inheritance, pick-me-ups, as well as related links.

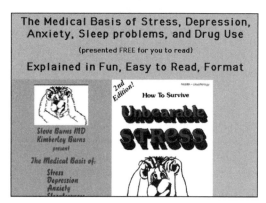

Mental Health InfoSource

http://www.mhsource.com/

Mental Health InfoSource provides a wide variety of mental health resources, including an interactive ask the expert feature, hundreds of articles, and an index of disorders. The **Disorders** section ranges from attention deficit hyperactivity disorder to sleep disorders. Each disorder includes an archive of expert answers, articles, diagnostic information, and related sites.

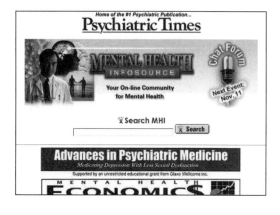

Mental Health Links

http://www.j.day.clara.net/mental.htm

Mental Health Links, organized by Jonathan Day, contains a catalog of mental health sites ranging from anxiety disorders to general mental health.

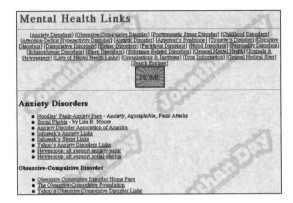

Mental Health Net

http://mhnet.org/

The Mental Health Net features over 6300 resources for disorders such as depression, anxiety, panic attacks, chronic fatigue syndrome, and substance abuse. Each category includes an annotated list of top-rated sites. In addition, the site has access to professional resources in psychology and psychiatry.

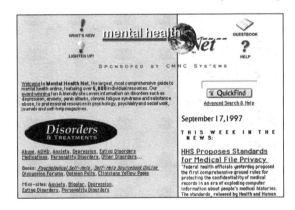

Mental Health Net
Eating Disorders

http://mhnet.org/guide/eating.htm

Mental Health Net Eating Disorders provides comprehensive resources on eating disorders, including anorexia nervosa and bulimia. The site includes an annotated list of related links, articles about eating disorders, and a newsgroup. The treatment and support services section offers an eating disorder quiz.

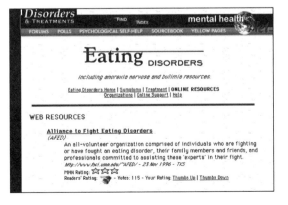

Mental Health Net Mental Disorders Symptoms and Treatments

http://mhnet.org/dxtx.htm

Mental Health Net Mental Disorders Symptoms and Treatments offers invaluable mental health resources for disorders and treatments. They include the American Clearinghouse's **Self-Help Sourcebook Online,** the American Academy of Child and Adolescent Psychiatry's **Facts for Families, Psychological Self-Help,** and **Mental Disorders Symptoms and Treatments.** In addition to these resources, the site provides an A to Z index to top-rated mental health sites reviewed by the readers.

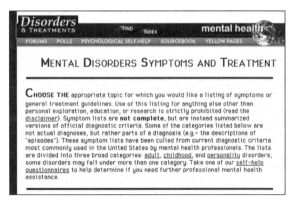

Mental Health Predictor

http://onthenet.com.au/~pict/mentpick.htm

Mental Health Predictor, from the Tweed Valley Health Service, is an online interactive calculator predicting the state of your mental health. You answer questions to present a personality profile of yourself.

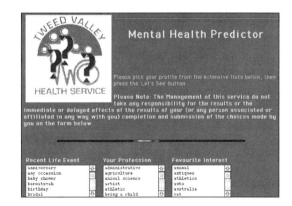

Mental Health Resources

http://mentalhealth.miningco.com/

Mental Health Resources, updated weekly by the Mining Company, provides an extensive online library of mental health resources categorized by topic. Topics consist of professional sites, child and adolescent resources, general resources, and anxiety, panic, and depression resources. The site also includes articles and a 24-hour chat room.

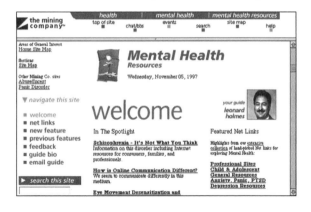

MentalWellness.com

http://www.mentalwellness.com/

MentalWellness.com provides patients, family members, and caregivers with mental health information. The site contains concise information about mental disorders, a glossary of commonly used terms, tips for saving money as the result of mental disability, and articles from Reuters News Service.

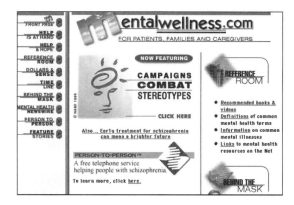

Metanoia Guide to Internet Mental Health Services

http://www.metanoia.org/imhs/

The Metanoia Guide to Internet Mental Health Services, in partnership with Mental Health Net, affords you the opportunity to talk online with psychotherapists and counselors who provide mental health services over the Internet.

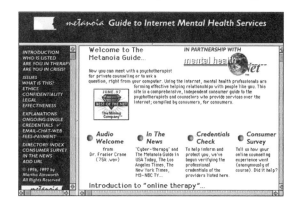

Mood Disorders

http://avocado.pc.helsinki.fi/~janne/mood/mood.html

Mood Disorders contains a wealth of information on mood disorders that disable millions of Americans every year and the various treatments available.

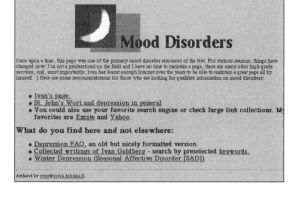

National Alliance for the Mentally Ill

http://www.nami.org/

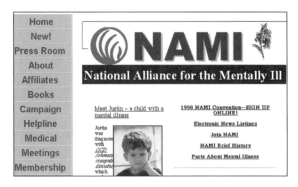

The National Alliance for the Mentally Ill, founded in 1979, provides quick facts about mental illness, a medical index with information on research, disorders, and medications, and links to other mental health sites. In addition, the site offers a toll-free helpline number 1-800-950-6264, a mailing list, and a search tool for finding information on mental illnesses or medications. For an overview of the site, click on **Index.**

National Institute of Mental Health

http://www.nimh.nih.gov/

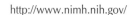
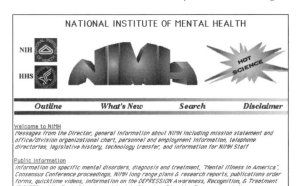

The National Institute of Mental Health, part of the National Institutes of Health, provides **Public Information,** in English and Spanish, on specific mental disorders, diagnosis, and treatment. The reading room of this section has articles on anxiety disorders, plain talk about depression, attention deficit hyperactivity disorder (ADHD), schizophrenia questions and answers, and other topics.

The National Mental Health Services Knowledge Exchange Network

http://www.mentalhealth.org

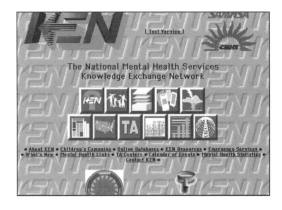

The National Mental Health Services Knowledge Exchange Network provides information about mental health via a toll-free telephone service, an electronic bulletin board, and online publications. Click on **Databases** to find mental health directories for consumer/survivors, organizations, and annotated bibliographies. The site also includes links to other mental health and federal sites.

NetPsychology

http://netpsych.com/

NetPsychology is one of the premiere mental health sites on the Web. The **Web** section contains an enormous collection of links to quality mental health sites. The site also includes a weekly featured article, chat rooms, news, and much more.

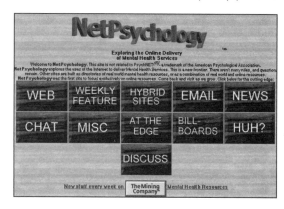

Obsessive-Compulsive Disorder

http://www.fairlite.com/ocd/

Obsessive-Compulsive Disorder contains definitions, abstracts and articles, information about medications, listings of medical and personal resources, a bulletin board, and links to related sites.

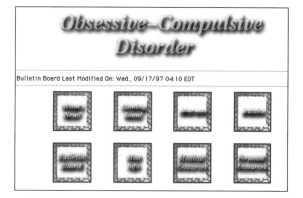

Online Psych

http://www.onlinepsych.com/

Online Psych provides the consumer with a comprehensive source of information about mental health. The **Mental Health Info** section has over 350 sites arranged by topic on various aspects of mental health.

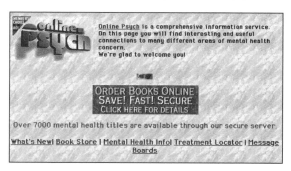

Other Psychiatry Sites on the Web

http://www.priory.co.uk/otherpsy.htm

Other Psychiatry Sites on the Web, from Yearbook of Psychiatry and Applied Mental Health, features a collection of psychiatry sites organized by category ranging from affective disorders to substance abuse for alcohol and drugs.

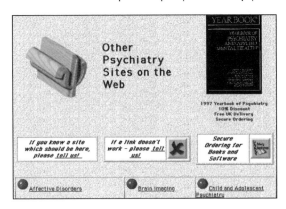

Pendulum Resources

http://www.pendulum.org/

Pendulum Resources is a comprehensive source of online information about bipolar disorders (manic-depression) and other mood disorders. The site contains articles, medication and support information, and a collection of related links.

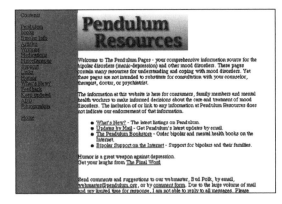

Personality Tests on the WWW

http://www.2h.com/Tests/personality.phtml

Personality Tests on the WWW features a collection of online mental health and psychological tests, including those for anxiety, self-esteem, stress, attention deficit disorder, and others. Among the tests are the Keirsey Temperament Sorter, a Coping With Stress Inventory, and Life-Style test.

Phantom Sleep Page

http://www.newtechpub.com/phantom/

The Phantom Sleep Page offers information about sleep apnea, snoring, and other sleep problems. The site includes a self-scoring sleep apnea quiz, articles, and related links.

Phantom Sleep Page™(Sleep apnea, snoring & other sleep problems)

We need to sleep well to enjoy being awake, thus we can live better if we overcome sleep disorders. Presenting useful information about sleep and sleep disorders including snoring and sleep apnea for the public, patients, and professionals. *The Phantom Sleep Newsletter™* Articles, bibliographies, newsletters, connections to research and support groups. Use the guide to *Sleeping on the Internet* (with links to other sites). **Incorporating S.N.O.R.E and the Sleep Apnea FAQ created by Doug Linder.**

Please do bookmark this page for ready reference, note this is a new URL: http://www.newtechpub.com/phantom This web site is a super-set of and includes material orginally posted at <world.std.com/~halberst>.

Phantom of the Night: Overcome Sleep Apnea & Snoring by T.S. Johnson M.D. & Jerry Halberstadt

The handbook for patients written by a sleep disorders expert and a patient. Second, revised edition (updated, April 1997) shipping by Priority Mail. Read more about this guide: Praise and reviews by readers (patients & professionals).

Psych Central

http://www.grohol.com/

Psych Central, Dr. John Grohol's mental health page, is an online guide to self-help and mental health resources. The site includes newsgroups, chat rooms, mailing lists, FAQs, and related Web links.

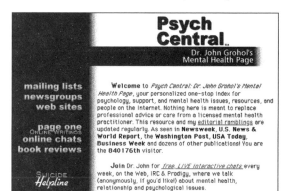

Psych Central™

Dr. John Grohol's Mental Health Page

mailing lists
newsgroups
web sites

page one
ONLINE WRITINGS
online chats
book reviews

SUICIDE
Helpline

Welcome to *Psych Central: Dr. John Grohol's Mental Health Page*, your personalized one-stop index for psychology, support, and mental health issues, resources, and people on the Internet. Nothing here is meant to replace professional advice or care from a licensed mental health practitioner. This resource and my editorial ramblings are updated regularly. As seen in **Newsweek, U.S. News & World Report**, the **Washington Post, USA Today, Business Week** and dozens of other publications! You are the 840176th visitor.

Join Dr. John for *free, LIVE interactive chats* every week, on the Web, IRC & Prodigy, where we talk (anonymously, if you'd like!) about mental health, relationship and psychological issues.

Psych Web

http://www.gasou.edu/psychweb/psychweb.htm

Psych Web, created by Russ Dewey, contains a rich collection of resources for psychology. Click on **Other Megalists of Psychology Resources** to find numerous mental health sites.

Welcome

Welcome to Psych Web! This Web site contains lots of psychology-related information for students and teachers of psychology. Check out What's New on Psych Web to see what has been added since your last visit. Sections of Psych Web include....

● Books
[Full-length, browsable web versions of two classics: *The Interpretation of Dreams (3rd ed)* by Sigmund Freud, and *Varieties of Religious Experience* by William James]
● Brochures and articles related to psychology
[Big lists of short articles...from counseling centers and on-line journals.]
● Commercial sites related to psychology
[If they ask for money anywhere on their pages, the link is listed here.]
● Discussion Pages
[Discuss any topic relevant to college-level psychology courses.]
● Find Anything
[Find web sites, e-mail addresses, telephone numbers...anything!]
● Georgia Southern Psychology Department Home Page
[Interviews with faculty, articles from our newsletter, information for our majors]
● Journals: Armin Guenther's Links to Psychological Journals
[A good, thorough list of English and German language psychology

Psychiatric Resources Arranged by Topic

http://www.hsls.pitt.edu/intres/mental/psyreso.html

Psychiatric Resources Arranged by Topic, from the University of Pittsburg's Internet Resources, contains an enormous mental health warehouse of information arranged by topics, ranging from addiction to violence.

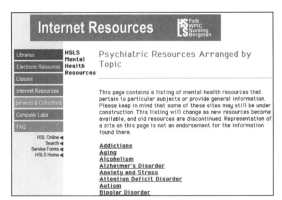

Self-Help & Psychology Magazine

http://www.cybertowers.com/selfhelp/

Self-Help & Psychology Magazine, an award-winning publication, offers articles on more than 20 self-help topics ranging from attention deficit to stress. In addition, the site offers FAQs, newsgroups, and cartoons.

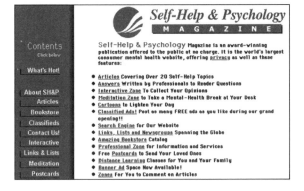

Self-Help Sourcebook OnLine

http://www.cmhc.com/selfhelp/

Self-Help Sourcebook OnLine, from the American Self-Help Clearinghouse and sponsored by Mental Health Net, offers a complete guide to organizations and people who will help you locate a support group in your community. The site contains 1000 pages of psychological self-help with over 2000 references to help you learn more about your problems and the valuable skills to fight them.

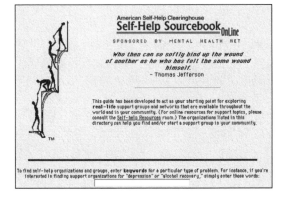

The Sleep Medicine Home Page

http://www.cloud9.net/~thorpy/

The Sleep Medicine Home Page provides a variety of sleep resources, including an alphabetical listing of sleep disorders, sleep-related newsgroups, federal and state information, and professional associations and foundations.

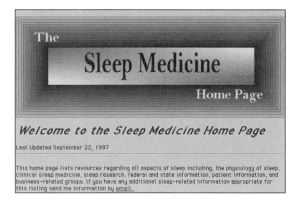

SleepNet

http://www.sleepnet.com/

SleepNet provides in-depth information on sleep. The site includes a forum, a guide to sleep disorders, sleep deprivation information, and over 130 sleep-related links.

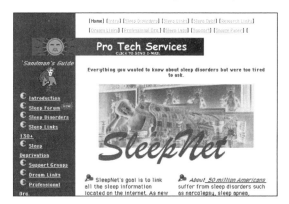

The Something Fishy Website on Eating Disorders

http://www.something-fishy.com/ed.htm

The Something Fishy Website on Eating Disorders is a comprehensive source of information on anorexia nervosa, bulimia, compulsive overeating, managing stress, and links to other eating disorder sites.

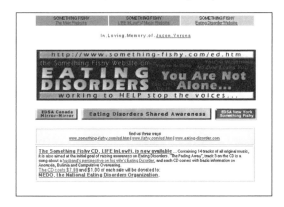

Specifica

http://www.realtime.net/~mmjw/

Specifica, an evolving resource of information and services for people in need, offers many articles and links to resources on mental illness and personality disorders.

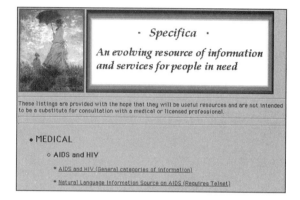

Stepping Stones

http://www.flpinstitute.com/steppingstones/

Stepping Stones, published by Bruce Wilson, is a monthly newsletter that features current information and practical tips to help you make permanent changes in your life. Topics include weight loss, smoking cessation, and career change. The site also includes updates on health-related news, an interactive reader's forum, and resources for change and a list of medical sites.

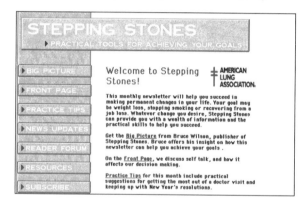

Stress Management

http://www.kaplan.com/games/chill/

Stress Management, from Kaplan, a major developer of college entrance examinations, offers a comprehensive online program for stress management. The site features information on overcoming stress, eating to avoid stress, and the top 10 tips for dealing with stress. In addition, there are relaxation exercises, meditation tips, thought exercises, a stress test, and stress-busting related links.

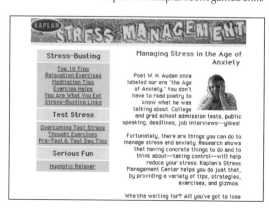

Suicide Awareness\Voices of Education

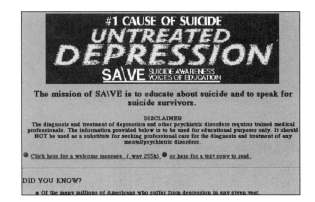

http://www.save.org/

Suicide Awareness\Voices of Education provides advice and information on teenage depression, suicide, and mental illnesses.

University of Alberta's Health Information Page

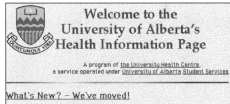

http://www.ualberta.ca/~jhancock/HealthEd.html

The University of Alberta's Health Information Page covers topics such as sexual health, stress and weight, and body image for young men and women. The site also includes pages written by students for students on topics such as "Living With HIV" and "Depression."

Web Psychologist

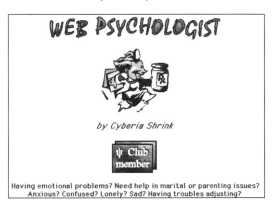

http://www.queendom.com/shrink.html

Web Psychologist, by Cyberia Shrink, offers therapist help or advice on emotional, marital, or parenting problems. You can read answers to previous problems or submit your own question.

WebPsych Partnership

http://www.cmhc.com/webpsych/

WebPsych Partnership is an index of annotated mental health sites arranged alphabetically.

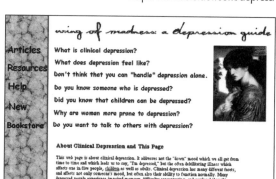

Wing of Madness

http://members.aol.com/depress/

Wing of Madness presents an online guide to clinical depression. The site represents one woman's struggle against depression and her findings serve as an invaluable source of information.

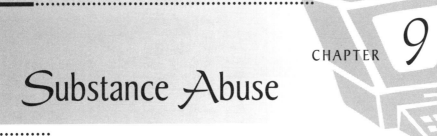

CHAPTER *9*

Substance Abuse

Alcohol/Drug Help Line

http://www.adhl.org/druglos.html

Alcohol/Drug Help Line is a street drug reference guide with information on common drugs from A to Z.

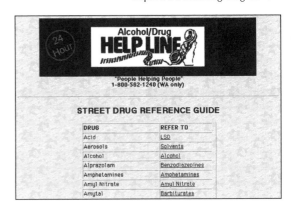

Connecticut Clearinghouse

http://www.ctclearinghouse.org/

Connecticut Clearinghouse, a program of Wheeler Clinic, offers research abstracts and hundreds of fact sheets related to alcohol, tobacco, and drugs. The site includes a search tool.

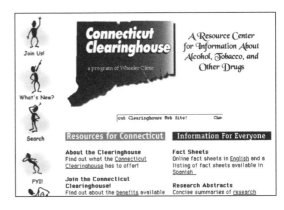

DARE-America.com

http://www.dare-america.com/

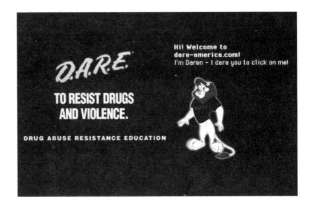

DARE-America.com is the Drug Abuse Resistance Education (D.A.R.E.) program designed to keep America's kids drug free. The site contains an online guide for parents and information for kids and teachers. To access this site, click on the lion **Daren.**

DEA

http://www.usdoj.gov/dea/

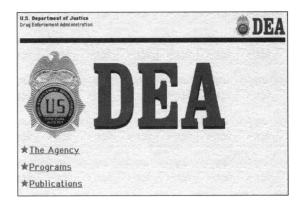

DEA, the U.S. Department of Justice Drug Enforcement Administration, provides the following online magazines about illegal drugs in the **Publications** section: *Drugs of Abuse, Get It Straight! A Drug Prevention Book,* and the *DEA Briefing Book.* The site also includes related sites and statistics.

Drug Policy Information

http://www.ncjrs.org/drgshome.htm

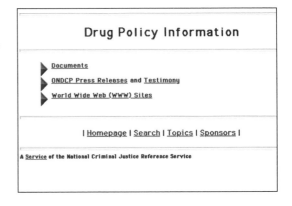

Drug Policy Information presents an extensive list of articles relating to such matters as community efforts, courts, drug treatments, and research. The site also contain numerous related links.

Drug-Free Resource Net

http://www.drugfreeamerica.org/

Drug-Free Resource Net, from the Partnership for a Drug-Free America, offers a comprehensive database to *illegal* drugs (but also to alcohol and tobacco): what they look like and what they do. The site also includes information about slang terms for drugs and how to recognize drug paraphernalia. Advice is offered to parents who are concerned that their children may be using illegal drugs.

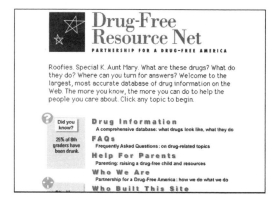

Drugs, Brains and Behavior

http://www.rci.rutgers.edu/~lwh/drugs/

Drugs, Brains and Behavior is an online version of a book written by C. Robin Timmons and Leonard W. Hamilton. Chapter titles include "Behavior and the Chemistry of the Brain" and "Tolerance, Drug Abuse and Habitual Behaviors."

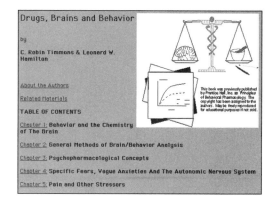

Florida Alcohol and Drug Abuse Association

http://www.fadaa.org/

The Florida Alcohol and Drug Abuse Association site contains a collection of fact sheets in the **Resource Center** section. Select **Just the Facts** in this section to find titles, including "African American Women: Cultural Norms and Prevention," "Designer Drugs," "Inhalants," and "Crisis Intervention."

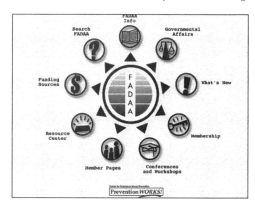

Hazelden

http://www.hazelden.org/

Hazelden is the home page of an alcoholism/drug abuse treatment center offering residential care to adults. Click on the **Resource Center** section to find useful links, interactive quizzes, and online articles.

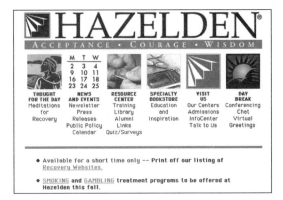

How to Raise Drug-Free Kids

http://www.drugfreekids.com/

How to Raise Drug-Free Kids, designed by *Reader's Digest,* presents an online family guide to help parents keep kids of all ages drug free. The site contains a printable booklet, a list of support groups, a quiz, and facts about drugs.

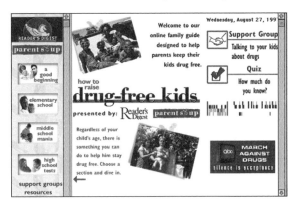

Indiana Prevention Resource Center

http://www.drugs.indiana.edu/

The Indiana Prevention Resource Center, at Indiana University, is a statewide clearinghouse for prevention and information about alcohol, tobacco, and other drugs. The site contains numerous resources about drugs, including a **Drug Info** feature with an online dictionary of street drug terms with over 3000 entries.

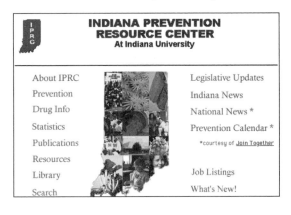

The Master Anti-Smoking Page

http://www.autonomy.com/smoke.htm

The Master Anti-Smoking Page is designed to help people QUIT smoking and to help people, especially young people, NOT START. The site provides a comprehensive collection of anti-smoking links, a Smoke No More Forum where people and organizations can share ideas, and tips for quitting smoking.

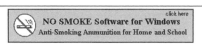

click here
NO SMOKE Software for Windows
Anti-Smoking Ammunition for Home and School

Sponsored by
NO SMOKE Software for Windows – NO SMOKE auf Deutsch

The Master Anti-Smoking Page

 Software to quit Smoking | Links | Smoke No More Forum | Student Queries | Tips On How to Quit

Email Us | Bright Ideas For Schools | Sign Our Guestbook

This page is designed to help people QUIT smoking and to helping people, especially young people, NOT START. It is administered by Elliot Essman, and dedicated to a cousin and two uncles who died prematurely from smoking.

We've got several major parts here. We'll start with the Links to any and every anti-smoking page on the web we can find. A major feature of these web pages is our Smoke No More Forum, where people and organizations can share ideas.

Minnesota Prevention Resource Center

http://www.miph.org/mprc/

The Minnesota Prevention Resource Center is a clearinghouse for alcohol, tobacco, drug, and violence prevention resources. The latest information is in the **What's New?** section, which contains numerous articles about abuse, treatment, and prevention. The site includes related links.

Minnesota Prevention
Resource Center

Welcome to the Minnesota Prevention Resource Center (MPRC) Web Site. We are a nonprofit organization funded through a grant from the Chemical Dependency Program Division, Minnesota Department of Human Services. We serve as a statewide clearinghouse for alcohol, tobacco, other drug and violence prevention resources. Our mission is to enhance the capacity of people interested in prevention in order to reduce problems resulting from alcohol, tobacco, other drugs and associated violence. MPRC provides an array of services and competent staff to meet your needs. We value your suggestions and comments and invite you to direct them to the address at the bottom of this page.

"We are excited about using this new technology as another way of providing you with the kinds of information you need. MPRC supports people, like you, who want to prevent the problems caused by misuse of alcohol, tobacco and other drugs. You can trust that we will make every effort to offer accurate and up to date information and

National Council on Alcoholism and Drug Dependence, Inc.

http://www.ncadd.org/

The National Council on Alcoholism and Drug Dependence, Inc. provides information to fight against alcoholism and other drug addictions. The site contains federal government advocacy information, awareness activities, parents and health information, and facts about alcoholism and other drug addictions. In addition, the site includes a toll-free hope line 1-800-NCA-CALL (1-800-622-2255).

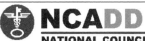 **NCADD**
NATIONAL COUNCIL ON ALCOHOLISM AND DRUG DEPENDENCE, INC.

12 WEST 21 STREET
NEW YORK, NY 10010
212.206.6770
FAX 212.645.1690

HOPE LINE: 800/NCA-CALL
(24 HOUR AFFILIATE REFERRAL)

EDUCATION, The National Council on Alcoholism and Drug Dependence provides education, information, help and hope in the fight against the chronic, often fatal disease of alcoholism and

National Families in Action Online!

http://www.emory.edu/NFIA/

National Families in Action Online! is a source of drug information for parents and young people. A number of drugs are discussed, including their effects, their common street names, and their legal status. The site also contains FAQs and a list of substance abuse–related organizations and resources.

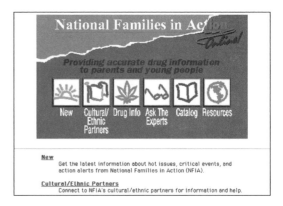

National Institute on Drug Abuse

http://www.nida.nih.gov/

The National Institute on Drug Abuse, part of the National Institutes of Health, provides information on drugs of abuse, online publications, and related Web sites.

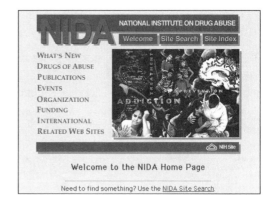

National Women's Health Resource Center

http://www.healthywomen.org/

The National Women's Health Resource Center is the national clearinghouse for women's health information. The site contains women's resources, including the *National Women's Health Report* newsletter and The Bod Squad. In addition, there are questions and answers to women's health concerns from the newsletter and a huge collection of links organized by topic.

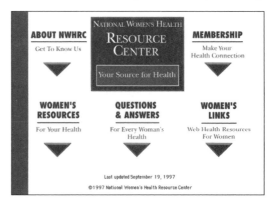

National Women's Resource Center

http://www.nwrc.org/

The National Women's Resource Center provides information on the prevention and treatment of alcohol, tobacco, and other drug abuse, as well as mental illness. The site has a **searchable bibliography database** on substance abuse and mental illness in women, an extensive **virtual library** for women's organizations, and other Web resources related to women's health and environment. The **document** section has reports and bibliographies on fetal alcohol syndrome (FAS), violence against women, gender-specific substance abuse treatment, and related subjects.

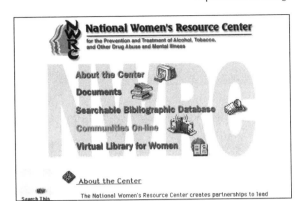

Nicotine and Tobacco Network

http://www.ahsc.arizona.edu/nicnet/

The Nicotine and Tobacco Network provides a multitude of resources about tobacco. The site contains articles on health and legal issues related to tobacco, links that emphasize prevention and cessation, the latest research updates, and discussion groups.

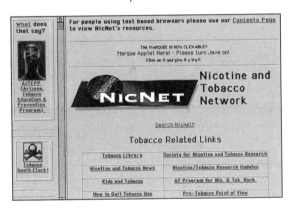

OncoLink Smoking and Tobacco

http://oncolink.upenn.edu/causeprevent/smoking/

OncoLink Smoking and Tobacco, from the University of Pennsylvania Cancer Center, provides a collection of articles on the hazards of smoking and tobacco from leading newspapers and media sources. The site includes other links to smoking and tobacco sites.

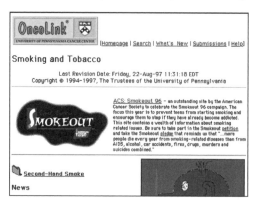

Prevline

http://www.health.org/

Prevline, from the National Clearinghouse for Alcohol and Drug Information, provides a wealth of information about the abuse of alcohol and drugs. Categories include Resources and Referrals, Research and Statistics, Searchable Databases, Discussion Forums, Online Publications, and Related Internet Links.

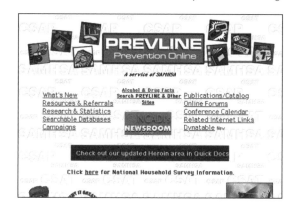

PRIDE USA

http://www.prideusa.org/

PRIDE USA (Parents Resource Institute for Drug Education) is an organization devoted to drug abuse prevention through education. The site provides information on a variety of topics ranging from alcohol to steroids. Each entry includes a brief description of the drug and its effects.

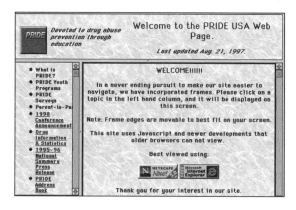

The QuitNet

http://www.quitnet.org/

The QuitNet, the Massachusetts Tobacco Control Program, offers a plethora of resources for those who want to quit smoking. Categories include news with many articles, a huge database of tobacco and smoking sites, an online support system/chat group, a reference library for quitting smoking, and much more.

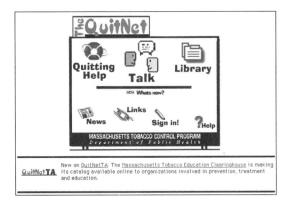

Reality Check

http://www.health.org/reality/

Reality Check provides a variety of online resources for marijuana use prevention, including publications, searchable databases, online forums, and related links. In addition, there is a parents section explaining why young people feel the need to use alcohol, tobacco, or illegal drugs.

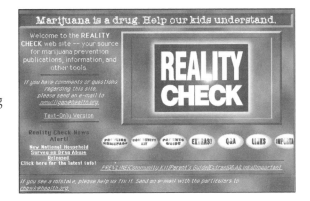

Smokeout

http://www.cancer.org/smokeout

Smokeout, provided by the American Cancer Society, is an entertaining resource for young adults on smoking issues. The site includes SmokeScream, with informative activities about the hazards of smoking, an FAQs section, related links, fun-filled games, and news.

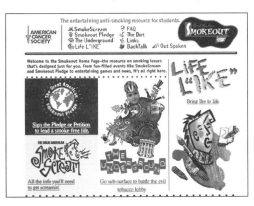

Smoking Cessation

http://quitsmoking.miningco.com/

Smoking Cessation, from the Mining Company, features a collection of weekly articles on the dangers of smoking and other related topics. The site also includes previous articles.

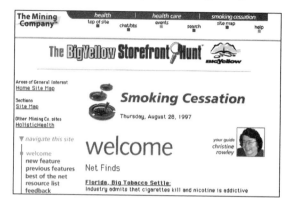

Tobacco BBS

http://www.tobacco.org/

Tobacco BBS is a free resource center focusing on tobacco and smoking issues. The site features news, information, assistance for smokers trying to quit, alerts for tobacco control advocates, and a forum for open debate on the wide spectrum of tobacco issues.

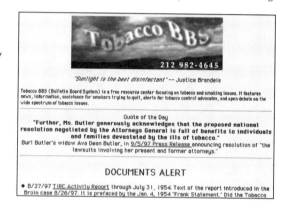

Tobacco Information & Prevention Sourcepage

http://www.cdc.gov/tobacco/

The Tobacco Information & Prevention Sourcepage, from the Centers for Disease Control and Prevention (CDC), provides a variety of resources and facts about the dangers of smoking. The site includes excerpts from the Surgeon General reports, practical tips for kids and teenagers, and other sources of information, including toll-free numbers and online consumer publications.

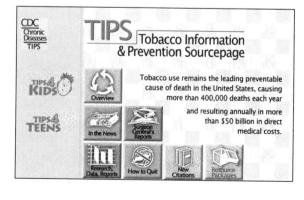

Web of Addictions

http://www.well.com/user/woa/

The Web of Addictions contains a large collection of fact sheets and links dealing with drug, tobacco, and alcohol abuse.

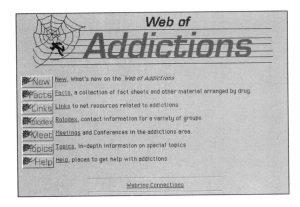

Aging, Long-Term Care, and Rehabilitation

Administration on Aging

http://www.aoa.dhhs.gov/

The Administration on Aging provides information on older persons and their families, practitioners and other professionals, the aging network, and researchers and students.

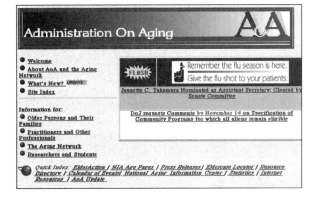

Aeiveos on Aging

http://www.aeiveos.com/library.htm

Aeiveos on Aging has a wide range of information about the science of aging, increasing longevity, health, and nutrition-related topics. To find more than 40,000 documents in this library, scroll to Resources to Learn More About Aging and Longevity and click on **Aeiveos Research Library** for information about diet and nutrition and how vitamins and nutrients affect the aging process. This section also contains the latest research news on aging and longevity.

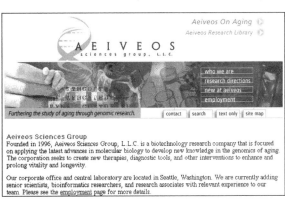

The Alzheimer Page

http://www.biostat.wustl.edu/alzheimer/

The Alzheimer Page, a service provided by Washington University in St. Louis, Missouri, offers a mailing list for anyone with an interest in Alzheimer's disease or related dementing disorders in older adults. In addition, the site includes a search tool to get advice, information, and references about Alzheimer's disease.

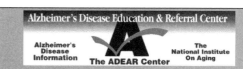

Alzheimer's Disease Education & Referral Center

http://www.alzheimers.org/

Alzheimer's Disease Education & Referral Center, a service of the National Institute on Aging, provides a variety of resources about Alzheimer's disease, including online publications such as "Alzheimer's Disease: Unraveling the Mystery" and numerous others.

Alzheimer's Disease Resource Page

http://www.cwru.edu/affil/adsc/intro.htm

Alzheimer's Disease Resource Page, sponsored by Case Western Reserve University in Cleveland, Ohio, has information for everyone on Alzheimer's disease, whether you are a caregiver, a practitioner, a researcher, or someone just interested in learning more.

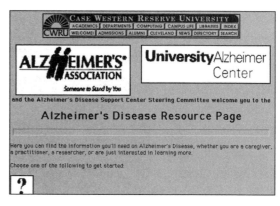

The Alzheimer's Disease Web Page

http://med-amsa.bu.edu/Alzheimer/

The Alzheimer's Disease Web Page, from Bedford Geriatrics Research Education Clinical Center at Boston University Medical School, offers information to families, caregivers, and others interested in Alzheimer's disease.

Bedford Geriatric Research Education Clinical Center, Bedford, MA

The Boston University Alzheimer's Disease Center

The Alzheimer's Disease Web Page

Bedford, MA

A Site dedicated to the distribution of information to Investigators, Families, Caregivers and others interested in Alzheimer's Disease.

Home of the First Veteran

Alzheimers.com

http://www.alzheimers.com/site/

Alzheimers.com, updated daily, is a gateway to information about Alzheimer's disease on the Internet. The resource provides a large online database of the the latest news and research on the disease, reviews of dozens of Alzheimer's-related sites in cyberspace, and an interactive forum for people who deal with it.

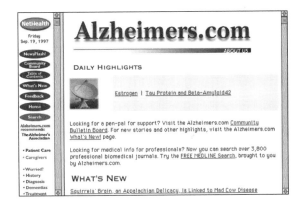

American Association of Retired Persons Webplace

http://www.aarp.org/

The American Association of Retired Persons (AARP) Webplace contains a wealth of online resources for the elderly. Click on **Getting Answers** to find caregiving and health information and a list of Internet resources.

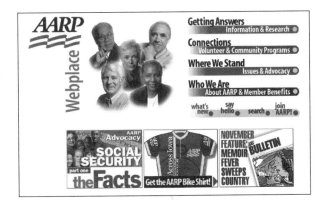

American Geriatrics Society

http://www.americangeriatrics.org/

The American Geriatrics Society is a professional organization of health care providers dedicated to improving the health and well-being of all older adults.

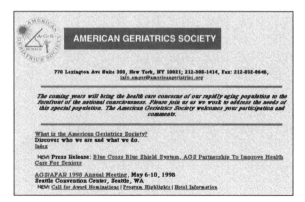

American Physical Therapy Association Section on Geriatrics

http://geriatricspt.org

The American Physical Therapy Association Section on Geriatrics contains information on health care, especially physical therapy, for older individuals. The site includes links of interest to physical therapists, those contemplating a career in the field, its own section members, and geriatric clients and their families.

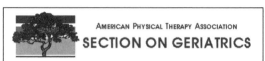

California Consumer HealthScope

http://www.healthscope.org/core.htm

HealthScope, sponsored by the Pacific Business Group on Health, compares health plans, hospitals, nursing homes, and health care services on the quality features that are important to you.

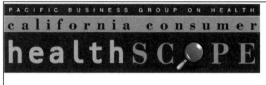

Caregiver Network Inc.

http://www.caregiver.on.ca/

The Caregiver Network Inc., developed by Karen Henderson, provides information on critical issues regarding caregiving. On the left side of the page, click on **Go Directly to Links** to find an index that includes caregiving information and Karen's Corner.

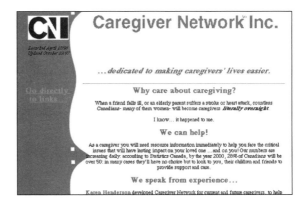

Caregiving Online

http://www.caregiving.com/

Caregiving Online is a monthly newsletter with useful information about emotional issues of caregiving, hiring home health help, purchasing home medical equipment supplies, and finding time for your own interests and hobbies.

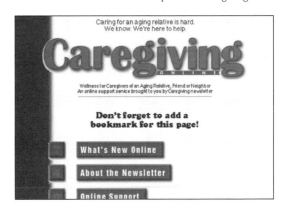

Directory of WEB and Gopher Sites on Aging

http://www.aoa.dhhs.gov/aoa/webres/craig.htm

Directory of WEB and Gopher Sites on Aging, maintained by the U.S. Administration on Aging, Department of Health and Human Services, contains over 2200 sites on more than 425 pages. The categories include aging, organizations, academic research, international sites, and other directories.

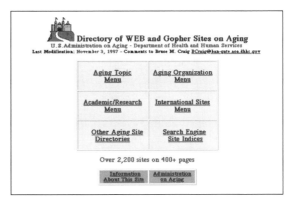

Dr. Frank On-Line!

http://www.drfrank.com/

Dr. Frank On-Line! is based on Dr. Frank MacInnis' successful syndicated newspaper column. The **Senior Clinic** section features weekly advice on social issues and medical, surgical, psychiatric, and other past middle age problems.

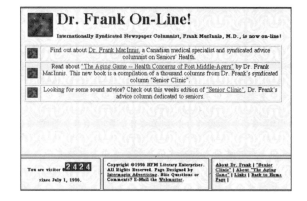

Eldercare Web

http://cube.ice.net/~kstevens/docs/

Eldercare Web, maintained by Karen Stevenson Brown, is a comprehensive senior health care information site.

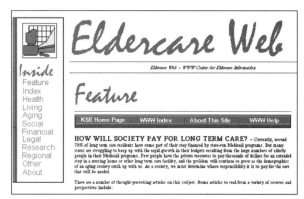

ElderConnect

http://www.ElderConnect.com/

The ElderConnect database contains information of over 33,000 acute rehabilitation providers, retirement communities, and providers specializing in all levels of long-term nursing care, as well as home health agencies.

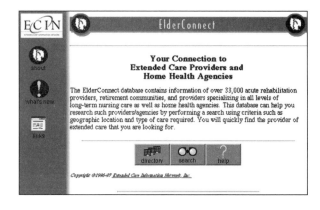

Family Caregiver Alliance

http://www.caregiver.org/

The Family Caregiver Alliance Web site is an information resource for long-term elder care. The site includes a clearinghouse with fact sheets, statistics, diagnosis, and research, a news bureau, a section on public policy issues, a resource center, online services, and links to related sites.

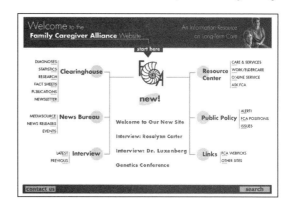

Gerisource

http://www.gerisource.com/

Gerisource, a clinical newsletter for long-term care, offers an online version that contains clinical tips, resources, citations, and abstracts of interest to direct care providers and administrators in geriatric care settings.

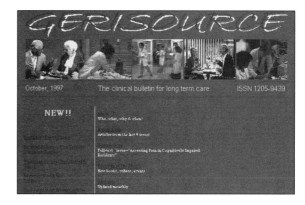

The Gerontological Society of America

http://www.geron.org

The Gerontological Society of America promotes multi- and interdisciplinary research in aging and disseminates gerontological research knowledge to researchers, practitioners, and decision and opinion makers.

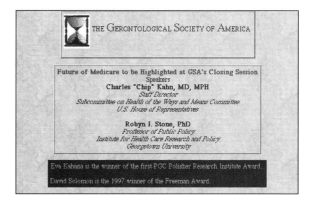

GeroWeb

http://www.iog.wayne.edu/GeroWebd/

GeroWeb, from the Institute of Gerontology at Wayne State University in Detroit, Michigan, is a directory of gerontology and aging sites.

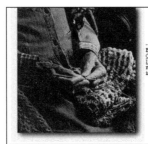

GoldenAge.Net

http://elo.mediasrv.swt.edu/goldenage/script.htm

GoldenAge.Net provides access to hundreds of related sites on health, caregivers, commercial products, government pages, and other essential services.

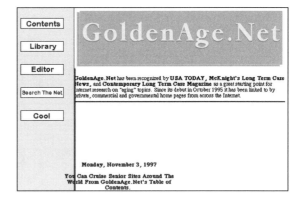

HealthAnswers Older Adult Resources Center

http://www.healthanswers.com/health_answers/oar/

HealthAnswers, developed by Orbis Broadcast Group, has an Older Adult Resources Center for locating home health and other long-term care services. For more information about geriatric care managers, click on **The Eldercare Locator** or contact the National Association of Professional Geriatric Care Managers, 1604 North Country Club Rd., Tucson, AZ 85716; 1-520-881-8008.

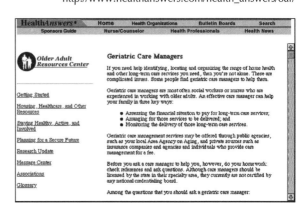

Horizon Adult Day Care

http://home.algorithms.net/horizon/

Horizon Adult Day Care provides long-term health care information for elderly and disabled people. The site is a warehouse of useful information containing resources and valuable links.

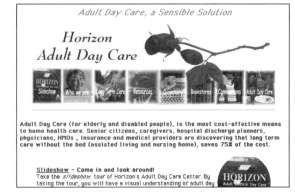

National Institute on Aging

http://www.nih.gov/nia/

The National Institute on Aging provides a variety of online health resources for Alzheimer's and cardiovascular diseases. The site also includes a directory of aging resources and brochures and fact sheets covering a wide range of topics related to health and aging.

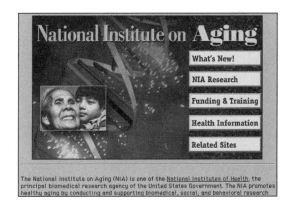

New Lifestyles

http://www2.newlifestyles.com/newlifestyles/

New Lifestyles is a directory of nursing centers, retirement communities, and residential care facilities for 29 major metropolitan areas across the United States.

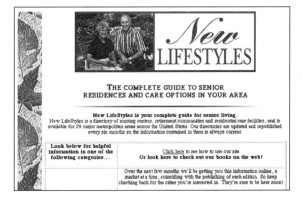

Older Americans

http://www.healthtouch.com/level1/leaflets/102179/102179.htm

Older Americans, from Healthtouch Online, provides a variety of resources for older Americans. Topics include aging and your body, aging and mental health, health and lifestyle issues, pressure sores (bed bores), home safety and taking medications, and pain treatment and control.

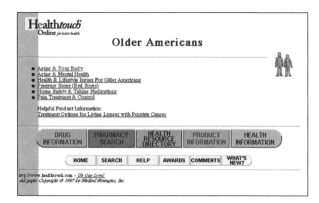

Osteoporosis and Related Bone Diseases

http://www.osteo.org

Osteoporosis and Related Bone Diseases, from the National Resource Center, provides a wealth of information about metabolic bone diseases, including clinical studies, news releases, and the latest research findings. The site offers prevention, early detection, and treatment information on Paget's disease, osteoporosis in men, osteogenesis imperfecta, and hyperparathyroidism.

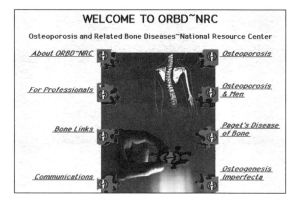

SeniorCom

http://www.senior.com/

SeniorCom contains a rich assortment of information for the elderly. In the **Senior News Network** use the pull-down menu and choose **Health and Wellness,** then click on **Go** to find a collection of health-related articles for seniors.

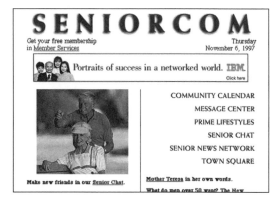

Today's Caregiver Online

http://www.caregiver.com

Today's Caregiver Online, like *Today's Caregiver* magazine, is dedicated to those caring for loved ones. It is written *by* caregivers *for* caregivers and covers all topics of importance to caregivers, regardless of the disease they are facing. The site offers resources, articles, support, information, advice, and more.

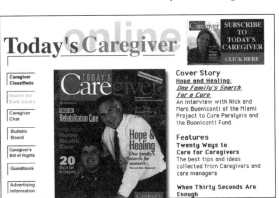

Biomedical Education

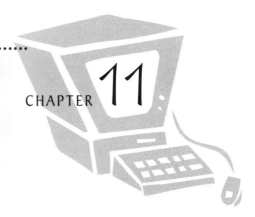

CHAPTER 11

Acronyms for Health Information Resources

http://www.ciesin.org/~mshams/acr.html

Acronyms for Health Information Resources provides an A to Z index of links to selected related Web sites. For example, click on the letter **F** to find a list of acronym health sites beginning with F.

ACRONYMS
FOR HEALTH INFORMATION RESOURCES

A * B * C * D * E * F * G * H * I * J
K * L * M * N * O * P * Q
R * S * T * U * V * W * X * Y * Z

FRANÇAIS

Acronyms for global information and data resources in the health sciences.
Linked acronyms point to selected related Web sites.
The acronyms and their expansions appear in the languages of origin.
This document is in progress, and is updated frequently. [Click on the "Reload" button to get the latest modifications of previously accessed pages.]

Comments and suggestions are very appreciated.
Send to Marie-Lise Shams: mshams@ciesin.org

Active Learning Centre Home Page

http://tyr.gdb.org:2001/quiz/home.cgi

The Active Learning Centre Home Page, created by Alex Turchin, a student at Johns Hopkins University School of Medicine, contains interactive self-assessment tests for microbiology, pharmacology and vaccines, and others. The site offers different test formats such as multiple choice, matching, or essay-type evaluations.

Active Learning Centre Home Page

Active Learning Centre is a compilation of self-assessment tests in different areas of knowledge. At present selection includes Microbiology, Pharmacology and Vaccines; others will follow (pending availability of spare time :). Currently available tests are based on (but not endorsed by) the Johns Hopkins University School of Medicine Pathology and Pharmacology courses.
All tests follow the same format and are capable of asking either multiple-choice, matching or essay-type (self-graded) questions.

Would you like to set up **YOUR OWN** quiz on ALC site? Check out this info!

MIRROR SITES:

● Brazil
Medstudents

The following databases are currently available:

1. Microbiology
  ○ Start the quiz
  ○ Microbiology Data Listing
  ○ Microbiology Data Query

241

Aeiveos on Aging

http://www.aeiveos.com/library.htm

Aeiveos on Aging has a wide range of information about the science of aging, increasing longevity, health, and nutrition-related topics. To find more than 40,000 documents in this library, scroll to Resources to Learn More About Aging and Longevity and click on **Aeiveos Research Library** for information about diet and nutrition and how vitamins and nutrients affect the aging process. This section also contains the latest research news on aging and longevity.

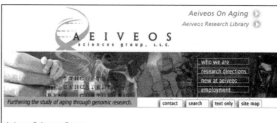

The Anatomy and Physiology Database

http://tqd.advanced.org/3007/

The Anatomy and Physiology Database provides an online crash course in anatomy and physiology. Select **Visit the Database** and scroll beyond the pictures to the text. At the text, click on the system you want to review (the pictures are *not* active links).

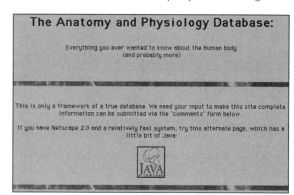

Breast Tutorial

http://www.biostat.wisc.edu/surgery/wolberg/breast.html

Breast Tutorial, written by Dr. William H. Wolberg, presents information and illustrations on breast problems for the layperson. Among the topics are breast anatomy, physiology, and examination, differential diagnosis and cancer types, role and type of definitive surgery, and self-help questions.

Cells Alive!

http://www.cellsalive.com/

Cells Alive! is a primer on cellular biology. It features a fascinating collection of pictures and animations with clear explanations. You can see how penicillin destroys bacteria, how cells keep their shape and how they communicate, you can view microscopic parasites, and learn much more.

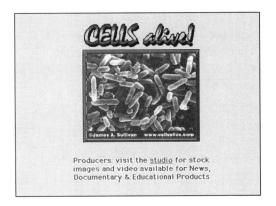

Center for Human Simulation

http://www.UCHSC.edu/sm/chs/

The Center for Human Simulation, from the University of Colorado Health Sciences Center, features both **Visible Human Male** and **Female** clickable digital figures for anatomical information.

Cochlear Fluids Research Laboratory

http://oto.wustl.edu/cochlea/

The Cochlear Fluids Research Laboratory, from Dr. Alec N. Salt in the Department of Otolaryngology at Washington University School of Medicine in St. Louis, Missouri, provides an illustrated description of the anatomy of the ear and its fluids.

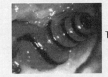

Cow's Eye Dissection

http://netra.exploratorium.edu/learning_studio/cow_eye/

Cow's Eye Dissection, from the Exploratorium as part of the Science Learning Network, is a step-by-step simulation for dissecting a cow's eye to learn about the parts of the eye.

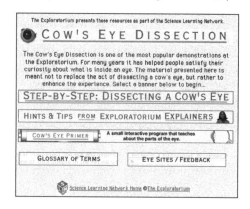

CyberMagazine

http://people.delphi.com/patrickdixon/

CyberMagazine, tomorrow's news today, presents Dr. Patrick Dixon's commentaries on biotechnology articles that he has culled from a variety of print sources. Article categories include Brave New World, Life and Death, and The Truth About AIDS.

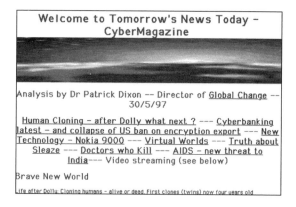

CyberPatient Simulator

http://www.netmedicine.com/cyberpt/cyber.htm

CyberPatient Simulator, from Net Medicine, is an interactive patient care simulator designed to help clinicians test and improve their skills. This is an excellent site for health professionals and those interested in learning more about treating diseases.

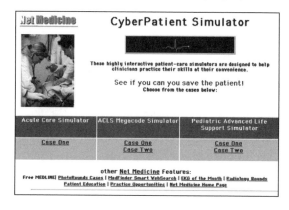

Digital Anatomist Program

http://www9.biostr.washington.edu/da.html

The Digital Anatomist Program, provided by the University of Washington Health Science Center for Educational Resources in Seattle, contains four online interactive atlases with two- and three-dimensional views of the following structures: the brain, the neurosystem, the thoracic organs, and the knee.

Interactive Atlases
Digital Anatomist Program

Awards

News: August 13, 1997... The search engine has been updated, so searches should be much faster now.

Search Atlases

Content: 2-D and 3-D views of the brain from cadaver sections, MRI scans, and computer reconstructions.
Author: John W. Sundsten
Institution: Digital Anatomist Program, Dept. Biological Structure, University of Washington, Seattle

Brain

Atlas is available on CD-ROM and similar motion materials on Videodisc from the University of Washington Health Science Center for Educational Resources.

Embryo Development

http://www.med.upenn.edu/embryo_project/embryo.html

Embryo Development presents a collection of pictures of the different parts of the embryo, including the ear, eye, heart, and nervous system.

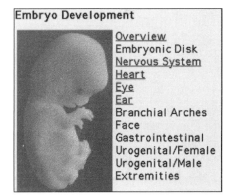

Embryo Development

Overview
Embryonic Disk
Nervous System
Heart
Eye
Ear
Branchial Arches
Face
Gastrointestinal
Urogenital/Female
Urogenital/Male
Extremities

Exercise Testing

http://www.mei.com/

Exercise Testing, from Marquette Medical Systems, provides online interactive cardiology tools for arrhythmia recognition, calculating heart attack survival, and evaluating chest pain.

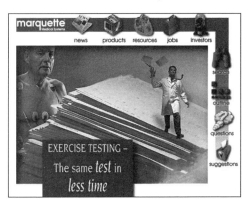

Finding-the-Path

http://www.med.harvard.edu/BWHRad/education/online/ftp/FTP.html

Finding-the-Path, developed by the Department of Radiology, Brigham and Women's Hospital/Harvard Medical School, is a problem-based guide to diagnostic imaging strategies in the emergency room. You, the emergency room physician, choose from a complex set of imaging modalities in evaluating your patients. The site has 50 cases to diagnose.

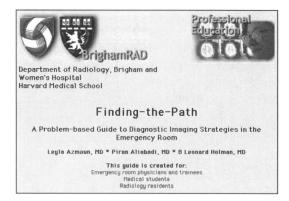

Healthfinder Medical Dictionaries

http://www.healthfinder.gov/meddict.htm

Healthfinder provides a collection of medical dictionaries with information on medical terms, various diseases, and treatments. The dictionaries included are MedicineNet, a medical dictionary, and CancerNet, from the National Cancer Institute.

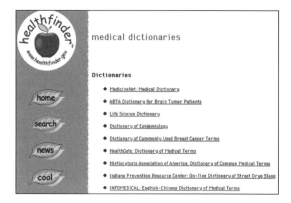

The Heart: An Online Exploration

http://sln.fi.edu/biosci/biosci.html

The Heart: An Online Exploration is an online tutorial about the heart. You can discover what makes it beat and what keeps it from beating. You can learn about the heart's functioning, what to expect when it doesn't function well, and what you can do to keep it from malfunctioning.

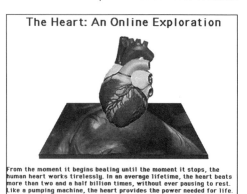

Heart Surgery Online

http://www.bharatonline.com/heart/

Heart Surgery Online is a comprehensive consumer resource for heart diseases and the structure of the heart. The site provides an overview on the anatomy of the heart and heart disease associated with each part of the heart.

WELCOME TO
"HEART SURGERY ONLINE"

The heart is truly the most fascinating part of the body. From the moment it begins beating, right until the moment it stops, the human heart works without a break. In an average lifetime, the heart beats **more than two and a half** *BILLION* times, without ever pausing to rest. *And as it beats, it gives LIFE.*

No other organ has caught the imagination of painters and poets alike. *The heart is purest theater*, throbbing in its cage palpably as any nightingale. Let danger threaten, and the thrilling heart skips a beat, and tight-rope walks arrhythmically. And all the while, we feel it, hear it even – **WE, its stage and its audience.**

It was not the livers or brains or entrails of saints that were lifted from the body in sublimest autopsy. It was the heart they cradled into worshipful palms, then soaked in wine and herbs and set into silver reliquaries for the veneration of the faithful.

It follows quite naturally that **Love should choose such an organ for its bower.** When Love blooms therein, the heart dances – and *tremor cordis* is upon one !

The heart has from time immemorial been surrounded by an aura of mystery and awe. Although some of this has been dispelled by the "cold reality" of modern science and technology, which has unravelled the mechanics of the heart, the air of fascination and wonder that the heart inspires in man has not diminished.

Human Anatomy On-line

http://www.innerbody.com./

Human Anatomy On-line features interactive views of the human body. The site contains over 100 illustrations of the human body with animations and thousands of descriptive links.

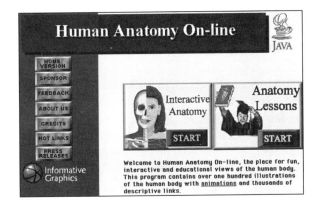

Human Genome Project Information

http://www.ornl.gov/hgmis/

The Human Genome Project Information is a worldwide research effort aimed at analyzing the structure of human DNA and determining the location of the estimated 100,000 human genes. The information site, maintained by the Oak Ridge National Laboratory, provides a variety of online genetics resources. including an **FAQs** section with basic information about the project, genetics information for everyone, publications such as *Your Genes, Your Choices,* and a collection of related links.

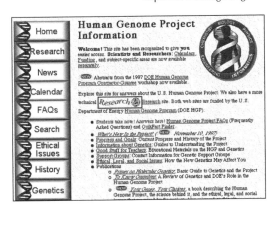

Infomedical

http://home.ipoline.com/~guoli/home/index.htm

Infomedical contains a collection of online medical dictionaries.

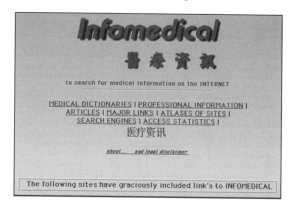

Information for Genetic Professionals

http://www.kumc.edu/gec/geneinfo.html

Information for Genetic Professionals, at the University of Kansas Medical Center, contains information for genetic counselors, clinical geneticists, and medical geneticists with links to a variety of clinical, research, and educational resources. To find genetic educational resources, click on **Genetics Education Center,** and to find a list of leading genetic centers, click on **Genome centers.**

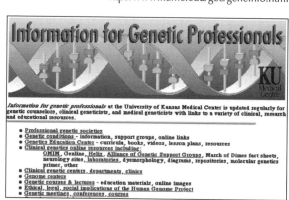

The Interactive Patient

http://medicus.marshall.edu/medicus.htm

The Interactive Patient, designed by Marshall University School of Medicine in West Virginia, allows you to simulate an actual patient encounter by examining an imaginary patient who complains of back pain. You can play doctor by asking questions, taking x-ray films, making a diagnosis, and prescribing medicine.

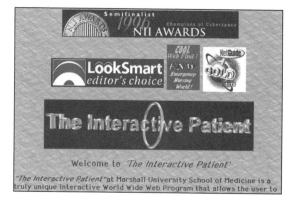

Layman's View on Brain Chemistry

http://aloha.net/~jms/brainuse.html

The Layman's View on Brain Chemistry provides clearly illustrated explanations about how the different parts of the brain function.

Layman's View on Brain Chemistry
This page is for entertainment purposes only

If the <u>doors of perception</u> were cleansed the world would appear to man as it is.....infinite.
– William Blake 1793

<u>Process</u> – Biochemical basis of Behavior, Personality, <u>Perception</u>

<u>Emotions</u> – neuropeptides attaching to receptors stimulating an electrical charge on <u>neurons</u>. Joy, grief, love are all biochemical;

The Levit Radiologic Pathologic Institute

http://rpiwww.mdacc.tmc.edu/

The Levit Radiologic Pathologic Institute, a section of the Division of Diagnostic Radiology at the University of Texas M.D. Anderson Cancer Center, contains interactive animated exhibits of the anatomy of the human body, the interactive ankle, and rotating foot and ankle.

THE UNIVERSITY OF TEXAS
MD ANDERSON
CANCER CENTER

Welcomes You To

THE LEVIT
Radiologic Pathologic
••••••••INSTITUTE

A Section of the Division of <u>Diagnostic Imaging</u>

Click on one of the items below to branch to that section.

Multimedia Exhibits about disease and anatomy, information about CD-ROMs, and other interactive teaching material.
Learning

Medical Dictionary from Merriam-Webster

http://www.medscape.com/mw/medical.htm

The Medical Dictionary from Merriam-Webster is provided through Medscape. With a click of your mouse, you can easily search for medical terms and information. To access this online dictionary, click on the **cancel** button and select **register** at the top of the page. It's FREE!

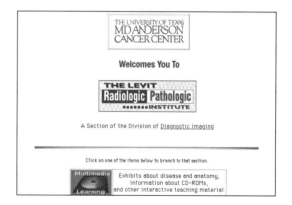

Medscape   Home | Search | Site Map | Talk to Us | Help ®

Medical Dictionary from Merriam-Webster
(Click here for help searching the dictionary.)

Enter your search term here, then click button:
[   ] [Perform search]
● Search for whole word
○ Search for partial word

© 1997 by Merriam-Webster, Incorporated

Search Site Map Help Talk to Us About Us   **Medscape**
For: [   ] [in Full-Text] [Search] ®
Advanced Searching: Full-Text | MEDLINE | TOXLINE | AIDSLINE | Bookstore | Dictionary | Drugs

Home Specialties News Journals Patient Info Exam Room Library Services
Produced by Medscape, Inc. All material on this server Copyright © 1994–1997 by the publishers involved.

MRI Image Map

MRI Image Map, created by the College of Medicine at the University of Kentucky, offers clickable images of the upper body of a male.

http://www.comed.uky.edu/body/mainbody.html

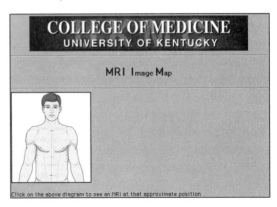

National Center for Biotechnology Information

The National Center for Biotechnology Information contains information about DNA and other related genetics topics, including a gene map that shows the chromosome location of over 16,000 human genes with links to the underlying sequence and map data.

http://www.ncbi.nlm.nih.gov/

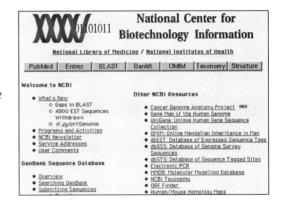

National Library of Medicine

The National Library of Medicine is an online guide offering an image archive of over 60,000 historical photographs and databases to a variety of medical information.

http://www.nlm.nih.gov/

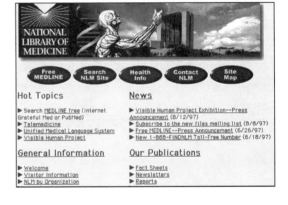

The Nobel Prize Internet Archive

http://www.almaz.com/nobel/

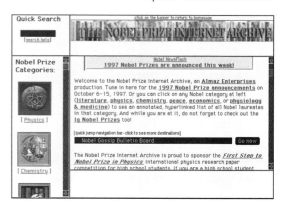

The Nobel Prize Internet Archive contains an annotated list of Nobel Laureats in physiology/medicine and in chemistry from 1901 to 1997. Click on **Physiology and Medicine** to learn about the 1997 winner Stanley B. Prusiner for his discovery of Prion, and click on **Chemistry** to learn about one of the 1997 winners Paul D. Boyer for his lifelong work on cell mechanisms.

The NPAC Visible Human Viewer

http://www.npac.syr.edu/projects/vishuman/VisibleHuman.html

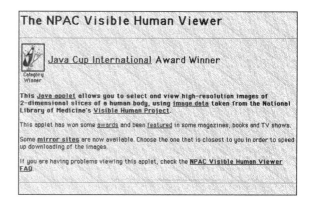

The NPAC Visible Human Viewer uses a Java applet, which allows you to select and view two-dimensional graphic images of a human body.

Obstetric Ultrasound

http://www.hkstar.com/~joewoo/joewoo2.html

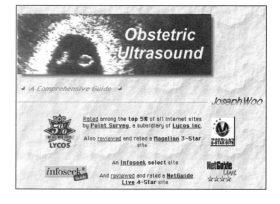

Obstetric Ultrasound contains dozens of ultrasound scans ranging from those of a five-week-old fetus to a fetus that is nearly five months old.

Orthopaedic Resident's CyberLink LaunchPad

http://www.telusplanet.net/public/jasmith/

The Orthopaedic Resident's CyberLink LaunchPad contains a comprehensive collection of orthopaedic resources, including online journals and articles, libraries, search engines, newsgroups, mailing lists, and related medical sites.

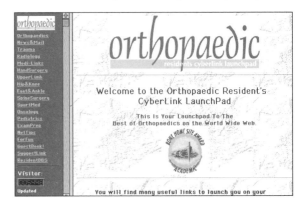

Pathology 703

http://www.biostat.wisc.edu/infolink/educ/path/slides-toc.html

The Pathology 703 home page, from the Department of Pathology and Laboratory Medicine at the University of Wisconsin Medical School, provides a library of over 40 pathology slides with descriptions.

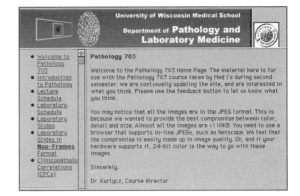

Royal Children's Hospital Cardiology Department

http://www.rch.unimelb.edu.au/Cardiology/index.htm

The Royal Children's Hospital Cardiology Department in Melbourne, Australia, contains a library of heart diagrams illustrating features of the normal cardiac structure and function, as well as cardiac defects.

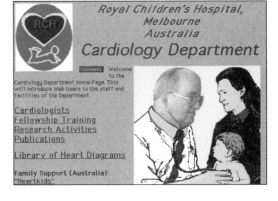

Select the Hand You Would Like to Diagnose

Select the Hand You Would Like to Diagnose, from the Stritch School of Medicine in Chicago, displays a series of hands with rheumatology-related disorders. You are asked to choose a hand and then make the diagnosis.

http://www.meddean.luc.edu/lumen/MedEd/medicine/Rheumatology/Hands/Handmain.html

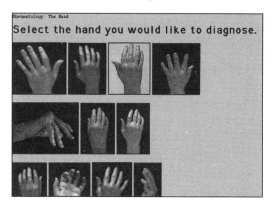

Three Dimensional Medical Reconstruction

Three Dimensional Medical Reconstruction is a collection of movie clips showing medical reconstructions of various parts of the body. There are animations for the colon, the skull, the brain, the lung, the torso, the heart, and the delivery of a baby.

http://www.crd.ge.com/esl/cgsp/projects/medical/

Three dimensional medical reconstruction

This is a collection of movie clips, showing various medical reconstructions. These images are derived from slice data from a variety of medical image modalities such as MR or CT. The two dimensional slice data from these scanners is used as input for the three dimensional reconstructions.

The data starts out as slices(images) taken at regular intervals throughout a portion of the body. The slices are first segmented to separate the various tissues. An algorithm developed at GE R&D known as marching cubes is then used to create a three dimensional representation of the structures. Once the 3D model is created, an animation package called LYMB is used to provide the visualization and animation.

Marching Through the Visible Man

The National Library of Medicine is creating a digital atlas of the human body. This project, called the Visible Human, has already produced computed tomography, magnetic resonance imaging and physical cross-sections of a human male cadaver. This paper describes a methodology and results for extracting surfaces from the Visible Male's CT data. We use surface connectivity and isosurface extraction techniques to create polygonal models of the skin, bone, muscle and bowels. Early experiments with the physical cross-sections are also reported.

Virtual Anatomy Project

Virtual Anatomy Project, at Colorado State University, contains an image browser that lets you view images and animations of the human body.

http://www.vis.colostate.edu/library/gva/

Virtual Anatomy Project

Description

The Virtual Anatomy (VA) project at Colorado State University (CSU) is working on generating a 3D geometric database of the human body. This database can be used for the creation of interactive and non-interactive forms of communication. A future goal of the project is to develop a virtual human anatomy lab for undergraduate anatomy instruction.

Press Release/Other Information

Researchers

Dr. Thomas Spurgeon, P.I. - CSU Dept. of Anatomy
Dr. David Alciatore, co-P.I. - CSU Dept. of Mechanical Engineering
Thomas McCracken, co-P.I. - Visible Productions
Dr. Rick Miranda, co-P.I. - CSU Dept. of Mathematics

Custom Software

David Alciatore - Sculpting Software
Rick Miranda and Chris Fedde - Triangulation Software
Jamison Gulden - Contouring/Segmentation Software
Dan Steward - Interactive Interface/Database Browser

The "Virtual"-Medical Center

http://www-sci.lib.uci.edu/~martindale/MedicalAnatomy.html

The "Virtual"-Medical Center, Martindale's Health Science Guide, is a comprehensive collection of sites for anatomy and histology. The site includes tutorials and encyclopedias, medical dictionaries and glossaries, online anatomy and histology exercises and examinations, and much more.

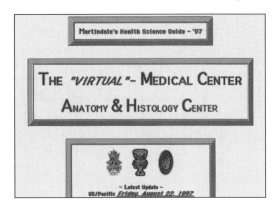

The Visible Embryo

http://visembryo.ucsf.edu/

The Visible Embryo is a tutorial that teaches the first four weeks of human development (pregnancy) from the fertilization to the somite stage. The tutorial offers beautiful graphics and clear descriptions.

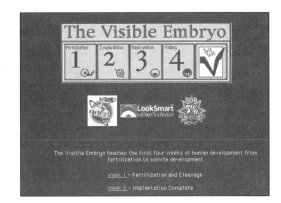

Visible Human Cross Sections

http://www.meddean.luc.edu/lumen/meded/grossanatomy/cross_section/

Visible Human Cross Sections, from Loyola University School of Medicine in Chicago, provides a clickable visualization of the male human body with accompanying descriptions and animations.

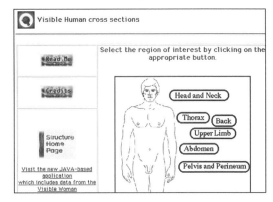

The Visible Human Project

http://www.nlm.nih.gov/research/visible/visible_human.html

The Visible Human Project, from the National Library of Medicine, provides detailed anatomical three-dimensional representations of the male and female human body. For viewing images from the project, scroll to **Projects Based on Visible Human Data.** To see animations, scroll to **Sources of Images and Animations.**

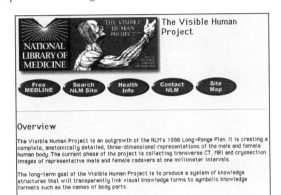

Visualizations of Viruses

http://www.bocklabs.wisc.edu/virusviztop.html

Visualizations of Viruses, from the Institute for Molecular Virology, provides a collection of images of virus structures and other molecular virology resources.

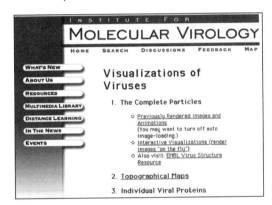

Web Path

http://medstat.med.utah.edu/WebPath/webpath.html

Web Path is an electronic laboratory of over 1800 pathologic images associated with human diseases. The site contains various online pathology minitutorials with illustrations and descriptions designed for medical students. Some of the tutorials provide consumer education for breast cancer, drug abuse pathology, firearms, and prostate pathology.

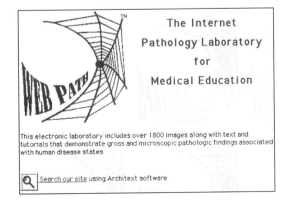

WelchWeb

http://www.welch.jhu.edu/internet/

WelchWeb, collected by the Johns Hopkins' William H. Welch Medical Library, contains a collection of biomedical Internet resources, including patient education resources.

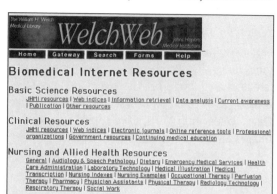

The Whole Brain Atlas

http://www.med.harvard.edu/AANLIB/home.html

The Whole Brain Atlas, created by physicians at the Harvard Medical School, provides hundreds of descriptive medical images of the brain under different conditions.

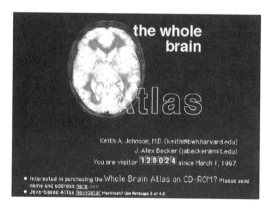

Diseases and Conditions

CHAPTER 12

General
Allergies and Asthma
Arthritis
Back Pain
Brain and Neurologic Disorders
Cancer
Cardiovascular Disease (Heart Attack, Stroke)
Chronic Fatigue Syndrome
Diabetes
Foot and Ankle Problems

Gastrointestinal Problems
Headache
HIV/AIDS and Other Sexually Transmitted
    Diseases
Infectious Diseases
Orthopaedic Problems
Skin Care and Skin Conditions
Urologic Disorders
Visual Disorders and Eye Care

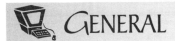

GENERAL

The ABCs of Safe and Healthy Child Care

http://www.cdc.gov/ncidod/hip/abc/abc.htm

The ABCs of Safe and Healthy Child Care, prepared by the Centers for Disease Control and Prevention (CDC), is an online handbook for child care providers, parents, or caregivers. The Handbook provides a whole alphabet of advice on keeping your child out of harm's way, including information on accident prevention, basic first aid, proper hygiene, common childhood diseases, and much more.

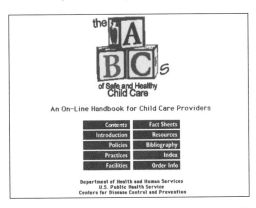

Amara's RSI Page

http://www.amara.com/aboutme/rsi.html

Amara's RSI Page provides ergonomic computing resources and information about repetitive strain injury (RSI).

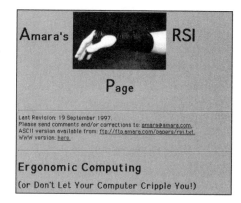

American Family Physician

http://www.aafp.org/family/afp/

American Family Physician is the official clinical bimonthly journal of the American Academy of Family Physicians. Each online issue contains a health article from the journal of interest to consumers. To find a list of these articles dating back to March 1993, scroll to the bottom of the page and click on **Patient Information Index.**

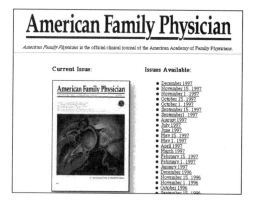

American Liver Foundation

http://sadieo.ucsf.edu/alf/alffinal/homepagealf.html

The American Liver Foundation home page provides a large collection of easy-to-read articles about hepatitis and other liver diseases. The information section contains over 60 topics with articles on diagnosis, epidemiology, drugs/procedures, transplants, clinical trials, treatment, pediatric concerns, gallstones, and cirrhosis.

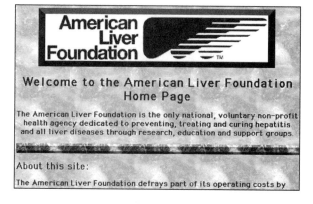

American Lung Association

http://www.lungusa.org/

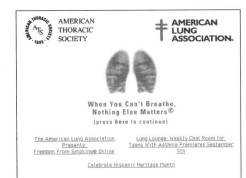

The American Lung Association provides information on asthma and other lung diseases, tobacco control, and environmental health. Click on **Learn about Lung** to access this information. The **ALA News** section features the latest news from the Association, medical update articles, a free subscription to an electronic newsletter, *Breathe Easy/ Asthma Digest,* and a reporter's corner with specific information on the various lung diseases. In addition, the site also includes a link to over 240 local Association offices in the United States, including Puerto Rico and the U.S. Virgin Islands.

The Bad Bug Book

http://vm.cfsan.fda.gov/~mow/intro.html

The Bad Bug Book, from the Center for Food Safety and Applied Nutrition of the Food and Drug Administration (FDA), provides a handbook of basic facts regarding foodborne pathogenic microorganisms and natural toxins.

U. S. Food and Drug Administration
Center for Food Safety and Applied Nutrition
Foodborne Pathogenic Microorganisms and Natural Toxins 1992 (Bad Bug Book)

The "Bad Bug Book"

This handbook provides basic facts regarding foodborne pathogenic microorganisms and natural toxins. Some technical terms have been linked to the National Library of Medicine's Entrez glossary. Recent articles from Morbidity and Mortality Weekly Reports have been added to selected chapters to update the handbook with information on later outbreaks or incidents of foodborne disease. At the end of selected chapters on pathogenic microorganisms, hypertext links are included to relevant Entrez abstracts and GenBank genetic loci. A more complete description of the handbook may be found in the Preface.

PATHOGENIC BACTERIA

- Salmonella spp.
- Clostridium botulinum
- Staphylococcus aureus
- Campylobacter jejuni
- Yersinia enterocolitica and Yersinia pseudotuberculosis
- Listeria monocytogenes
- Vibrio cholerae O1

Balance, Dizziness & Vestibular Disorders

http://www.familyvillage.wisc.edu/lib_bala.htm

Balance, Dizziness & Vestibular Disorders, from the Vestibular Disorders Association, presents an overview of vestibular disorders and offers a glossary of terms, lists of educational materials, and links to other related sites.

Balance, Dizziness & Vestibular Disorders

- Who to Contact
- Where to Go to Chat with Others
- Learn More About It
- Web Sites

Who to Contact

Vestibular Disorders Association (VEDA)
PO Box 4467
Portland, Oregon, USA 97208-4467
(503) 229-7705
(800) 837-8428
Fax: (503) 229-8064
e-mail: veda@teleport.com

BloodLine

http://www.cjp.com/blood/

BloodLine, the online hematology resource, provides the most current original articles, continuous medical education offerings, grants and fellowships, links, meetings, organization information, and publications.

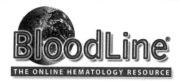

Celiac Support Page

http://shoga.wwa.com/~pej/cfaq.html

The Celiac Support Page provides people who have celiac disease (gluten intolerance) and are not aware of it with a means to determine what is wrong, and to help those who know to lead more comfortable and healthy lives.

Centers for Disease Control and Prevention

http://www.cdc.gov/

The Centers for Disease Control and Prevention (CDC), an agency of the U.S. Department of Health and Human Services, provides a ton of information for chronic disease prevention, environmental health, infectious diseases, injury prevention, and occupational safety. Each area includes numerous subdivisions and its own search tool.

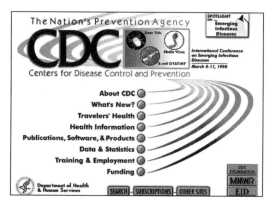

CenterWatch

http://www.centerwatch.com/

CenterWatch has a collection of approximately 2000 clinical trials on a wide range of diseases along with contact names for each trial. You can use this service to search for clinical findings, discover physicians and medical centers performing clinical research, and learn about drug therapies recently approved by the Food and Drug Administration (FDA).

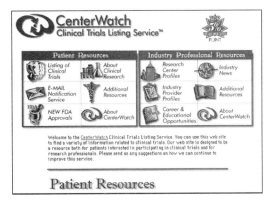

CF-Web

http://cf-web.mit.edu/

CF-Web has extensive information on cystic fibrosis, including medical information in CF-FAQ, discussion and support groups, newspaper articles, a bibliography, and links to related sites.

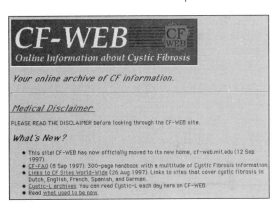

Chronic Autoimmune Liver Disease Support Group

http://members.aol.com/pbcers/liverdis.htm

The Chronic Autoimmune Liver Disease Support Group home page provides a wealth of medical resources about liver diseases, including information about medications, new research, pain management, diagnostic tests, and clinical trials. The site includes support groups, organizations, related links, and a search tool.

The Chronic Candidiasis Syndrome

http://members.aol.com/docdarren/med/candida.html

The Chronic Candidiasis Syndrome (yeast infection) page is a well-organized index that includes the symptoms, diagnosis, treatment, a doctor referral list, what to do after treatment, and related links.

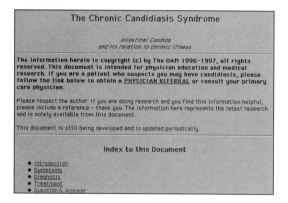

ChronicIllNet

http://www.chronicillnet.org/

ChronicIllNet is a leading multimedia information source on the Internet dedicated to chronic illnesses, including AIDS, cancer, Persian Gulf War syndrome, autoimmune diseases, chronic fatigue syndrome, heart disease, and neurological diseases. The site also features online news from the correspondents, T.J. Moriarty and Neenyah Ostrom.

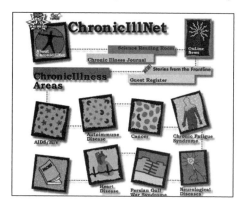

CLD Information Resource

http://www.cheshire-med.com/programs/pulrehab/rehinfo.html

CLD Information Resource, from the Cheshire Medical Center, provides a collection of articles related to chronic lung disease (CLD) and conditions. Topics include chronic obstructive pulmonary disease, asthma, interstitial lung disease, respiratory infections, and cystic fibrosis. The site also includes a discussion group, search tools, and related links.

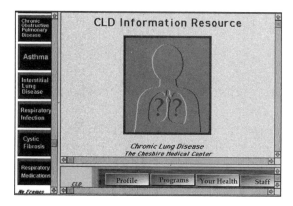

Colorado Health Net

http://bcn.boulder.co.us/health/chn/

Colorado Health Net has treatment and symptom information for a variety of chronic illnesses ranging from minor to life-threatening. The site includes a search tool and other health resources.

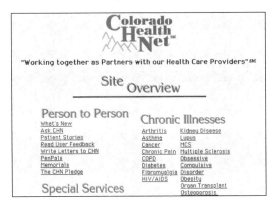

CoMed Communications Internet Health Forum

http://www.comed.com/

CoMed Communications Internet Health Forum provides a collection of selected health-related sites organized by disease and topic indexes. The topics include allergies, diabetes, Crohn's disease, and non-traditional medicine.

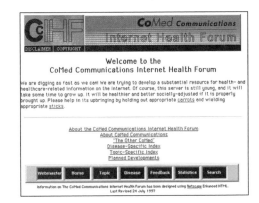

The Complete Canadian Health Guide

http://www1.sympatico.ca/healthyway/HGUIDE/hguide.html

The Complete Canadian Health Guide, a bestselling health reference book, provides information on a variety of health conditions. The site contains excerpts from Chapter 16, "Some Specific Diseases and Disorders," which deal with conditions of special concern in North America today. The diseases range from AIDS to urinary tract infections.

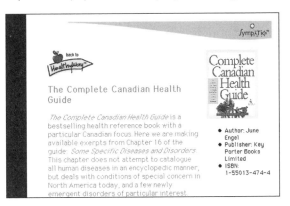

Computer Related Repetitive Strain Injury

Computer Related Repetitive Strain Injury discusses repetitive strain injury (RSI), commonly known as carpal tunnel syndrome. Topics include symptoms, prevention, and recuperation. The site includes a bibliography and related links.

http://engr-www.unl.edu/ee/eeshop/rsi.html

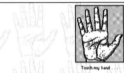

Computer Related Repetitive Strain Injury

Copyright © 1996 Paul Marxhausen. THIS DOCUMENT IS NOT AN OFFICIAL PUBLICATION OF THE UNIVERSITY OF NEBRASKA-LINCOLN.

As more and more work, education and recreation involves computers, everyone needs to be aware of the hazard of *Repetitive Strain Injury* to the hands and arms resulting from the use of computer keyboards and mice. This can be a serious and very painful condition that is far easier to **prevent** than to cure once contracted, and can occur even in young physically fit individuals. It is not uncommon for people to have to leave computer-dependent careers as a result, or **even to be permanently disabled and unable to perform tasks such as**

Computer-Related Ergonomics Information and Products

The Computer-Related Ergonomics Information and Products home page provides computer-related information about ergonomics problems and solutions for eyestrain, visual impairment, musculoskeletal discomforts, and stress symptoms. The site also demonstrates a model workstation design and includes other Internet ergonomics resources.

http://www.distrib.com/ergonomics/homepage.html

Computer-Related Ergonomics Information and Products

Welcome to the Ergonomics Home Page.*

If this is your first visit, a good starting point is the web page "About Computer-Related Ergonomics and this Web Site."

You may also wish to read the "Workstation Design Ergonomics Diagrams and Checklist."

The rest of this web page is divided into an overview of common computer-related ergonomics problems and solutions, and a meta-index of ergonomics resources on the net.

COMPUTER-RELATED ERGONOMIC PROBLEMS & SOLUTIONS

Eyes

Department of Human Services Public Health Division

The Department of Human Services Public Health Division, from Melbourne, Victoria, Australia, provides an A to Z index of public health information with a wide range of documents on topics such as drugs, communicable diseases, and infectious diseases.

http://hna.ffh.vic.gov.au/phb/

Department of Human Services ☆☆

PUBLIC HEALTH DIVISION

A Victorian Government Department
555 Collins Street, Melbourne, Victoria, AUSTRALIA

(Last updated: August 25th 1997)

● Indices

 • A-Z of Public Health Information and Publications
 • Archived Documents

Please sign our Visitors Book after you browse our site.
Your comments are welcome!

● New Documents

 Towards a Safer Choice: The Practice of Traditional Chinese Medicine in Australia
  - This report is the first comprehensive review of the practice of traditional Chinese Medicine in Australia - detailing the need for regulation.

 Review of Traditional Chinese Medicine - Discussion Paper
  Sets out occupational options for regulation of the profession of Traditional

Diseases & Treatments

http://www.medicinenet.com/mainmenu/encyclop/med_a.htm

Diseases & Treatments, from MedicineNet, is an encyclopedic diseases and conditions index written in plain language by board-certified physicians. Among the diseases and conditions included are acne, meningitis, shingles, writer's cramp, and urethra infection.

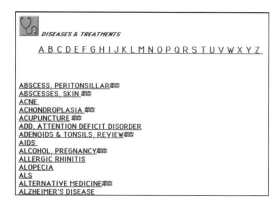

Diseases and Conditions

http://www.nerdworld.com/cgi-bin/page.cgi?cat=1460

Diseases and Conditions, by Nerd World Media, is a mega-index of sites. The disease categories range from AIDS to Tuberculosis.

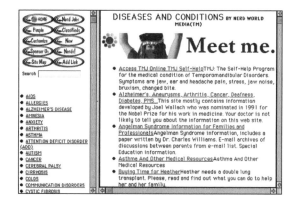

Diseases, Disorders and Related Topics

http://www.mic.ki.se/Diseases/

Diseases, Disorders and Related Topics, prepared by the Library of Karolinska Institute in Stockholm, Sweden, for its Medical Information Center, offers a gigantic and comprehensive collection of links to sites for diseases, disorders, and illnesses organized by topic, including bacterial and fungal, respiratory tract, urologic and male genital, cardiovascular, and many others. Each topic features the National Library of Medicine's Medline database to further search for medical information. The site also provides a search tool and an alphabetical list of diseases.

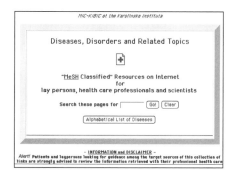

Diseases of the Liver

http://cpmcnet.columbia.edu/dept/gi/disliv.html

Diseases of the Liver presents a collection of articles on liver diseases and conditions organized in an alphabetical list. The articles contain links to information at this site and relevant sites elsewhere.

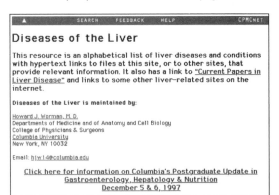

Dr. Grossan

http://www.ent-consult.com/

Dr. Grossan, an ear, nose, and throat specialist, offers online medical advice for a wide range of ailments, including allergies and swimming-related ear infections.

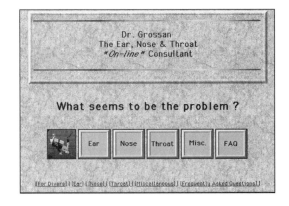

General Practice and Medical Specialties

http://www.mit.edu/afs/athena/user/p/a/pandre/
www/General-Practice.html

General Practice and Medical Specialties, part of the MD InterActive Web site, provides easy-to-understand articles on diseases and conditions written by doctors from MIT and three major hospitals in the Boston area. Categories include AIDS, cancer, eye diseases, neurology, gastroenterology, parasitic diseases, and skin diseases.

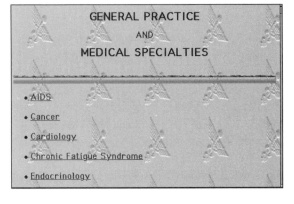

Health

http://www.whitehouse.gov/WH/pointers/html/health.html

Health provides a vast pool of information about the leading causes of death in America, health care issues, health and the environment, and alcohol, smoking, and drugs.

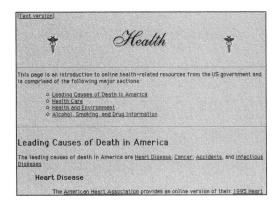

Health Care

http://www.med.upenn.edu/health/hi.html

Health Care, from the University of Pennsylvania Health System (UPHS), provides a variety of online resources and publications for the consumer. The **Health Topics** section contains tips and information on asthma, diabetes, hypertension, and safety; the **Managing Chronic Conditions** offers help in managing asthma, diabetes and other chronic conditions; and the **Publications** section features articles on healthy living for the whole family. In addition, the site includes health **Self-tests and Quizzes.**

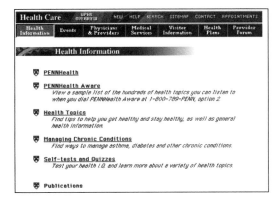

Health Guides

http://www.bimc.edu/netscape2/guides.html

Health Guides, from Beth Israel Health Care System and St. Luke's-Roosevelt Hospital Center in New York, contains extensive patient information on breast cancer, cancer and chronic pain management, colon and rectal cancer, and a dietary fiber guide.

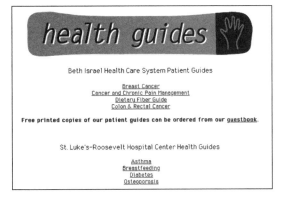

HealthFinder

http://www.health-connect.com/

The HealthFinder database, featured in the Health Connection Guide, provides thousands of health care resources on the Internet. The diseases and conditions directory in the database contains over 6000 sites with topics ranging from AIDS and HIV to von Hippel-Lindau disease.

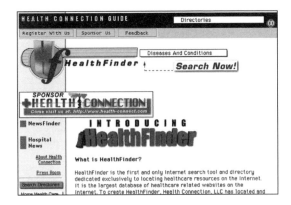

HealthGate Wellness Center

http://www.healthgate.com/HealthGate/hic/

The HealthGate Wellness Center provides health information on a variety of diseases ranging from allergies to skin cancer. Each disease area includes treatment information, references, and a chat group.

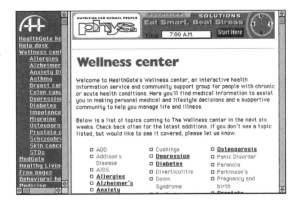

Healthy Lives

http://www.healthylives.com/

Healthy Lives, a service of GlaxoWellcome, offers a source of disease-specific information for both patients and health professionals. Its online magazine, *Healthy Lives,* discusses many diseases, health-related issues, trends, treatment programs, and research. The site includes information on asthma, migraine headaches, shingles, and other diseases.

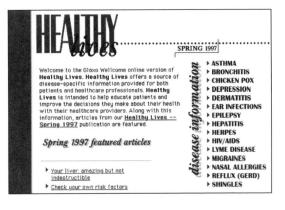

Hemophilia Home Page

http://www.web-depot.com/hemophilia/

The Hemophilia Home Page is a comprehensive resource for bleeding disorders. Topics include information about hemophilia and AIDS, gene therapy, hepatitis C, women with bleeding disorders, and other topics.

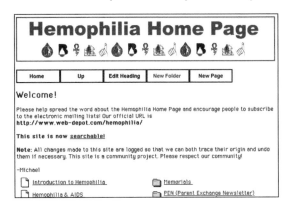

Home Page for Hernia Information

http://www.hernia.org/

Home Page for Hernia Information provides a variety of hernia resources, including an explanation of a hernia, methods of repair, complex and stomach hernias, and other topics.

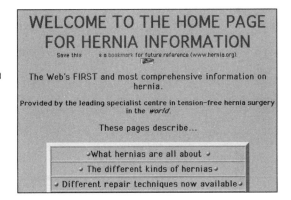

Homepage for the Immune Mailing List

http://www.best.com/~immune/

Homepage for the Immune Mailing List provides information about various diseases and conditions, as well as allergies. The site offers a mailing list subscription, a mailing list archives since 1990, information about immune-related illnesses, and links to related sites.

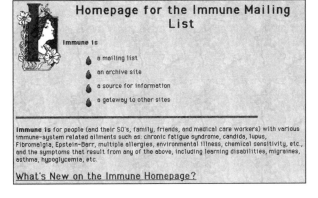

A Hyperpedia of Disease and Health Related Topics

http://www.urmc.rochester.edu/Miner/Docs/PATED1/hy.htm

A Hyperpedia of Disease and Health Related Topics, from the University of Rochester Medical Center, is a clickable electronic encyclopedia containing information on diseases from A to Z.

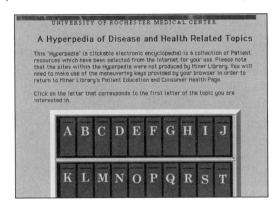

Information for Patients

http://www.aafp.org/patientinfo/

Information for Patients, developed by the American Academy of Family Physicians, contains a collection of handouts covering more than 200 health topics. The handout categories consist of the body, common conditions/diseases/disorders, treatments, and healthy living.

Infoseek Diseases & Conditions

http://www.infoseek.com/Health/Diseases_and_conditions

Infoseek has an alphabetical directory of diseases and conditions organized into 25 categories. Some of the categories include Arthritis, Foot Problems, Inner Ear Disorders, Hernias, and Tuberculosis.

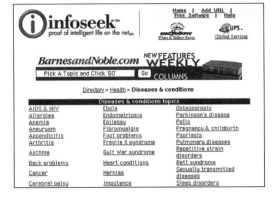

Inside Medicine

http://www.lifestages.com/health/

Inside Medicine, an online publication of the Center for Current Research, features free background information on a wide range of medical problems for any given disease, condition, or treatment.

Lerner Lymphedema Services

http://204.91.84.126/

Lerner Lymphedema Services is a network of treatment facilities exclusively dedicated to the treatment of lymphedema. The site contains patient information about lymphedema, its etiology, prevention, and treatment.

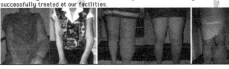

Louis A. Dvonch MD

http://www.webcom.com/ldvonch

The Louis A. Dvonch MD home page provides information on the prevention of stroke, heart attack, and the symptoms of Alzheimer's disease.

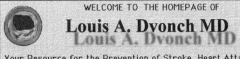

Mayo Health O@sis Library References Diseases & Conditions

http://www.mayohealth.org/mayo/library/htm/disease.htm

The Mayo Health O@sis Library provides a comprehensive reference library on diseases and conditions ranging from allergies to skin conditions.

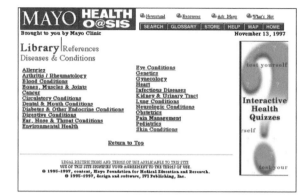

Medicine Box Ailment Center

http://www.medicinebox.com/ailment.htm

The Medicine Box has an Ailment Center providing treatment/remedy information and related links for a variety of conditions, including AIDS, chronic back pain, Alzheimer's disease, cancer, dementia, and others.

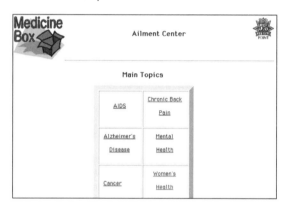

Medscape Patient Information Page

http://www.medscape.com/home/Patient/PatientInfo.html

Medscape Patient Information Page has information about a variety of medical conditions, among them AIDS, allergy and allergic diseases, leukemia, Hodgkin's disease, diabetes, eye disorders, inherited disorders, and digestive disorders.

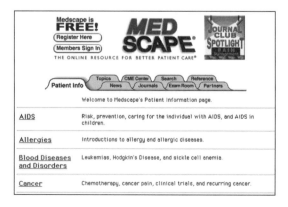

The Merck Manual

http://www.merck.com/pubs/mmanual/

The Merck Manual is a huge department store of medical and health information featuring an online edition of the *Merck Manual of Diagnosis and Therapy* in the **Publications** section. Its **Table of Contents** lists over 20 medical categories of disorders addressing symptoms, common clinical procedures, and laboratory tests. The **News** section has puzzles and quizzes and the **Disease InfoPark** has information about glaucoma, heart disease, osteoporosis, and other conditions.

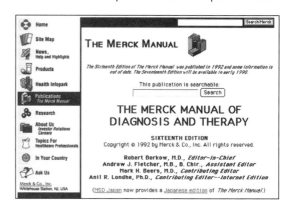

Michigan Electronic Library Disease and Condition Specific Resources

http://mel.lib.mi.us/health/health-disease.html

The Michigan Electronic Library provides an A to Z index to specific disease and condition sites ranging from AIDS and HIV to urologic disorders.

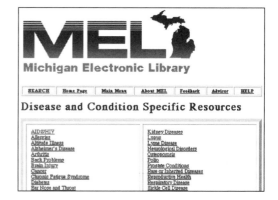

Morbidity and Mortality Weekly Report

http://www.cdc.gov/epo/mmwr/mmwr.html

The Morbidity and Mortality Weekly Report, prepared by the Centers for Disease Control and Prevention (CDC), is a series of weekly health reports to the CDC from state health departments. The site also provides a searchable documents index dating back to 1993.

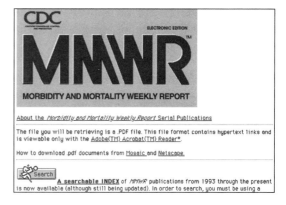

National Center for Chronic Disease Prevention and Health Promotion

http://www.cdc.gov/nccdphp/nccdhome.htm

The National Center for Chronic Disease Prevention and Health Promotion is a huge government site that offers information relating to its major program areas, arranged in the following categories: Maternal and Infant Health, Comprehensive Approaches, Disease and Prevention Control, Modifying Risk Factors, and Surveillance. All articles are easy to read.

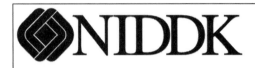

CDC   Search

**National Center for
Chronic Disease Prevention and Health Promotion**

Welcome to the National Center for Chronic Disease Prevention and Health Promotion (NCCDPHP) World Wide Web home page. NCCDPHP was established in 1988 to consolidate Centers for Disease Control and Prevention (CDC) efforts in chronic disease prevention and health promotion.

Chronic Disease Information

- Vision Statement/Mission
- NCCDPHP Organization Chart
- Chronic Disease and Chronic Disease Risk Factors (Graph)
- Burden of Chronic Disease and Infant Mortality
- Cost-Effectiveness of Prevention
- CDC's Partnership with States
- Prevention Priorities
- State Participation in NCCDPHP Grant Programs (Graph)
- Publications

The National Institute of Diabetes and Digestive and Kidney Diseases

http://www.niddk.nih.gov/

The National Institute of Diabetes and Digestive and Kidney Diseases of the National Institutes of Health contains public health information on a variety of diseases, including diabetes, digestive diseases, endocrine and metabolic diseases, hematologic disorders, and kidney diseases.

NIDDK

The National Institute of Diabetes
and Digestive and Kidney Diseases
of the
National Institutes of Health

Welcome

Health Information for the Public

- Diabetes
- Digestive Diseases
- Endocrine and Metabolic Diseases
- Hematologic Disorders
- Kidney Diseases
- Nutrition and Obesity
- Urologic Diseases

NIH Health Information Index 1997

http://www.nih.gov/news/96index/pubincov.htm

The NIH Health Information Index 1997 is a quick referral guide for finding answers to your health questions. The 1997 Index provides information on major research areas, important health-related topics, and diseases currently under investigation by the National Institutes of Health or their scientists. In addition, the site helps identify the institute(s) responsible for the area of interest, with links directly to the home page of that institute.

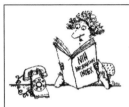

NIH
Health Information
Index
1997

Go to: [A-E] [F-J] [K-O] [P-T] [U-Z] [Abbreviations]

Where can you find information on diseases currently under investigation by NIH or NIH-supported scientists, major NIH research areas, and important health-related topics?

Right here in the *NIH Information Index* use this referral guide as a quick way to find answers to your health-related questions.

Each listing includes the abbreviated name(s) of the NIH institute, center, division, or

Osteoporosis and Related Bone Diseases

http://www.osteo.org

Osteoporosis and Related Bone Diseases, from the National Resource Center, provides a wealth of information about metabolic bone diseases, including clinical studies, news releases, and the latest research findings. The site offers prevention, early detection, and treatment information on Paget's disease, osteoporosis in men, osteogenesis imperfecta, and hyperparathyroidism.

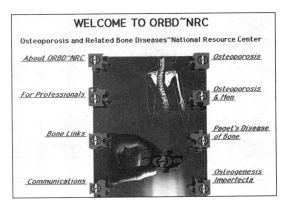

Otolaryngology Resources on the Internet

http://www.bcm.tmc.edu/oto/othersa1.html

Otolaryngology Resources on the Internet, from the Bobby R. Alford Department of Otorhinolaryngology and Communicative Sciences at the Baylor College of Medicine, provides a collection of patient education resources for head and neck medicine. For another 12 related topics, click on the **Baylor Patient Education Center.**

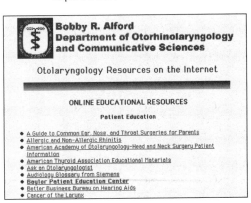

Patient Education Center

http://www.netmedicine.com/pt/patient.htm

The Patient Education Center, from NetMedicine, has easy-to-understand articles on common illnesses ranging from abdominal and gastrointestinal diseases to skin diseases.

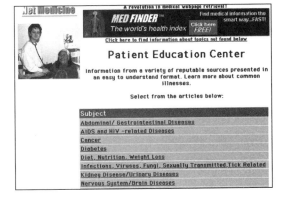

A Patient's Guide to Carpal Tunnel Syndrome

http://www.sechrest.com/mmg/cts/ctsintro.html

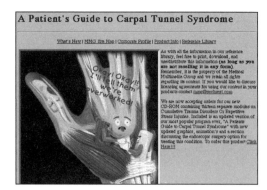

A Patient's Guide to Carpal Tunnel Syndrome provides basic information on the anatomy of the hands and wrists, diagnosis of carpal tunnel syndrome, and available treatments for sufferers of this repetitive motion injury. The site includes step-by-step pictures, diagrams, and animation of the surgical procedure that relieves the symptom. In addition, a reference library has similar information about lower back pain, knee problems, cumulative trauma disorders, and shoulder problems.

RenalNet

http://www.renalnet.org/

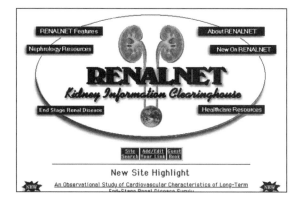

RenalNet is an information clearinghouse for the cause, treatment, and management of kidney disease and end-stage renal disease (ESRD).

Saint Francis Osteoporosis Center at Warren Clinic

http://www.warrencl.com/ocosteo.html

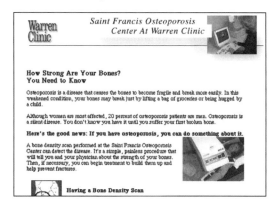

Saint Francis Osteoporosis Center at Warren Clinic provides a variety of osteoporosis resources for women. Scroll to the bottom of the page for an online osteoporosis risk questionnaire and information about calcium and vitamin D, exercise and osteoporosis, osteoporosis therapy, and home safety.

Sapient Health Network

http://www.shn.net/

The Sapient Health Network provides free health information and resources for a variety of serious and chronic illnesses, including asthma, breast cancer, diabetes, and others. Each illness area contains a Newsstand, a Library, a section on Your Health, and an interactive Community. To access this free service, complete an online registration form.

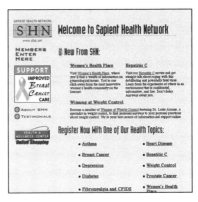

Self Healthsite

http://www1.sympatico.ca/healthyway/BAYER/Home.htm

Self Healthsite, from Bayer, provides information and answers to questions about heart disease, strokes, and arthritis. There are also tips and reminders on how to achieve or maintain a healthy lifestyle.

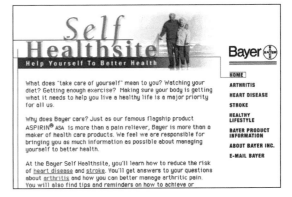

Thyroid Foundation of Canada

http://home.ican.net/~thyroid/Canada.html

The Thyroid Foundation of Canada Web site, available in English and French, provides thyroid disease health guides for patients and their families. This series of 12 pamphlets give an overview of the main thyroid conditions. The site also includes links to other health- and thyroid-related organizations and resources.

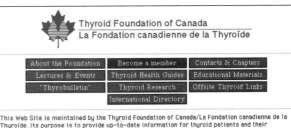

Thyroid Home Page

http://www.thyroid.com/

The Thyroid Home Page, maintained by the Santa Monica Thyroid Diagnostic Center, provides patient information about thyroid disease. In addition, the site offers **Need a Second Opinion** feature where you can e-mail your thyroid disease question to Dr. Richard B. Guttler.

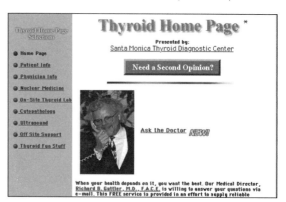

Tinnitus FAQ

http://www.cccd.edu/faq/tinnitus.html

Tinnitus FAQ, a resource for understanding tinnitus, provides information for learning about tinnitus, head noises such as a ringing, rushing, or buzzing in the ears.

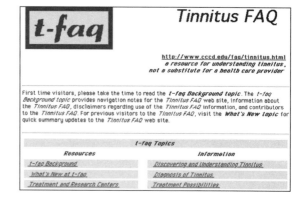

UCLA MedNet Patient Learning Series

http://www.mednet.ucla.edu/healthtopics/Ptlearn/PLSLIST.HTM

UCLA MedNet offers a series of patient learning articles that explain various disorders ranging from acne to vaginitis. The articles include the latest medical approaches to diagnosis and treatment.

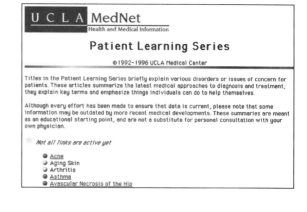

The Virtual Hospital
Iowa Health Book

http://www.vh.org/Patients/Patients.html

The Virtual Hospital presents the online *Iowa Health Book,* which contains a huge collection of patient educational materials for treating a wide variety of medical problems ranging from controlling pain to family safety. You can find patient information in the *Iowa Health Book* by searching for it or by browsing by department or by organ system. The site also provides an annotated list of these *Iowa Health Book* materials.

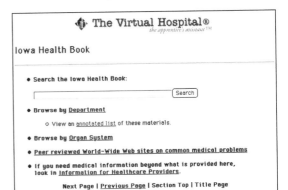

The Virtual Hospital
University of Iowa
Family Practice Handbook

http://indy.radiology.uiowa.edu/Providers/
ClinRef/FPHandbook/FPContents.html

The Virtual Hospital presents the *University of Iowa Family Practice Handbook,* which contains information on a variety of diseases ranging from heart disease to dermatitis.

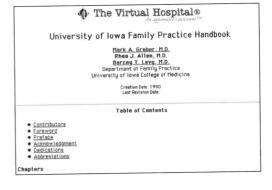

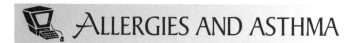 ALLERGIES AND ASTHMA

AllerDays

http://www.allerdays.com/

AllerDays contains features on allergies, allergy treatments, therapies, medications, and home remedies. The site includes a glossary of allergy terms, a search tool, and links to related resources.

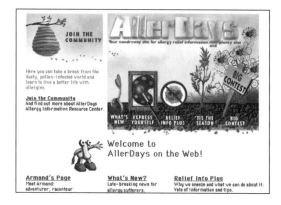

Allergy & Asthma Rochester Resource Center

http://www.eznet.net/aarrc/

The Allergy & Asthma Rochester Resource Center has information about allergies and asthma. Consumers will be interested in topics such as allergy and asthma management, triggers, and participation in studies. A search tool is offered, as are links to related sites.

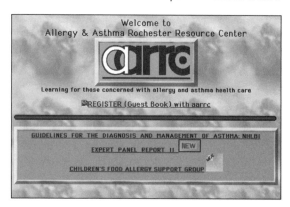

Allergy and Asthma Network Mothers of Asthmatics, Inc.

http://www.podi.com/health/aanma/

Allergy and Asthma Network Mothers of Asthmatics, Inc. provides basic information, FAQs, and the latest news about allergies and asthma.

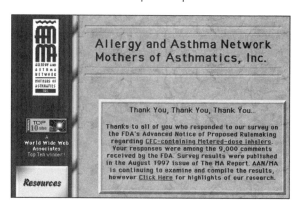

Allergy, Asthma & Immunology Online

http://allergy.mcg.edu/

Allergy, Asthma & Immunology Online provides a wealth of general information about asthma and allergies. The site includes a glossary and an asthma self-test.

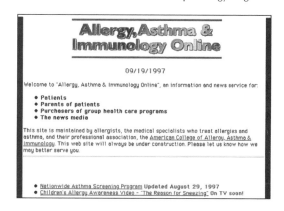

Allergy Asthma Technology Ltd.

http://www.allergyasthmatech.com/

Allergy Asthma Technology Ltd. is a supplier of medically approved and fully-tested products for allergy and asthma sufferers. The site provides information on causes, diagnoses, and treatments of allergies and asthma.

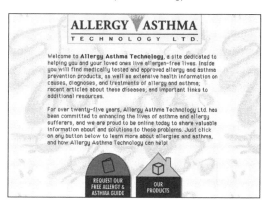

Allergy CyberCenter

http://www.allergycentre.com.au/

Allergy CyberCenter provides a variety of allergy resources, including an alphabetical list of information about allergy treatments and symptoms. In addition, the site includes an e-mail service for answers to your allergy problems, journalist information to various allergy topics, and specialized diets for different allergies.

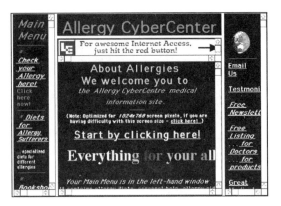

Allergy Glossary

http://www.hon.ch/Library/Theme/Allergy/Glossary/allergy.html

Allergy Glossary, from the Health On the Net Foundation, provides a comprehensive glossary featuring treatment and symptom information for allergies. The site also includes MedHunt, Alta Vista Europe, and Alta Vista USA search engines to help find additional allergy information.

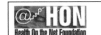

Allergy Home Page

http://www.cmh.edu/allergy/

The Allergy Home Page, from the Children's Mercy Hospital in Kansas City, provides an index of information to allergy/asthma medications ranging from antihistamines to nose sprays.

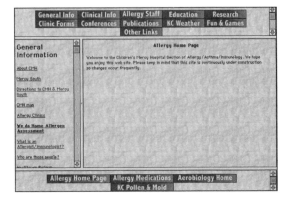

Allergy Internet Resources

http://www.io.com/~kinnaman/allabc.html

Allergy Internet Resources contains numerous articles about asthma and common and uncommon allergies. The allergy topics include food, children, skin, and specific substances.

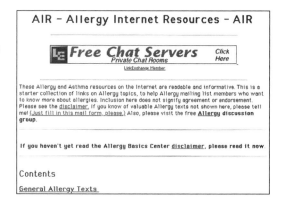

Allergy Relief Zone

http://www.allergy-relief.com/

The Allergy Relief Zone provides general information for allergy sufferers. Topics include gardening for allergy sufferers, allergy sufferer's sneeze page, the allergy sufferer's dream house, and the office allergy guide.

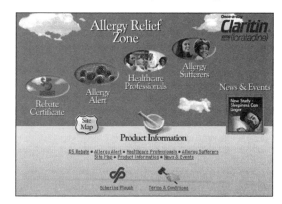

The Allergy Shop

http://www.allergyshop.com/

The Allergy Shop provides a wealth of information about allergies and protecting against allergies. The site includes links for allergies, asthma, asthma medications, and general medical resources.

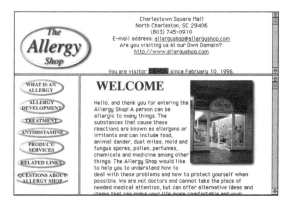

Allergy-Info.com

http://www.zyrtec.com/

Allergy-Info.com, from Pfizer, has an **Info Center** with lots of allergy information and a **Pollen Count** feature.

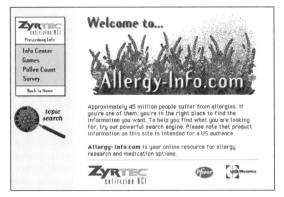

Allernet

http://www.allernet.com/

Allernet, an allergy and asthma Web site, provides useful information for allergy sufferers in the categories All About Allergy, Helpful Hints for Allergy Sufferers, and Allergy FAQ.

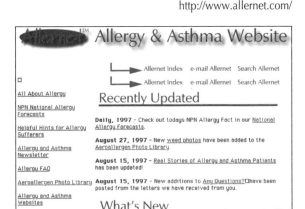

American Academy of Allergy, Asthma, & Immunology

http://www.aaaai.org/

The American Academy of Allergy, Asthma, & Immunology offers online articles for the public about immunology, asthma, rhinitis, and other allergic diseases. The site also includes an In the News feature providing up-to-date immunology and allergy news.

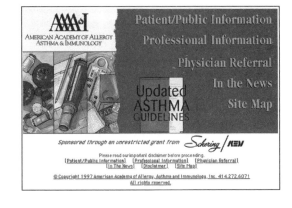

Asthma Management Handbook

http://hna.ffh.vic.gov.au/asthma/amh/amh.html

Asthma Management Handbook 1996, part of the National Asthma Campaign in Australia, provides a wealth of resources and patient information sheets about asthma. Topics included are diagnosis, widely prescribed medications, and methods of measuring lung function.

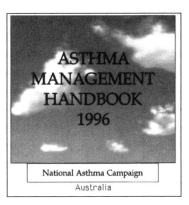

Asthma Under Control

http://www.asthmacontrol.com/

Asthma Under Control, from GlaxoWellcome, contains information on controlling asthma.

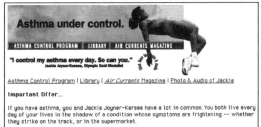

Better Health USA

http://www.betterhealthusa.com

Better Health USA discusses the age-old adage you are really what you eat. Is your life even slightly affected by allergies? A mystery ailment of yours may be caused by the food you eat.

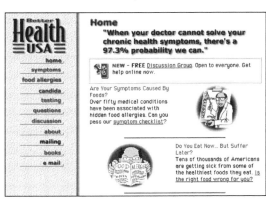

Education for Latex Allergy/Support Team & Information Coalition

http://pw2.netcom.com/~ecbdmd/elastic.html

The Education for Latex Allergy/Support Team & Information Coalition (ELASTIC) provides information about latex allergy and a comprehensive listing of sites. Among the categories are tire dust, television (with transcripts of programs), safe sex, gloves, and support groups.

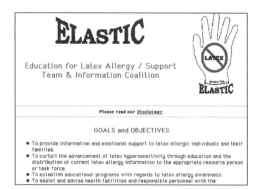

The Food Allergy Network

http://www.foodallergy.org/

The Food Allergy Network offers consumer information about food allergies. The site presents little-known facts, dispels myths, provides empirical studies, and has information about product alerts.

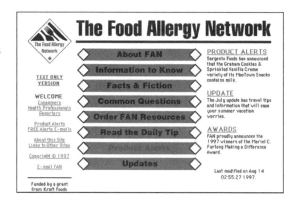

National Institute of Allergy and Infectious Diseases

http://www.niaid.nih.gov/publications/publications.htm

The National Institute of Allergy and Infectious Diseases, from the National Institutes of Health, provides a collection of online publications about allergies and infectious diseases. The publication categories include AIDS information, asthma and allergies, chronic fatigue syndrome, sexually transmitted diseases, and other diseases.

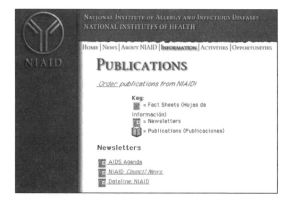

National Jewish Medical and Research Center

The National Jewish Medical and Research Center publishes Med Facts, online information for a variety of medical topics ranging from air pollutants to vocal cords. Scroll to **Table of Contents** to find a list of Med Facts topics.

http://www.njc.org/MFhtml/MFlist_subj.html

NATIONAL JEWISH
Medical and Research Center

Global Leader in Lung, Allergic and Immune Diseases

1400 Jackson St., Denver, Colorado 80206 - 303/388-4461
Call for information: LUNG LINE® - - 800/222-LUNG (5864)

Med Facts

From <u>National Jewish Medical and Research Center</u>
1400 Jackson Street, Denver, Colorado 80206

Subject List

The On-Line Allergy Center

The On-Line Allergy Center has helpful information on the relief of a variety of symptoms, including nasal congestion, eye redness/soreness, itching, sneezing, wheezing, coughing, and skin rashes/irritation.

http://www.sig.net/~allergy/

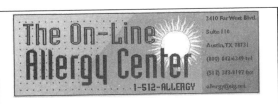

The On-Line Allergy Center
3410 FarWest Blvd.
Suite 110
Austin, TX 78731
(800) 842-6349 tel
(512) 343-8197 fax
allergy@sig.net

1-512-ALLERGY

The On-Line Allergy Center is an information service provided by **Russell Roby, LL.B., M.D.** Browse through the following pages for helpful information on the relief of a variety of symptoms including: ... *nasal congestion* ... *eye redness/soreness* ... *sneezing* ... *wheezing* ... *coughing* ... *joint pain* ... *intestinal pain* ... *skin rashes/irritation* ... *itching* ... *yeast infections* ... *mood swings* ... *hyperactivity* ... *attention deficit disorder* ... *fatigue* Check back each month for new information on how to combat the symptoms of allergies.

MAGELLAN
3 STAR SITE

ichat You can now chat on our website with Dr. Roby. Dr. Roby will be scheduling office hours soon.
<u>Simply click here to chat</u>.

Patricia Wrean's Asthma and Allergy WWW Resources Page

Patricia Wrean's Asthma and Allergy WWW Resources Page is an enormous collection of annotated asthma and allergy sites. Categories include general medical resources, related diseases and conditions, medications, and allergy and asthma.

http://www.cco.caltech.edu/~wrean/resources.html

Patricia <u>Wrean</u>'s Asthma and Allergy WWW Resources Page

Here is a listing of some asthma and allergy WWW resources I think may be of interest to those wanting to educate themselves about asthma and allergies. <u>Comments, additions, and corrections are requested</u> I will accept additions upon my own judgement -- I'll warn you right now that I'm a confirmed skeptic and am not a great believer in alternative medicine. As this resources list is intended for general educational purposes directed at the layman, sites containing only product/ordering information with no educational material are unlikely to be added. Inclusion of a Web resource on this page does not imply any endorsement of its contents. For anyone who preferred the <u>old version of this resources list</u>, it's still available.

For a complete list of resources for asthmatics, please see the alt.support.asthma Reading/Resource List. It is maintained by Lynn Short / lfshort@europa.com, and is posted periodically to <u>alt.support.asthma</u>, <u>alt.med.allergy</u>, <u>sci.med</u>, and <u>misc.kids</u>. I highly recommend it!

Asthma

<u>alt.support.asthma FAQ: General Information</u>
    This is the html version of the general information FAQ for the newsgroup <u>alt.support.asthma</u>, containing information in a question-and-answer format about asthma, symptoms, triggers, forms of treatment, related conditions and diseases, and asthma medications.

Sniffles & Sneezes

http://www.allergyasthma.com/

Sniffles & Sneezes is a quarterly public service newsletter, currently offering 25 articles on a wide variety of issues related to allergy and asthma care and prevention. The site also provides a list of names and addresses of asthma and allergy organizations.

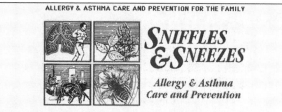

Teach Your Patients About Asthma: A Clinician's Guide

http://www.meddean.luc.edu/lumen/MedEd/
medicine/Allergy/Asthma/asthtoc.html

Teach Your Patients About Asthma: A Clinician's Guide, from the National Asthma Education Program, is a practical and flexible guide designed to help clinicians teach adults and children with asthma and parents of children with asthma about their disease and its management.

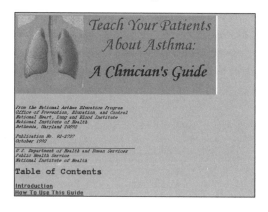

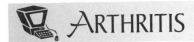 ARTHRITIS

American College of Rheumatology

http://www.rheumatology.org/find.html

The American College of Rheumatology specializes in arthritis care and research. The **Patient Information** section offers general fact sheets on a number of rheumatologic disorders and the **Publications** section offers summaries of articles. For the site's table of contents, click on **Search/Site Index.**

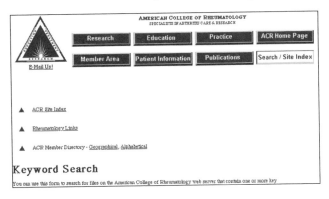

Arthritis Foundation

http://www.arthritis.org/

The Arthritis Foundation is a plentiful source of information about arthritis, using news articles and fact sheets, as well as items from the magazine *Arthritis Today.* The site presents patient-oriented briefs on exercise and arthritis, gout, joint surgery, living with arthritis, osteoarthritis, arthritis research, and rheumatoid arthritis.

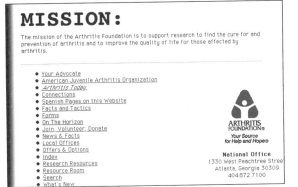

ArthritisHelp

http://rheuma.bham.ac.uk/primer.html

ArthritisHelp, from the Department of Rheumatology at the University of Birmingham in the United Kingdom, is a primer for consumers on rheumatic diseases, including rheumatoid arthritis.

arthritishelp
ah!

This primer is a short description of rheumatic diseases, aimed at people with no prior knowledge of medical subjects, but who are interested in this subject for any reason. They, or a relative or friend, may suffer from a rheumatic complaint, for example. It is not a comprehensive review, but attempts to make sense of a complex topic that even doctors find confusing! It contains links to other sites which publish items of related interest.

Rheumatic diseases include a variety of different conditions. However, the common feature is that they all involve joints and the surrounding tissues such as ligaments, tendons and muscles. They can involve other, seemingly unrelated organs as well, such as eyes, skin and glands. Rheumatic diseases are usually divided into those that primarily involve joints, known as Arthritis, and those involving other tissues, called Connective Tissue Diseases. Arthritis is further subdivided into Inflammatory and Non-Inflammatory Arthritis.

Ask Dr. Bones

http://bunny.lek.net/~fed/

Ask Dr. Bones, created by a rheumatologist, contains extensive medical information about musculoskeletal conditions. The site includes case studies, a sports section, tips of the week, questions and answers, and a bone-up section with articles on arthritic-related conditions. Dr. Bones invites you to submit your medical question.

Ask Dr. Bones

About the author

Case Studies
Case 1~ This condition may cause death
Case 2~ 35 year old man with skin rash and arthritis
Case 3~ This treatment is for what common condition?
Case 4~62 year old man who walks with pain
Case 5~Sudden onset of a swollen painful knee
Case 6~What is the diagnosis?
Case 7~A type of chronic arthritis
Case 8~A bad case of sunburn?
Case 9~Can you do this?
Case 10~No, these are not UFO's

Sports Section

Late score on "rub ons"
Warning...women athletes beware!
Look who is pumping iron
Rice for an ankle sprain?

Tips Of The Week

National Institute of Arthritis and Musculoskeletal and Skin Diseases

http://www.nih.gov/niams/

The National Institute of Arthritis and Musculoskeletal and Skin Diseases provides health information and a variety of fact sheets on arthritis, musculoskeletal, and skin diseases.

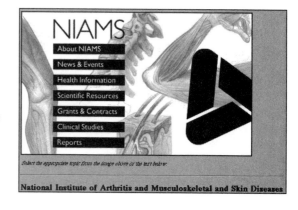

NIAMS
About NIAMS
News & Events
Health Information
Scientific Resources
Grants & Contracts
Clinical Studies
Reports

Select the appropriate topic from the image above or the text below

National Institute of Arthritis and Musculoskeletal and Skin Diseases

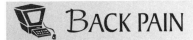

BACK PAIN

A Guide for Care of Your Back

http://www.halcyon.com/moonbeam/back/

A Guide for Care of Your Back has useful information from the doctors and therapists at the Virginia Mason Medical Center.

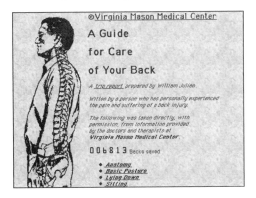

Kaiser Permanente Health Reference: Back Pain Information

http://www.scl.ncal.kaiperm.org/medadvice/backpain/
backpaininfo.html

The Kaiser Permanente Health Reference, provided by the Santa Clara Medical Center, has back pain information and advice on how to alleviate back problems.

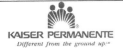

Oh, My Aching Back

http://www.achingback.com/

Oh, My Aching Back is an investigative guide to maintaining a healthy back. It is based on a CD-ROM and contains a wealth of helpful information on human anatomy, back problems, exercise, prevention techniques, lifestyle choices, and back-related links.

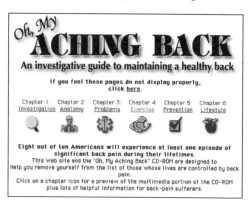

A Patient's Guide to Low Back Pain

http://www.sechrest.com/mmg/back/backpain.html

A Patient's Guide to Low Back Pain, from the Medical Multimedia Group (MMG), presents an illustrated guide to low back pain with information on anatomy, symptoms, diagnosis, and treatment.

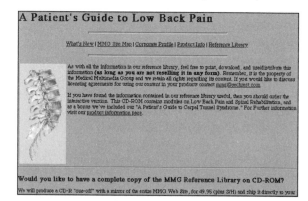

Understanding Acute Low Back Problems in Adults

http://www.medaccess.com/guides/cpgs/CPG_14.htm

Understanding Acute Low Back Problems in Adults, an online booklet, is provided by MedAccess. Topics include cause of low back problems, things to do about low back problems, getting relief, physical activity, exercise, and much more.

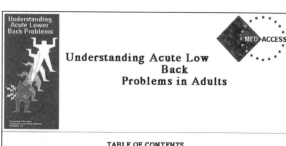

The Virtual Hospital Acute Low Back Problems in Adults

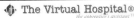

http://www.vh.org/Patients/IHB/Ortho/BackPatient/Contents.html

Acute Low Back Problems in Adults, from The Virtual Hospital's *Iowa Health Book,* is a collection of 15 concise articles on causes, management, and prevention of low back pain. The **Things To Do About Low Back Problems** section is especially helpful for anyone suffering from this common ailment.

> ### ⬥ The Virtual Hospital®
> *the apprentice i assistant™*
>
> ### Acute Low Back Problems in Adults
>
> Published by a non-Federal panel of experts sponsored by the Agency for Health Care Policy and Research
> Peer Review Status: Externally reviewed by the AHCPR
> Creation Date: December 1994
> Last Revision Date: Unknown
>
> **Consumer Version**
> **Clinical Practice Guideline**
> **Number 14**
>
> ### Table of Contents
>
> ● About the Back and Back Problems
> ● Purpose
> ● Causes of Low Back Problems
> ● Things To Do About Low Back Problems
> ● Getting Relief
> ● Physical Activity
> ● Bed Rest
> ● About Work and Family

BRAIN AND NEUROLOGIC DISORDERS

The Alzheimer Page

http://www.biostat.wustl.edu/alzheimer/

The Alzheimer Page, a service provided by Washington University in St. Louis, Missouri, offers a mailing list for anyone with an interest in Alzheimer's disease or related dementing disorders in older adults. In addition, the site includes a search tool to get advice, information, and references about Alzheimer's disease.

> ### *Washington University in St. Louis*
> ### The **ALZHEIMER Page**
>
> http://www.biostat.wustl.edu/ALZHEIMER
>
> The ALZHEIMER Page is an educational service created and sponsored by the **Washington University** Alzheimer's Disease Research Center (**ADRC**) in **St. Louis, Missouri** and supported by a grant from the **National Institute on Aging** (**NIA**) (#AG05681). Opinions expressed are not necessarily those of the ADRC or NIA.
>
> **What is the ALZHEIMER list all about?**
> Answers to some frequently asked questions about the **ALZHEIMER** mailing list and its digest, **ALZHEIMER-digest**.
> **How do I subscribe to the ALZHEIMER list?**
> Simple instructions on how to join the **ALZHEIMER** or **ALZHEIMER-digest** mailing lists.
> **How many people are subscribed to ALZHEIMER?**
> Everyone of these subscribers is here to share questions, answers, suggestions and tips on Alzheimer disease and related dementing disorders.

Alzheimer's Disease Education & Referral Center

http://www.alzheimers.org/

The Alzheimer's Disease Education & Referral Center, a service of the National Institute on Aging, provides a variety of resources about Alzheimer's disease, including online publications such as "Alzheimer's Disease: Unraveling the Mystery" and numerous others.

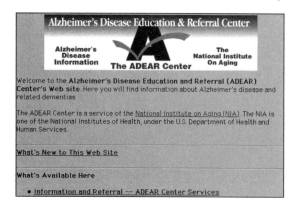

Alzheimer's Disease Resource Page

http://www.cwru.edu/affil/adsc/intro.htm

Alzheimer's Disease Resource Page, sponsored by Case Western Reserve University in Cleveland, Ohio, has information for everyone on Alzheimer's disease, whether you are a caregiver, a practitioner, a researcher, or someone just interested in learning more.

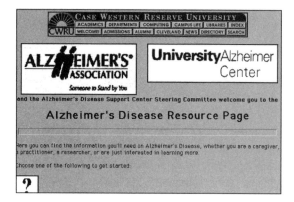

The Alzheimer's Disease Web Page

http://med-amsa.bu.edu/Alzheimer/

The Alzheimer's Disease Web Page, from Bedford Geriatrics Research Education Clinical Center at Boston University Medical School, offers information to families, caregivers, and others interested in Alzheimer's disease.

Bedford Geriatric Research Education Clinical Center, Bedford, MA

The Boston University Alzheimer's Disease Center

The Alzheimer's Disease Web Page

A Site dedicated to the distribution of information to Investigators, Families, Caregivers and others interested in Alzheimer's Disease.

Alzheimers.com

http://www.alzheimers.com/site/

Alzheimers.com, updated daily, is a gateway to information about Alzheimer's disease on the Internet. The resource provides a large online database of the the latest news and research on the disease, reviews of dozens of Alzheimer's-related sites in cyberspace, and an interactive forum for people who deal with it.

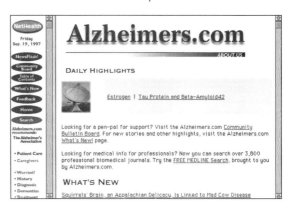

Aneurysm & AVM Support Page

http://www.westga.edu/~wmaples/aneurysm1.html

The Aneurysm & AVM Support Page contains medical/research aspects of aortic aneurysms in both a professional and layperson's style. The **Introduction** section has sites devoted to various vascular problems.

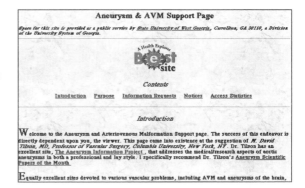

Brain Surgery Information Center

http://www.brain-surgery.com/

The Brain Surgery Information Center describes various medical conditions that might require brain surgery and then describes the process of brain surgery itself—what you might expect in the preoperative stage, the operative stage, and the postoperative stage.

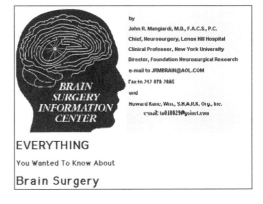

Caring for People with Huntington's Disease

Caring for People with Huntington's Disease has information for caring for people with Huntington's disease. The site includes articles on specific care issues, as well as a list of other sites related to Huntington's disease.

http://www.kumc.edu/hospital/huntingtons/

Caring for People with Huntington's Disease

This page is meant to be a source of information for those with Huntington's disease, those at risk, their families, caregivers and those just wanting to know more. It is best viewed with Netscape or Microsoft Internet Browser. If you have visited here before and things do not seem to look right or work, try reloading the page.

Huntington's Disease is an inherited degenerative neuropsychiatric disorder which affects both body and mind. Symptoms most commonly begin between the ages of 35 and 50, although onset may occur any time from childhood to old age. Research is progressing rapidly, but there is currently no cure.

Huntington's disease is inherited in an autosommal dominant fashion. Each child of an affected parent has a 50 % chance of inheriting the disease and is said to be at risk. The discovery of the HD gene in 1993 has made it possible to test at-risk individuals for Huntington's disease before symptoms occur. In the absence of a cure, however, the decision to be tested or not remains a difficult one, and there are many important legal, financial and personal considerations. For more information about the genetic basis of Huntington's disease, you may wish to visit the Online Mendellian Inheritance in Man (OMIN) to learn about the genetic basis or the DNA library at the National Library of Medicine to see the actual gene sequence.

The Comprehensive Epilepsy Center

The Comprehensive Epilepsy Center, of New York Hospital–Cornell Medical Center, provides treatment information for adult and pediatric patients with intractable (hard-to-treat) seizures, as well as those with other epilepsy-related diagnostic and management problems. For more information on treatment options available through the Center, call 1-212-746-2359.

http://neuro.med.cornell.edu/NYH-CMC/res19a.html

**CORNELL MEDICAL CENTER
NEW YORK HOSPITAL**

The Comprehensive Epilepsy Center of New York Hospital – Cornell Medical Center provides a multidisciplinary approach to the complex medical and social needs of patients with **seizures**. The program serves **adult and pediatric patients with intractable (hard to treat) seizures,** as well as those with other epilepsy-related diagnostic and management problems.

- Treatment of Epilepsy
- Surgery for Epilepsy
- Investigational Drug Trials
- Vagal Nerve Stimulator
- Pediatric Epilepsy Surgery
- Comprehensive Patient Care
- Areas of Special Interest

  - Pediatric Epilepsy Program
  - Pregnancy - Epilepsy
  - Seizures Affected by Menstruation
  - Menopause - Epilepsy

For more information on treatment options available through the Comprehensive Epilepsy Center, please call: **(212) 746-2359**

Dana BrainWeb

Dana BrainWeb reviews common brain diseases from Alzheimer's disease to manic depression and stroke. The site offers basic information, support, and sources of further information.

http://www.dana.org/brainweb/

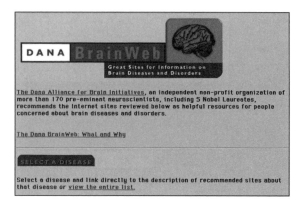

DANA BrainWeb
Great Sites for Information on Brain Diseases and Disorders

The Dana Alliance for Brain Initiatives, an independent non-profit organization of more than 170 pre-eminent neuroscientists, including 5 Nobel Laureates, recommends the Internet sites reviewed below as helpful resources for people concerned about brain diseases and disorders.

The Dana BrainWeb: What and Why

SELECT A DISEASE

Select a disease and link directly to the description of recommended sites about that disease or view the entire list.

The EpiCentre

http://137.172.248.46/epilepsy.htm

The EpiCentre provides information about epilepsy and its treatment. The site is divided into sections: What It's All About, Investigation, Treatment, Seizures, and FAQs with related links.

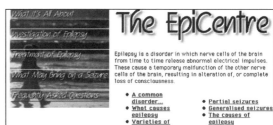

Institute of Neurotoxicology and Neurological Disorders

http://www.innd.org/

The Institute of Neurotoxicology and Neurological Disorders provides the current news and information about neurotoxicology and neurological disorders from a wide variety of consumer health resources on the Internet. The categories include hazardous substances, neurological disorders, and online articles from the *NeuroToxicology Journal.*

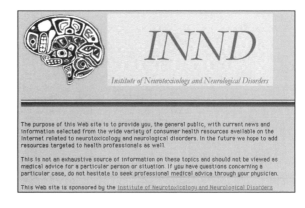

International MS Support Foundation

http://aspin.asu.edu/msnews/

The International MS Support Foundation, created by Jean Sumption, offers something for everyone. The page contains over 200 articles and a wide variety of related links ranging from nutrition to a doctor's corner and medical information.

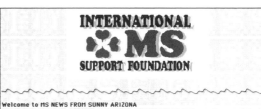

The MS Resource Center

http://www.betaseron.com/

The MS Resource Center, from Betaseron, is an interactive online information source, designed to link you to the latest MS-related resources and services. This online database of information provides the opportunity to access FAQs about MS and MS therapy and read MS-related publications and newsletters and inspiring profiles of MS sufferers.

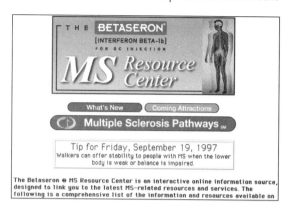

Multiple Sclerosis Society of Canada

http://www.mssoc.ca/

The Multiple Sclerosis Society of Canada provides information about MS. The Frequently Asked Questions section, based on its comprehensive booklet, *Multiple Sclerosis: Its Effects on You and Those You Love,* has a list of questions ranging from general areas (e.g., "What is multiple sclerosis?") to specific ones (e.g., "Should I give up alcohol?" "Is bowel function affected by multiple sclerosis?" and "What are the effects of pregnancy?").

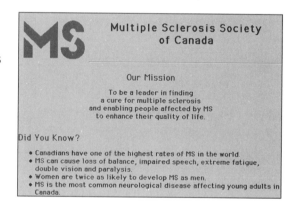

National Institute of Neurological Disorders and Stroke

http://www.ninds.nih.gov/

The National Institute of Neurological Disorders and Stroke provides information on a wide variety of neurological diseases and conditions in both the **Health Information** and the **Health Publications** sections. The sections contain articles and guides to epilepsy, Parkinson's disease, clinical alerts, advisories, and much more.

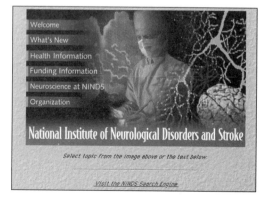

National Institute on Aging

http://www.nih.gov/nia/

The National Institute on Aging provides a variety of online health resources for Alzheimer's and cardiovascular diseases. The site also includes a directory of aging resources and brochures and fact sheets covering a wide range of topics related to health and aging.

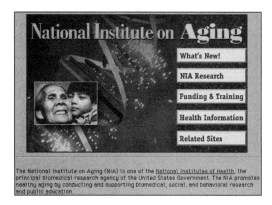

Parkinson's Disease

http://www.clearlight.com/~morph/present/park0.htm

Parkinson's Disease is a teaching presentation on Parkinson's disease that includes a brief history, epidemiology, drug management, rehabilitation, and surgical intervention.

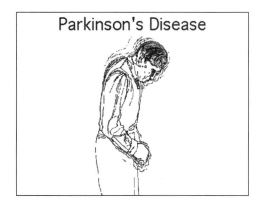

The Parkinson's Web

http://pdweb.mgh.harvard.edu/

The Parkinson's Web provides a variety of resources for this disease, including a primer, medical treatment information, and related links.

The Race to Erase MS

http://www.erasems.org/

The Race to Erase MS is a celebrity benefit supporting aggressive research to find a cure for multiple sclerosis (MS). The site includes information on MS, an e-mail feature where Dr. Brian Morgan answers questions about MS online, and related MS news and links.

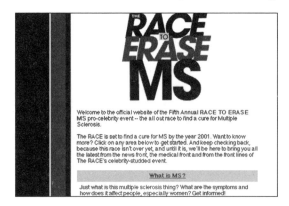

VHL Family Alliance Home Page

http://www.vhl.org/healthcare/handbook.htm

VHL Family Alliance Home Page is a comprehensive resource for people with von Hippel-Lindau disease, their families, and support personnel. The reference material emphasizes conversations and personal advice about questions of treatment. More objective data are provided in the sections Possible Manifestations of VHL; Diagnosis, Treatment, and Research; Living with VHL; and Reference.

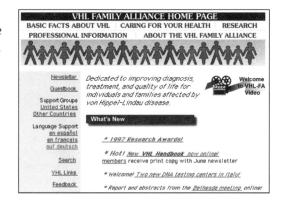

The World of Multiple Sclerosis

http://www.ifmss.org.uk/

The World of Multiple Sclerosis serves as a clearinghouse for educational and scientific information about MS. It is the Web site for the International Federation of Multiple Sclerosis Societies (IFMSS), a nonprofit umbrella organization for the 35 established national MS member societies throughout the world. The site provides a **Frequently Asked Questions** section, available in six languages, with information about MS. The site also includes a list of the major and national MS organizations around the world.

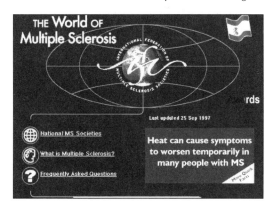

Worldwide Congress on Pain

http://www.pain.com

The Worldwide Congress on Pain, sponsored by the Dannemiller Memorial Educational Foundation, has a variety of resources for pain, including consumer information, an ask the pain doctor feature, and links to related sites.

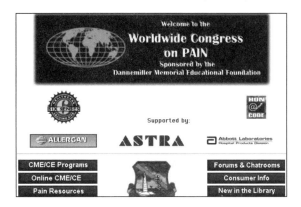

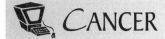 CANCER

American Cancer Society

http://www.cancer.org/

The American Cancer Society provides a variety of cancer resources for prevention, detection, and treatment. The **Cancer Info** section has a wealth of information for specific cancers, patients and families, statistics, guidelines, and tobacco information. The site also contains the latest research progress, news, and extensive links to other cancer sites in the **WWW Directory** section. Furthermore, you can jump directly to a site category using a pull-down menu to find a link to a local ACS chapter.

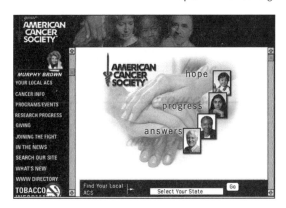

Arizona Cancer Center

http://www.azcc.arizona.edu/

The Arizona Cancer Center, a National Cancer Institute-Designated Comprehensive Cancer Center at the University of Arizona Health Sciences Center in Tucson, provides a wealth of information about the different kinds of cancer in the public education section. The section includes information on prostate, colon, skin, and breast cancers.

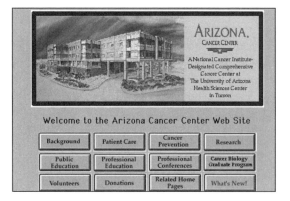

Ask NOAH About: Cancer

http://www.cuny.edu/cancer/cancer.html

The New York Online Access to Health (NOAH) is the combined effort of the New York Public Library and other educational institutions. Ask NOAH About: Cancer is a giant warehouse of information about cancer, care and treatment, statistics, information resources, symptoms, and types. All information is well organized, thorough, and easy to read. A search tool is offered, as are links to related sites on the Internet.

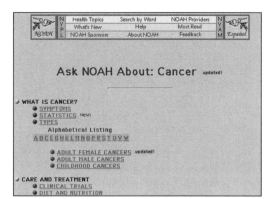

BACUP

http://www.cancerbacup.org.uk/

The BACUP Web site contains a variety of online booklets and fact sheets with cancer information for patients. The site also includes the *BACUP News,* a publication featuring stories of interest to cancer patients.

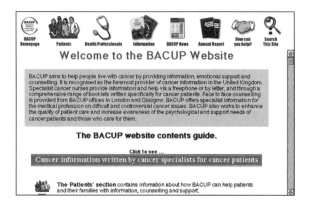

Bone Marrow Transplants

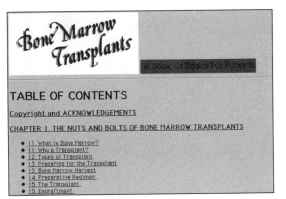

http://nysernet.org/bcic/bmy/bmt.book/toc.html

Bone Marrow Transplants, an online book written in plain language, tells you everything you ever wanted to know about bone marrow transplants. It contains over 130 articles that address every aspect of transplants.

Breast Cancer Awareness

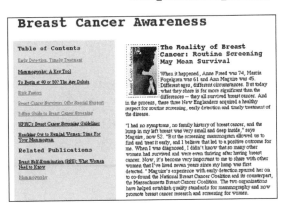

http://www.harvardpilgrim.org/html/frontpage/
breast_cancer/breast_cancer.htm

Breast Cancer Awareness, from the Harvard Pilgrim HMO, offers a variety of breast cancer resources, including breast self-examination, mammography information, a breast cancer screening guide, and survival stories.

Breast Cancer Network

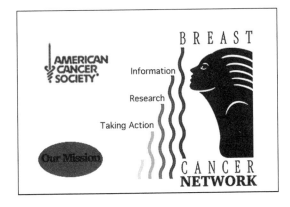

http://www.cancer.org/bcn/bcn.html

The Breast Cancer Network, part of the American Cancer Society home page, provides reliable information on breast cancer and breast reconstruction and includes the latest breast cancer news and an easy-to-understand glossary.

Can.Survive

http://www.avonlink.co.uk/amanda/

Can.Survive, Amanda Gee's home page, is a tribute to people suffering from all kinds of illnesses and injuries. The site contains copious cancer resources for Hodgkin's disease, non-Hodgkin's disease, treatment information, and links to all the major online cancer resources. To find information on this site, click on **Alphabetical Index** or use the search tool.

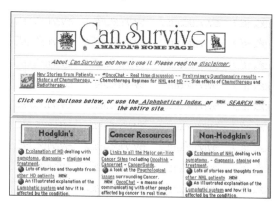

Cancer Care, Inc.

http://www.cancercareinc.org

Cancer Care, Inc. provides assistance to people with any type of cancer, at any stage of illness. The services include support groups, cancer and treatment information, referral help, patient and family education programs, information on financial assistance, and more. All of Cancer Care's services are free of charge. For more information on the services, call 1-800-813-HOPE (1-800-813-4673) from anywhere in the United States.

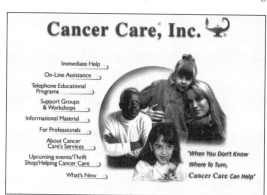

Cancer News on the Net

http://www.cancernews.com/

Cancer News on the Net, edited by Dr. Richard K.J. Brown, has more than 15 categories of information about cancer. In addition, the site includes home pages created by cancer patients.

Cancer Related Links

http://seidata.com/~marriage/rcancer.html

Cancer Related Links provides a comprehensive collection of cancer resources divided into categories.

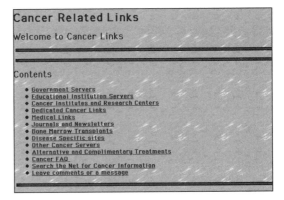

Cancer Web

http://infoventures.com/cancer/

Cancer Web, a service of Information Venture, Inc., contains the *CancerWeb Report,* a monthly online publication with the latest cancer information from leading research and medical journals. The site also offers other cancer-related resources.

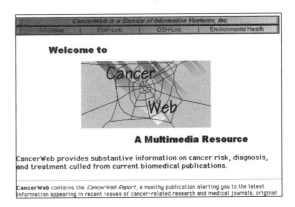

CancerGuide: Steve Dunn's Cancer Information Page

http://cancerguide.org/

CancerGuide, prepared by Steve Dunn, contains a consumer's reference library with articles on cancer ranging from fundamentals to more specialized areas. The Guide also includes articles on alternative therapies not approved by mainstream medicine.

CancerNet

http://wwwicic.nci.nih.gov/

CancerNet, sponsored by the National Cancer Institute, provides a wide range of cancer resources, including information about treatment, detection and prevention, supportive care, clinical trials, breast cancer research, a glossary of cancer terms, and links to other cancer sites. In addition, the site focuses on information about cancer in general.

CanSearch: Online Guide to Cancer Resources

http://www.cansearch.org/canserch/canserch.htm

Marshall Kragen's CanSearch, sponsored by the National Coalition for Cancer Survivorship, walks you through CancerNet and OncoLink and provides helpful tips for using these sites most effectively. His site also includes links to support groups for specific cancers.

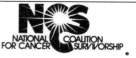

Guide to Internet Resources for Cancer

http://www.ncl.ac.uk/~nchwww/guides/clinks1.htm

The Guide to Internet Resources for Cancer, from the University of Newcastle, contains over 30 pages of links to cancer-related information for both the public and health professionals. For an overview of the site, click on **Alphabetical Index of Diseases and Topics.**

The International Myeloma Foundation

http://myeloma.org/

The International Myeloma Foundation provides online resources for patients with multiple myeloma, their families, and the professionals who help to manage this form of cancer.

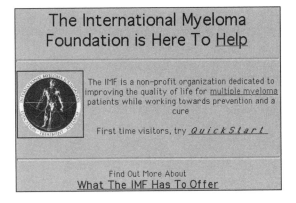

An Introduction to Skin Cancer

http://www.maui.net/~southsky/introto.html

An Introduction to Skin Cancer contains a collection of topics related to skin cancer.

Leukemia Links

http://www.acor.org/diseases/hematology/Leukemia/leukemia.html

GrannyBarb and Art's Leukemia Links is the place for everything you ever wanted to know about leukemia. The resource contains an enormous collection of links to leukemia-related sites with information for research, treatment, bone marrow transplants, the relationship between leukemia and genetics, online journals, clinical trials, and much more.

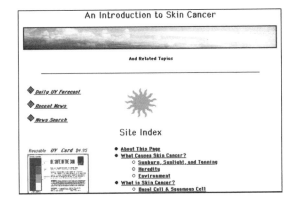

Lung Cancer

http://www.erinet.com/fnadoc/lung.htm

Lung Cancer provides information about the main types of lung cancer and the specific diagnosis and treatment of each type. The site also includes related links.

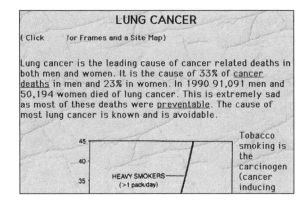

Mammograms

http://rex.nci.nih.gov/MAMMOG_WEB/MAMMOG_DOC.html

Mammograms, from the National Cancer Institute, offers women a resource on mammograms. Topics range from background information to an index of printable materials.

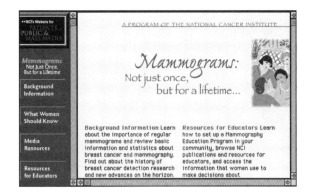

Medicine Online

http://www.meds.com/

Medicine Online provides extensive medical resources about colon cancer, lung cancer, and leukemia. The site includes articles from the *Daily Oncology News Digest,* reports from the *Conrad Notes* medical meetings, cancer forums, discussion groups, related links, and a search tool.

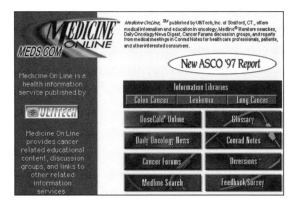

Mediconsult.com Chemotherapy and You

http://www.mediconsult.com/noframes/general/shareware/chemo/

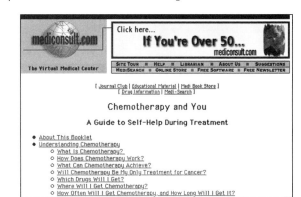

Mediconsult.com Chemotherapy and You is an online version of the National Cancer Institute publication No. 94-1136, a self-help guide to chemotherapy for cancer patients and their families. The site provides information on understanding chemotherapy, coping with side effects, eating well during chemotherapy, and other topics.

Medinfo.org

http://cure.medinfo.org/

Medinfo.org provides cancer information from a variety of online oncology resources, including mailing lists, patients' Web sites, ReutersHealth, CancerNet, and organizations. You can also find and search for cancer information in medical journals and specialized Web sites.

Melanoma Patients' Information Page

http://www.sonic.net/~jpat/getwell/

The Melanoma Patients' Information Page contains information for melanoma patients and others interested in melanoma. The site includes a searchable research abstracts database, a bulletin board, a glossary of terms, and a medical dictionary.

Memorial Sloan-Kettering Cancer Center

http://www.mskcc.org/

The Memorial Sloan-Kettering Cancer Center Web site offers a variety of cancer resources, including news of the latest developments in cancer research in the **Just In** section. The **Prevention & Detection** section contains cancer information about protection, prevention, and screening, and the **Treatment** section provides overviews of the various cancers and includes also a list of other related cancer sites. For a table of contents, click on **Site Guide.**

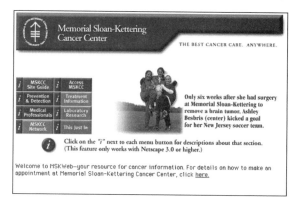

National Cancer Institute PDQ Patient Treatment

http://cancernet.nci.nih.gov/clinpdq/pif.html

PDQ Patient Treatment documents, prepared by the National Cancer Institute, are A to Z cancer indexes covering patient treatment information on diseases ranging from AIDS-related lymphoma to vulvar cancer. All PDQ patient treatment documents are written in easy-to-understand, nontechnical language.

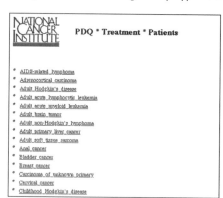

National Comprehensive Cancer Network

http://www.cancer.med.umich.edu/NCCN/NCCN.html

The National Comprehensive Cancer Network contains links to the nation's 15 leading cancer centers and provides an enormous amount of information about cancer in the form of search tools, articles, news magazines, and links to other cancer sites.

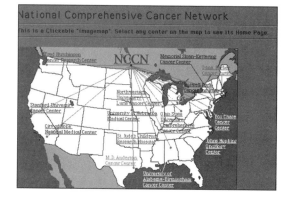

National Marrow Donor Program

http://www.marrow.org/

The National Marrow Donor Program provides a wealth of information about bone marrow transplants and links to related sites. You can also register to become a marrow donor and learn how the process of finding a match occurs.

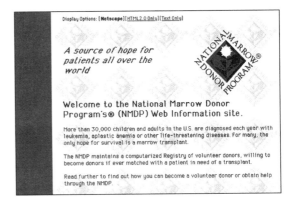

OncoLink

http://oncolink.upenn.edu/

OncoLink, from the University of Pennsylvania Cancer Center, is one of the premiere cancer sites on the Internet. The site provides a variety of cancer resources, including the latest cancer news from a number of media sources, disease-oriented menus for specific types of cancer, clinical trials for new treatments, cancer FAQs with answers, global resources for cancer information, and much more.

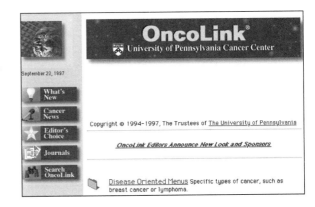

OncoLink NCI/PDQ Patient Statements

http://oncolink.upenn.edu/pdq_html/2/engl/

OncoLink NCI/PDQ Patient Statements, from the University of Pennsylvania Cancer Center, is a fund of knowledge with up-to-date summary information for the treatment of various cancers. Disease topics range from adrenocortical carcinoma to Wilms' tumor. Click on the **Table of Contents** for each disease to find a complete list of information.

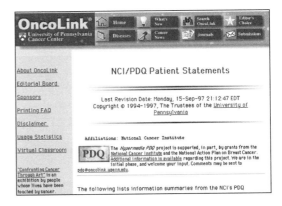

Oncology Clinical Studies

http://www.tapholdings.com/

Oncology Clinical Studies, from TAP Holdings, Inc., a pharmaceutical company, provides extensive patient information on breast cancer, cervical cancer, pancreatic cancer, and brain cancer. Each type of cancer includes links to related sites.

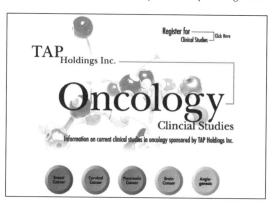

Pathology Simplified

http://www.erinet.com/fnadoc/path.htm

Pathology Simplified, written by pathologist Pat Connelly, is a nontechnical reference on lung cancer, breast cancer, and the Pap smear.

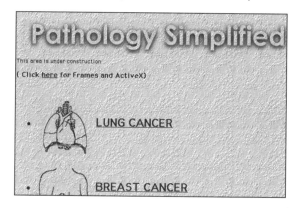

Patient Resource Center

http://www.salick.com/resource/

Patient Resource Center, provided by Salick Health Care, Inc., features online consumer cancer resources, including an extensive, alphabetical index of cancer sites.

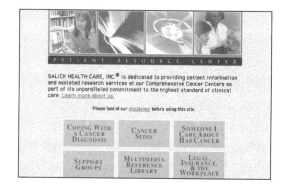

Patients and Public

http://rex.nci.nih.gov/INTRFCE_GIFS/INFO_PATS_INTR_DOC.htm

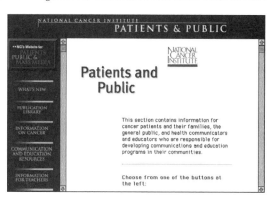

Patients and Public, from the National Cancer Institute and the National Institutes of Health, provides a wealth of online resources for cancer patients, their families, and educators. The **Publication Library** section features a variety of articles in the browsing rooms. The **Information on Cancer** section contains topics such as the 100 types of cancer, the prevention, detection, and treatment of cancer, a glossary of cancer-related terms, and a series of fact sheets organized in an alphabetical index. The **Communication and Education Resources** section offers copy-ready materials and hundreds of patient education resources in a searchable database.

University of Michigan Comprehensive Cancer Center

http://www.cancer.med.umich.edu/

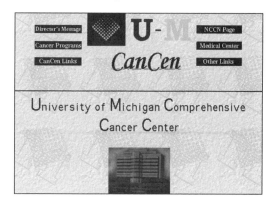

The University of Michigan Comprehensive Cancer Center is a mega-source of cancer information, including resources for prevention, diagnosis, and treatment, and a multitude of related cancer sites. The site also includes links to the nation's 15 leading cancer centers and offers a toll-free cancer information line 1-800-865-1125.

University of Texas M.D. Anderson Cancer Center

http://utmdacc.uth.tmc.edu/

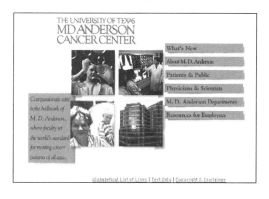

The University of Texas M.D. Anderson Cancer Center contains a patients and public section with information on hospice organizations, cancer-related publications, and other cancer sites.

CARDIOVASCULAR DISEASE (HEART ATTACK, STROKE)

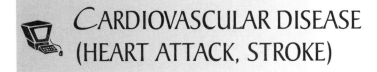

American Heart Association Heart & Stroke A-Z Guide

http://www.amhrt.org/Heart_and_Stroke_A_Z_Guide/

The American Heart Association site contains an enormous resource, the **Heart & Stroke A-Z Guide,** an index to hundreds of topics related to conditions and factors associated with heart problems and stroke. The Guide also includes a search tool.

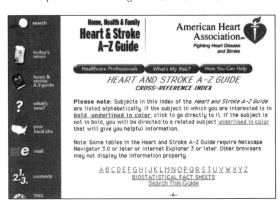

Cardiology Compass

http://osler.wustl.edu/~murphy/cardiology/compass.html

Cardiology Compass, supported by the Washington University School of Medicine in St. Louis, Missouri, contains a variety of cardiovascular resources, including patient and education information.

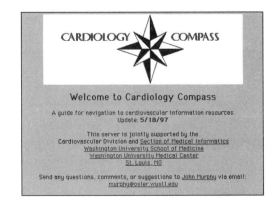

Cardiovascular Institute of the South

http://www.cardio.com/

The Cardiovascular Institute of the South contains many articles about heart and circulatory problems, including prevention, diagnosis, and surgical and nonsurgical treatments. The site also includes a search tool, related cancer links, and medical indexes.

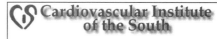

CIS (Cardiovascular Institute of the South), a leading center for the advanced diagnosis and treatment of heart and circulatory disease, presents for your education and republication, a wide-ranging library of doctor column-style reports on this vital and rapidly evolving aspect of medicine.

These reports cover the full spectrum of prevention, diagnosis, nonsurgical and surgical treatment of circulatory problems. They are updated regularly, and constitute one of the Internet's most-accessible and current sources for lay audiences on heart-related illness.

Search the CIS site:

Cholesterol & the Heart

http://www.medicinenet.com/mainmenu/encyclop/
article/art_c/choleste.htm

Cholesterol & the Heart, from MedicineNet, is a highly informative article about cholesterol and its role as a cause of heart disease. The article also discusses treatment of high cholesterol levels and the part played by triglycerides.

DISEASES & TREATMENTS

CHOLESTEROL & THE HEART

MedicineNet POWER POINTS about CHOLESTEROL AND THE HEART:

- Cholesterol is produced in the liver and carried in the bloodstream by lipoproteins.
- LDL cholesterol is associated with an increased risk of coronary artery disease.
- Coronary heart disease is the most common cause of death in the U.S.
- Risk factors for coronary heart disease have been identified.
- After 20 years of age, cholesterol level testing is recommended every 5 years.
- Treatment recommendations for elevated cholesterol are based on the levels of total cholesterol, LDL cholesterol, HDL cholesterol, and other risk factors for coronary heart disease.
- Diets high in cholesterol and saturated fats can increase blood

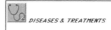

Cleveland Clinic Heart Center

http://www.heartcenter.ccf.org:8080/

The Cleveland Clinic Heart Center publishes *Heartline,* a cardiac health awareness news magazine for consumers. The **Quality Indicators** section provides invaluable patient information on coronary artery disease, heart failure, heart rhythm disorders, and heart valve disease.

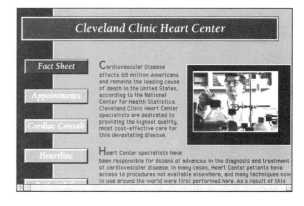

Cleveland Clinic Heart Center

Fact Sheet

Appointments

Cardiac Consult

Heartline

Cardiovascular Disease affects 68 million Americans and remains the leading cause of death in the United States, according to the National Center for Health Statistics. Cleveland Clinic Heart Center specialists are dedicated to providing the highest quality, most cost-effective care for this devastating disease.

Heart Center specialists have been responsible for dozens of advances in the diagnosis and treatment of cardiovascular disease. In many cases, Heart Center patients have access to procedures not available elsewhere, and many techniques now in use around the world were first performed here. As a result of this

The General Education Site for Cardiovascular Diseases

http://www.arrhythmia.com/

The General Education Site for Cardiovascular Diseases, a public service of Internet Medical Education, contains a consumer section with articles on a variety of cardiovascular disorders. The information is presented in the language that your own doctor might use to help you understand each disorder. To find the articles, click on **Patients, Family, and Concerned Laymen** and then on **Subject reviews.** The site also includes an online patient cardiovascular diseases glossary.

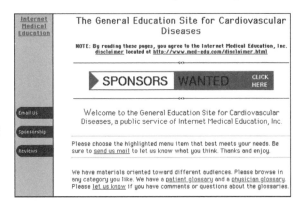

Heart Home Page

http://www.hearthome.com/

The Heart Home Page, sponsored by Galichia Medical Group, is a source of information about the prevention and treatment of heart disease. Scroll and click on **answers** to FAQs about heart disease. For a free subscription to a quarterly newsletter, click on **Take Your Health to Heart.**

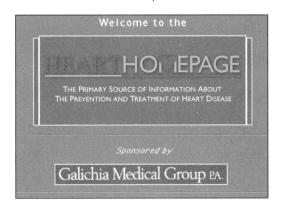

Heart Information Network

http://www.heartinfo.com/

The Heart Information Network provides a wide range of information and services to heart patients and others interested in learning about lowering risk factors for heart disease. The site includes heart news, a lengthy FAQs section, related heart links, and a section to post your own experiences with heart problems.

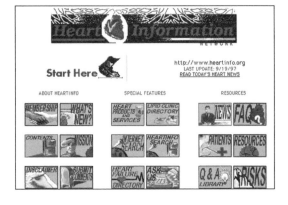

Hypertension Network

http://www.bloodpressure.com/

The Hypertension Network provides cardiovascular information about blood pressure in the **Question and Answer (Q & A)** section. Topics covered are basic facts, lifestyle, treatment, and home monitoring. The site also features drug and research news, clinical trial information, and a search engine for tracking down doctors who specialize in treating hypertension.

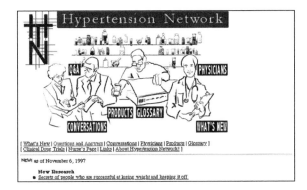

Jon's Place

http://www.geocities.com/Heartland/Hills/2571/jonsplace.htm

Jon's Place provides heart information for all those who have heart failure or know someone who does. The site includes everything from coping with heart failure to diet information.

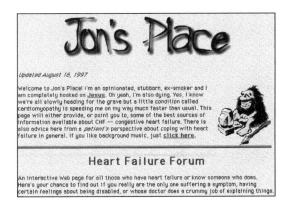

The National Heart, Lung, and Blood Institute

http://www.nhlbi.nih.gov/nhlbi/nhlbi.htm

The National Heart, Lung, and Blood Institute offers a collection of online articles about health information for cardiovascular, lung, blood, and sleep disorders. The articles cover topics ranging from obesity and cholesterol to high blood pressure.

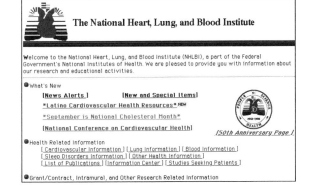

Stroke

http://www.clearlight.com/~morph/present/strk0.htm

Stroke is an online manual for strokes with a brief history and epidemiology, etiology, the clinical picture, acute care, and rehabilitation.

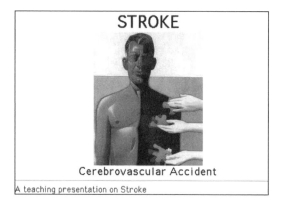

Stroke and Cerebrovascular Disease

http://www-med.stanford.edu/school/stroke/

Stroke and Cerebrovascular Disease is an online guide for patients and their families offered by the Stanford Stroke Center. This handbook provides information on the different types of stroke, the warning signs and risk factors for stroke, suggestions to reduce risk for stroke, and an overview of the techniques for diagnosis and treatment.

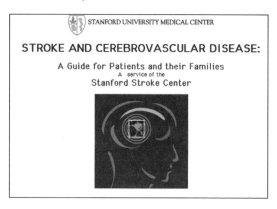

The Women's Heart Disease and Stroke Quiz

http://www.hsf.ca/test/4quiz.htm

The Women's Heart Disease and Stroke Quiz, from the Heart and Stroke Foundation of Canada, is designed to test and increase women's knowledge of their risk for heart disease and stroke. Links at the end of the quiz provide more information about risk factors you can control (e.g., cholesterol, high blood pressure, smoking, stress), as well as three broad questions women should ask their doctors to help identify and lower risk for these diseases.

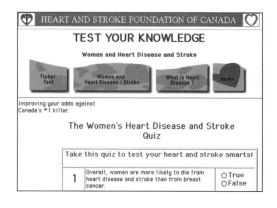

CHRONIC FATIGUE SYNDROME

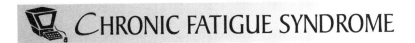

The CFS Home Page

http://www.cdc.gov/ncidod/diseases/cfs/cfshome.htm

The CFS Home Page, from the Centers for
Disease Control and Prevention (CDC),
provides facts about chronic fatigue syndrome
(CFS), information about support groups, and
summaries of CDC publications on CFS.

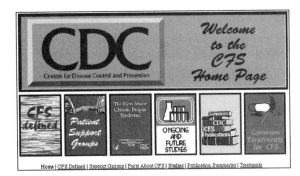

The Cheney Clinic Information Services

http://www.fnmedcenter.com/ccis/

The Cheney Clinic Information Services features
an online consultation and information service for
chronic fatigue syndrome (CFS). In addition, the
site offers an interactive test for CFS, FAQs,
interactive pharmaceutical and supplement
databases, and monthly e-mail subscription
seminars.

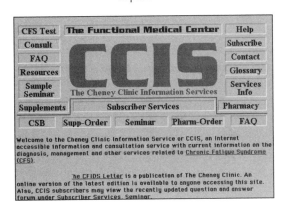

Chronic Fatigue Syndrome/ Myalgic Encephalomyelitis

http://www.cais.com/cfs-news/

The Chronic Fatigue Syndrome/Myalgic Encephalomyelitis Web site, created by Roger Burns, provides a large collection of links to chronic fatigue syndrome resources on the Internet.

Chronic Fatigue Syndrome / Myalgic encephalomyelitis

[Quick Index]   [General info about CFS]   [Frequently Asked Questions]

- News about CFS / M.E.
- Information files, and resources for doctors
- Discussion groups
- CFS-related web pages
- Gateway to the Rest of the World

This web page is provided by Roger Burns. See also the introductory essays about CFS. There is an alternate site for this page at http://www.alternatives.com/cfs-news/index.htm. Latest version: 97/07/21

NEWS   [CFS-NEWS]
   [QUICK Index]

Due to compatibility problems, the CFS-NEWS TICKER has been discontinued for the time being. However, the latest news about CFS can be found in the LATEST NEWS segment of the CFS-NEWS page.

YPWCNet's Info Source

http://www.ypwcnet.org/resource/

YPWCnet's Info Source contains information about childhood diseases, including chronic fatigue syndrome. The site also offers toll-free numbers in the **Charitable Organizations** section and a rich variety of pediatric sites in the **Children's Health** section.

YPWCNET'S
INFO SOURCE

The main idea of our site revolves around sick kids with Chronic Fatigue Syndrome, but that does not mean that we are blind to all the other diseases. The truth is, CFS has many things in common with other diseases, and some of these on the list below are not related at all. But because of the tie that we share, no matter what the reason for that is, our site is like a "sister site" to other sick kids sites.

This page has what we hope to be a very complete list of sites all over the net on all different diseases, places for more information, newsgroups, mailing lists etc. If you have something to contribute, please contact us, we are trying to build a comprehensive list, but it is going to take some time, and we could use all the help we can get.

Charitable Organizations - Toll Free Number Listing

Children's Health - List of Pediatric Sites

- AIDS and HIV
- Attention Deficit Disorder (ADD)
- Cancer
- Chronic Fatigue and Immune Dysfunction Syndrome (CFIDS/CFS/ME)
- Epilepsy

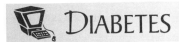

DIABETES

American Diabetes Association

http://www.diabetes.org

The American Diabetes Association site provides an extensive collection of articles, presenting reliable diabetes information under headings such as Living with Diabetes, Legislation, Sex, Nutrition and Fitness, Pregnancy, and Medical Treatment. In addition, the site includes issues of the Association's *Diabetes Forecast* magazine, related links to diabetes sites, an interactive "Are You at Risk?" diabetes test, and daily recipes.

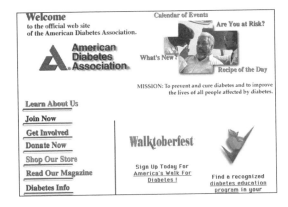

Canadian Diabetes Association

http://www.diabetes.ca/

The Canadian Diabetes Association Web site, available in English and French, provides useful information for people who have diabetes and anyone with an interest in this disease. Topics include What Is Diabetes, Diabetes and Driving, and Diabetes and Impotence. The site also has an interactive diabetes quiz.

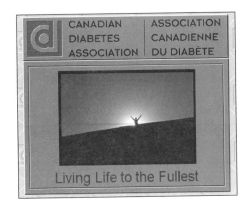

Children with Diabetes

http://www.castleweb.com/diabetes

Children with Diabetes tells you everything you might want to know about diabetes, whether in children or in adults, briefly, concisely, and in language that is easy to understand. Naturally, many articles discuss diet, but other offerings include diet camps, a diabetes dictionary, related Web sites, and a search tool.

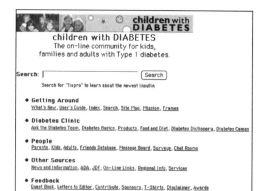

The Diabetes Homepage

http://www.nd.edu/~npippin/diabetes/diabetes.html

The Diabetes Homepage, created and maintained by Harry J. Howisen, provides consumer resources about diabetes to dispel common misconceptions surrounding diabetes. Topics include Managing Your Diabetes, Diabetes Information, and Virtual Diabetic Games.

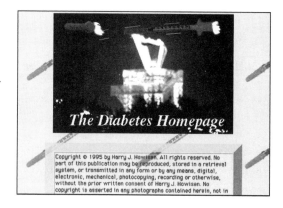

Diabetes Mall

http://www.diabetesnet.com/

The Diabetes Mall provides patient information on exercise, diet, weight loss, and useful links to diabetes sites. The site includes supplies, books, and services for effectively managing diabetes.

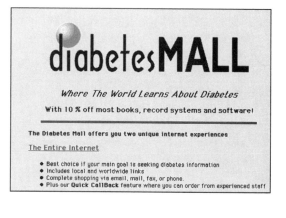

Diabetes Monitor

http://www.mdcc.com/

The Diabetes Monitor provides consumer-oriented information about diabetes in three ways: (1) a listing of resources on the Internet, (2) Diabetes Mentor, a large and eclectic collection of articles, handouts, and announcements, and (3) a search tool.

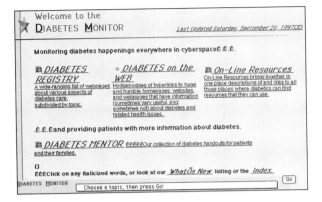

The Family's Guide to Diabetes

http://diabetes.cbyc.com/

The Family's Guide to Diabetes contains a variety of topics providing information on diabetes. The topics include a child's diabetes survey, information on hypoglycemia and hyperglycemia, autobiographical stories, and other related diabetes pages.

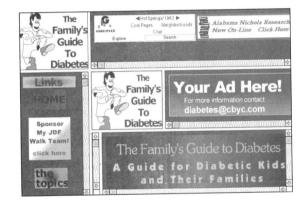

Joslin Diabetes Center

http://www.joslin.harvard.edu/

Joslin Diabetes Center, at Harvard University, provides an extensive online diabetes library. Topics include general facts and information, prevention of diabetes, high blood sugar, a diabetes checklist, nutrition information, and others.

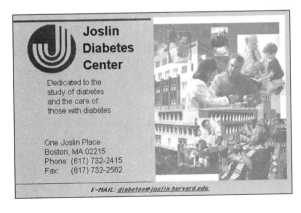

Juvenile Diabetes Foundation International

http://www.jdfcure.com/

The Juvenile Diabetes Foundation International, a non-profit health agency, supports and funds diabetes research. The site contains a mail-order pharmacy, information and online publications about diabetes, and related sites.

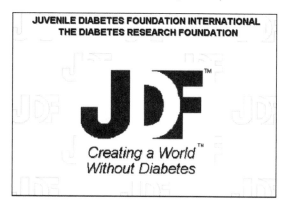

Managing Your Diabetes

http://www.lilly.com/diabetes/

Managing Your Diabetes, from Lilly, is divided into three areas: (1) an education center, which provides specific information about the nature of diabetes, the use of insulin, and the role of nutrition; (2) a question and answer category, which provides answers to FAQs; and (3) a search tool for accessing further information.

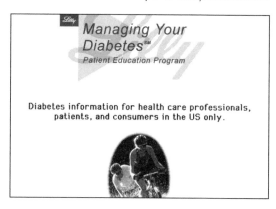

Patient Information on Diabetes

http://www.niddk.nih.gov/diabetesdocs.html

Patient Information on Diabetes, from the National Institute of Diabetes and Digestive and Kidney Diseases (NIDDK) home page, contains a collection of patient information articles on diabetes. Among the topics are noninsulin-dependent diabetes, diabetic eye disease, diabetes in African Americans, diabetic neuropathy, and diabetes recipes and cookbooks.

Personal Diabetes Center

http://www.medilife.com/medilife/diabetes/

Personal Diabetes Center, from MediLife, provides a rich assortment of information about diabetes for patients and their families in five categories: (1) Interactive Tests, where you visit the testing clinic to determine your stress level, your risk of developing heart disease over the next ten years, your fitness level, and your risk of developing diabetes in the future; (2) Ask the Educator, where you can pose questions you may have about diabetes; (3) Diabetes Health University, which features courses that address aspects of preventing, dealing with, and understanding diabetes; (4) Library of Reference Materials, which has over 250 articles addressing a wide array of diabetes issues; and (5) Diabetes Yellow Pages, which includes over 50 external links to online diabetes resources.

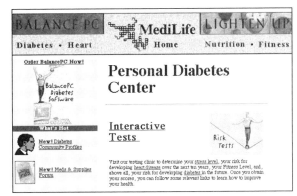

Reducing the Burden of Diabetes

http://www.cdc.gov/nccdphp/ddt/ddthome.htm

Reducing the Burden of Diabetes, the Centers for Disease Control and Prevention (CDC) diabetes home page, focuses on health promotion, disease prevention, and treatment strategies. The site contains articles and fact sheets, information from each state, FAQs, and related diabetes links.

FOOT AND ANKLE PROBLEMS

The American Podiatric Medical Association

http://www.apma.org/

The American Podiatric Medical Association, the leading podiatric medical association, provides a wealth of resources about foot afflictions and infirmities and their treatments. The **Foot Information** section has health topics ranging from aging to women's feet and a list of sports-related foot care topics.

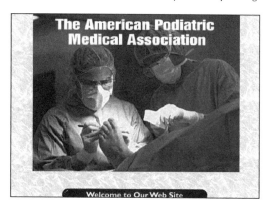

Center for Podiatric Information

http://www.infowest.com/podiatry/

The Center for Podiatric Information provides information about foot problems in two general areas: (1) general foot care (calluses, corns, bunions, etc.) and (2) medical information (heel spurs and other more serious conditions). The site includes resources for diagnosing and treating foot and ankle disorders.

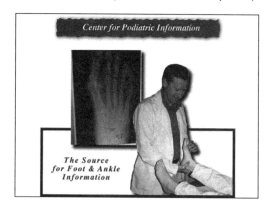

Foot & Ankle Affiliates of Central NJ

http://inetserv1.medicalexchange.com/podiatry/faa/topics.html

Foot & Ankle Affiliates of Central NJ provides consumer information on a variety of common foot and ankle disorders.

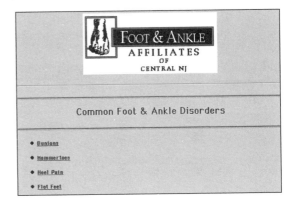

Foot & Ankle Web Index

http://www.footandankle.com

Foot & Ankle Web Index offers numerous podiatry resources, including patient information about foot ailments, a referral service for patients, and links to a wealth of podiatry-related information on the Internet.

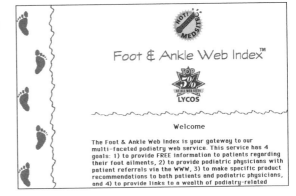

Foot Web

http://www.footweb.com/

Foot Web has been created as a network and information resource for all foot problems and conditions. The site includes a podiatry service that connects you with foot specialists around the world and an information source where all your foot problem questions on flat feet, bunions, corns, arthritis, foot odor, surgery, and more are answered.

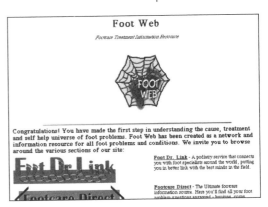

Podiatry Online

http://207.158.247.38/footman/pdonline.html

Podiatry Online provides a comprehensive collection of podiatry sites, including those dealing with common foot problems. In addition, there are sites for live chat, articles from *Podiatry Today Magazine,* an e-mail newsletter, and a list of podiatrists' offices.

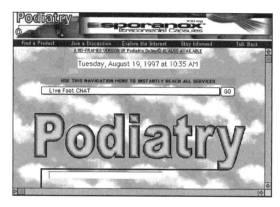

Podiatry Quick Reference

http://pages.ripco.com:8080/~haddon/

Podiatry Quick Reference provides a comprehensive collection of podiatry sites.

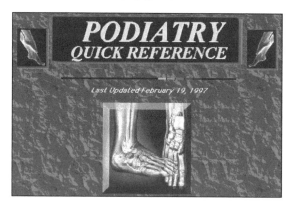

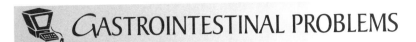 GASTROINTESTINAL PROBLEMS

Columbia University Gastroenterology Web

http://cpmcnet.columbia.edu/dept/gi/

The Columbia University Gastroenterology Web page provides a collection of articles on 13 medical conditions in the **Information on Specific Diseases.** The conditions include cholera, constipation, gallstones, hemorrhoids, and liver disease. All articles address the condition in general, then discuss symptoms, diagnosis, treatment, and prevention.

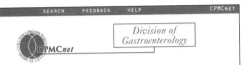

Crohn's Disease Web Page

http://members.aol.com/bospol/homepage/crohns.htm

The Crohn's Disease Web Page is a comprehensive resource with general information, illustrations, articles, and answers to FAQs about Crohn's disease. The site includes extensive related links and medical search tools.

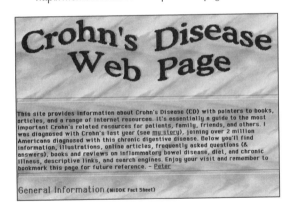

Gastro Online

http://www.gastronews.com/

Gastro Online provides comprehensive gastrointestinal tract and liver resources for professionals and nonprofessionals. The **Lay Public** area contains articles, support groups, a bulletin board for posting questions to specialists, and a Web section with related sites.

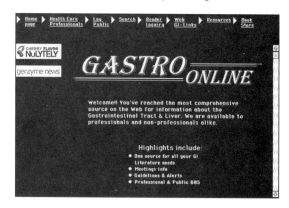

The Kidney Stone Web Site

http://members.aol.com/rogerbaxtr/pages/Kidney_Stone_Page.html

The Kidney Stone Web Site has comprehensive information on diagnosing, treating, and preventing kidney stones.

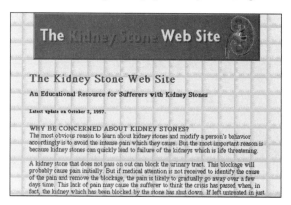

Patient Information on Digestive Diseases

http://www.niddk.nih.gov/digestivedocs.html

Patient Information on Digestive Diseases, from the National Institute of Diabetes and Digestive and Kidney Diseases (NIDDK) home page, contains a collection of patient information articles on digestive diseases and disorders. Among the topics are constipation, Crohn's disease, gallstones, heartburn, lactose intolerance, and ulcerative colitis.

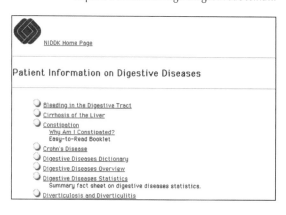

Temple University School of Medicine Gastroenterology Section

http://www.temple.edu/gisection/

Temple University School of Medicine Gastroenterology Section provides useful resources for patients, physicians, and researchers. The patient information topics range from "How your digestive system works" to "cirrhosis of the liver." The patient information also offers another collection of articles on digestive diseases from the National Institute of Diabetes and Digestive and Kidney Diseases (NIDDK).

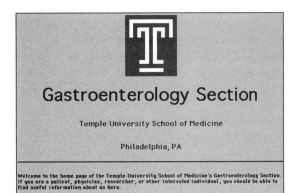

Gastroenterology Section

Temple University School of Medicine

Philadelphia, PA

Welcome to the home page of the Temple University School of Medicine's Gastroenterology Section. If you are a patient, physician, researcher, or other interested individual, you should be able to find useful information about us here.

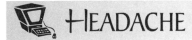 HEADACHE

American Council for Headache Education

http://www.achenet.org/

The American Council for Headache Education (ACHE) provides headache education and information for headache sufferers and their families. ACHE's support group network meets in over 50 cities and online via the Internet and online commercial services such as America On Line, CompuServe, and Prodigy.

American Council for Headache Education

A Non-Profit Physician-Patient Partnership to Advance Headache Prevention and Treatment.

- About ACHE
- Understanding Headache
- Prevention & Treatment
- Members Only
- Join ACHE
- Physician Referrals

This site looks best and is most effective when viewed with the Netscape or Microsoft Internet browsers. If you are using AOL, Prodigy, CompuServe, Mosaic or another browser, what you see here (*and on other sites*) may not include all of the pictures or appear in a distorted layout, and you may have trouble with the members only forums and on-line forms.

The Diagnosis and Treatment of Headache and Migraine

http://www.hscsyr.edu/~haasd/

The Diagnosis and Treatment of Headache and Migraine, by Dr. David C. Haas, serves as a primer for treating and diagnosing the major types of headaches.

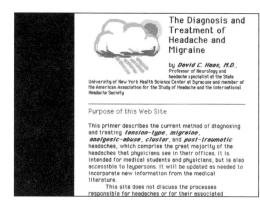

The Head Pain Primer

http://www.thriveonline.com/thrive/health/headache.primer.html

The Head Pain Primer, provided by Thrive Online, contains information and fact sheets on the major headache types, including migraine, cluster, and tension.

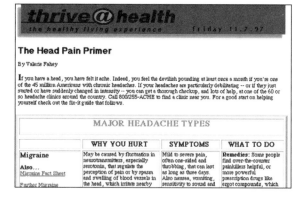

Headache Advice for Patients

http://www.bayer.com/Bayer2/EAuswahl.html

Headache Advice for Patients, provided by Bayer Aspirin, is an online questionnaire designed to differentiate between a tension-type headache and a migraine headache.

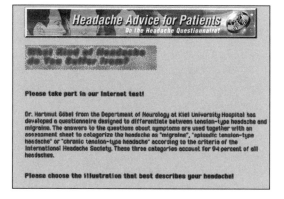

Headache Resource Center

http://www.womenslink.com/health/excedrin/

The Headache Resource Center, sponsored by Excedrin, provides advice on how to better manage headache pain.

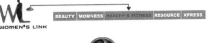
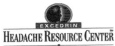

Migraine Resource Center

http://www.migrainehelp.com/

The Migraine Resource Center, a service of GlaxoWellcome, provides a wealth of resources for headache suffers. The site defines a migraine headache, contains a simple self-diagnosis tool to help determine if your headaches are migraine, discusses the common triggers that might bring on a migraine, offers suggestions for coping with a migraine, and includes a list of support services.

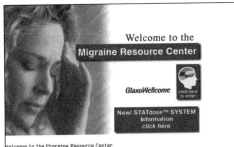

National Headache Foundation

http://www.headaches.org/homepage.htm

The National Headache Foundation home page offers topic sheets for specific headache conditions and sample articles from its quarterly newsletter, *NHF Head Lines.*

Ronda's Migraine Page

http://www.msn.fullfeed.com/~ronda/

Ronda's Migraine Page offers information and resources for sufferers of migraine and other headaches. The site includes an online journal of migraine experiences and concerns posted by migraine sufferers.

Ronda's Migraine Page

What's New

Journal of Sufferers

Help and Support

Definitions

Medicine

Images of Migraine

Advice

Other Resources

Painting by Sean McHone

You Are Not Alone

http://www.softcom.net/users/wavsrus/karen.html

You Are Not Alone, created by Karen Cohen, provides a collection of informative personal chronic pain disorder pages with resources for migraine headaches, fibromyalgia, post-traumatic stress, depression, and endometriosis. The site also includes online medical references to check out your doctor's prescriptions.

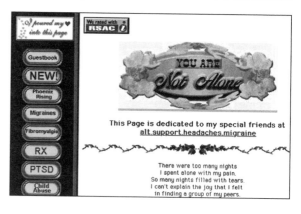

I poured my ♥ into this page

We rated with
RSAC

Guestbook

NEW!

Phoenix Rising

Migraines

Fibromyalgia

RX

PTSD

Child Abuse

YOU ARE Not Alone

This Page is dedicated to my special friends at alt.support.headaches.migraine

There were too many nights
I spent alone with my pain.
So many nights filled with tears.
I can't explain the joy that I felt
in finding a group of my peers.

HIV/AIDS AND OTHER SEXUALLY TRANSMITTED DISEASES

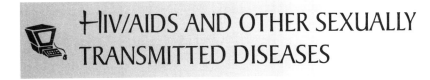

AIDS Education Global Information System

http://www.aegis.com/

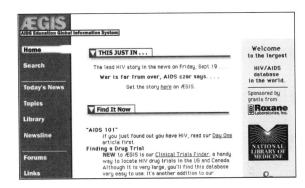

The AIDS Education Global Information System, operated by the Sisters of St. Elizabeth of Hungary, is one of the largest HIV/AIDS databases on the Web. The site provides a powerful search engine to find information about HIV/AIDS from a variety of sources. In addition, the site offers an online library categorized by topic with more than 350,000 publications. Among its other resources is a **Today's News** feature, updated daily, which includes a comprehensive summary of the major HIV/AIDS news articles.

AIDS Research Information Center

http://www.critpath.org/aric/aricinc.htm

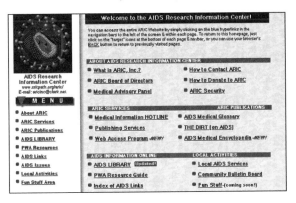

The AIDS Research Information Center provides a large collection of online articles in its **AIDS Information Library,** medical information and mail/phone contacts in the **PWA Resource Guide,** and an **Index of AIDS Links.**

AIDS Virtual Library

http://planetq.com/aidsvl/

The AIDS Virtual Library, updated monthly, contains an immense collection of resources dealing with the social, political, and medical aspects of AIDS, HIV, and related issues. Among the topics are alternative treatments, document archives and indices, health care topics, safer sex information, and links to other AIDS/HIV sites.

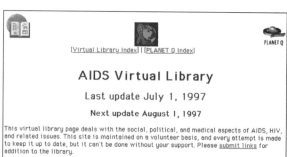

Ask NOAH About: AIDS and HIV

http://www.noah.cuny.edu/aids/aids.html

The New York Online Access to Health (NOAH) is the combined effort of the New York Public Library and other educational institutions. Ask NOAH About: AIDS and HIV contains a well-organized synopsis of AIDS, women and AIDS, treatment for AIDS, AIDS-related illnesses, news media reports, clinical trials, and much more.

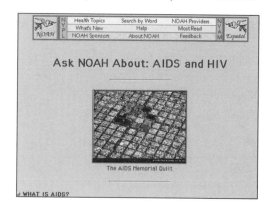

The Body

http://www.thebody.com/

The Body, an AIDS and HIV information resource, provides a collection of AIDS and HIV educational articles on treatment, quality of life, and issues related to the role of government. The site includes a search tool.

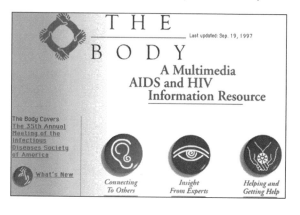

CAT HIV/AIDS Info

http://www.qcfurball.com/cat/aids.html

CAT HIV/AIDS Info, from Children's Animated Television (CAT), has many informative documents regarding AIDS prevention, AIDS testing, condom usage, food safety advice for people with AIDS, caring for people with AIDS, AIDS hotline numbers, an Ask Dr. Rick feature, exercise and HIV, women and AIDS, and needle exchange. The site also includes a list of other AIDS links.

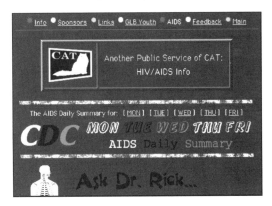

Centers for Disease Control and Prevention National AIDS Clearinghouse

http://www.cdcnac.org/

The Centers for Disease Control and Prevention (CDC) National AIDS Clearinghouse provides a wealth of online HIV/AIDS and sexually transmitted diseases (STDs) resources, including published reports, news, and research findings that focus on education and prevention. The site includes searchable databases and related links.

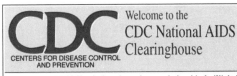

Department of STD Control

http://biomed.nus.sg/dsc/dsc.html

The Department of STD Control, in Singapore, provides illustrated educational information on sexually transmitted diseases (STDs) and AIDS. The site contains topics on genital growths, discharges, rashes, and ulcers.

HIV InfoWeb

http://www.infoweb.org/

HIV InfoWeb contains a variety of HIV/AIDS resources with treatment information and newsletters, agencies or groups, online discussion groups, and a list of premiere HIV/AIDS sites.

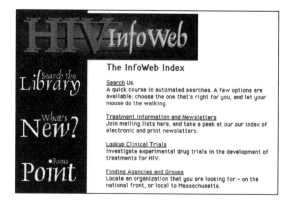

HIV InSite

http://hivinsite.ucsf.edu/

HIV InSite, from the University of California at San Francisco, provides the late-breaking news on AIDS/HIV-related medical research, prevention strategies, legal issues, social issues, and current events. The site also includes state-by-state resources, statistics, and contacts.

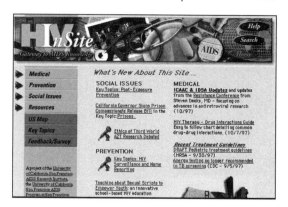

HIV/AIDS Prevention

http://www.cdc.gov/nchstp/hiv_aids/dhap.htm

HIV/AIDS Prevention, from the Centers for Disease Control and Prevention (CDC) Division of HIV/AIDS Prevention, contains links about basic HIV/AIDS information, funding oppor-tunities, AIDS software, AIDS training, demo-graphic slides, press releases, and much more. For the latest information and fact sheets about AIDS, click on **New.**

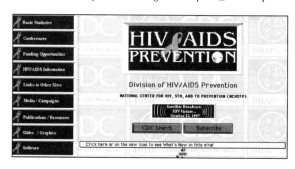

HIV/AIDS Surveillance Data Base

http://www.census.gov/ftp/pub/ipc/www/hivaidsn.html

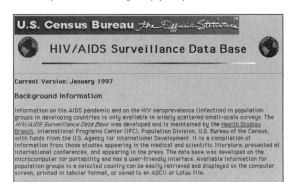

The HIV/AIDS Surveillance Data Base, compiled by the U.S. Census Bureau, contains information of HIV infection in developing countries. It is a compilation, updated semiannually, from studies in the medical and scientific literature, presented at international conferences, and published in the press.

HIV/AIDS Treatment Information Service

http://www.hivatis.org/

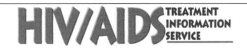

The HIV/AIDS Treatment Information Service provides information about federally approved treatment guidelines for HIV and AIDS. The Service is staffed by bilingual (English and Spanish) health information specialists who answer questions on HIV treatment options. The health information specialists can also refer callers to an extensive network of federal information services and national and community-based organizations for treatment-related information.

HIVemir

http://florey.biosci.uq.oz.au/hiv/HIV_EMIR.html

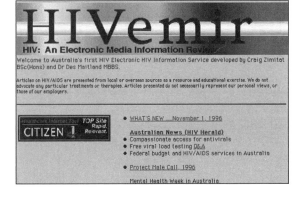

HIVemir, an electronic media information review from Australia, reviews HIV information. Articles include information about HIV/AIDS, fact sheets, clinical trials, community support groups, and other topics.

HIVPositive.com

http://www.HIVpositive.com/

HIVPositive.com provides informative resources about AIDS and HIV for consumers. To learn more about HIV and AIDS, click on **HIV & You,** which includes a glossary.

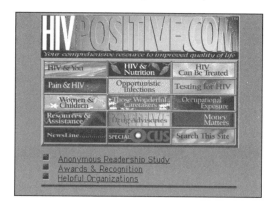

Johns Hopkins AIDS Service

http://www.hopkins-aids.edu/

The Johns Hopkins AIDS Service is a comprehensive, reliable, and timely source of information for HIV/AIDS care providers. Among its online resources is John Bartlett's book, *Medical Management of HIV Infection,* which is a pocket guide to the care and management of patients with HIV.

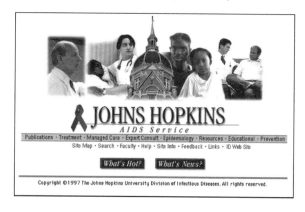

Marty Howard's HIV/AIDS HomePage

http://www.smartlink.net/~martinjh/

Marty Howard's HIV/AIDS HomePage provides a variety of HIV/AIDS resources, educational programs, an autosubscribe area for HIV/AIDS-related mailing lists, a listing of HIV/AIDS-related online "chat type" support groups, Social Security information, and links to related sites.

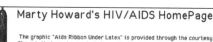

National AIDS Treatment Information Project

http://www.kff.org/archive/aids_hiv/natip/html/

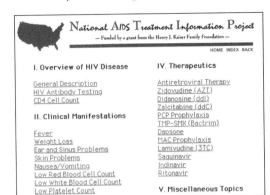

The National AIDS Treatment Information Project, funded by the Henry J. Kaiser Family Foundation, provides information about HIV and AIDS. Topics include an overview of the HIV disease, clinical manifestations, opportunistic diseases, and therapeutics.

The Relationship between the Human Immunodeficiency Virus and the Acquired Immunodeficiency Syndrome

http://math-www.uni-paderborn.de/~axel/aids/etiology.html

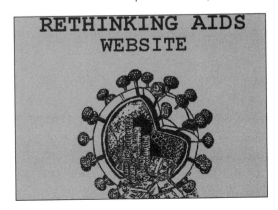

The Relationship between the Human Immunodeficiency Virus and the Acquired Immunodeficiency Syndrome is a significant report published by the National Institutes of Health in September 1995. The research paper, complete with all relevant references, contains the mainstream scientific evidence for a causative role of HIV for AIDS.

Rethinking AIDS Website

http://www.virusmyth.com/aids/

The Rethinking AIDS Website claims that there is another cause of AIDS and even that HIV is not involved. A growing eminent group of biomedical scientists maintain that the cause of AIDS is still unknown. To find these scientists' papers online, click on the **Author Index.**

Sci.med.aids FAQ

http://www.aids.wustl.edu/

Sci.med.aids FAQ contains answers to questions from the sci.med.aids newsgroup members and other AIDS resources. AIDS topics include causes and opportunistic infections, vaccines, treatments or cures, and prevention and education. The site also includes a search tool.

sci.med.aids FAQ

Frequently Asked Questions

Welcome to sci.med.aids, the international newsgroup on the Acquired Immune Deficiency Syndrome ('What is sci.med.aids?'for more details).

This article, called the sci.med.aids "FAQ", answers frequently asked questions about AIDS and the sci.med.aids newsgroup. If you are new to sci.med.aids, please read this FAQ before posting articles or responses. If you are a sci.med.aids veteran, please skim the FAQ occasionally. You may find something new here.

This document is in process. We will continue to update it. Many parts are somewhat out of date. *Please* contribute to the sci.med.aids FAQ. Currently there are some gaping holes. Send suggested changes and additions to us. You don't have to format it: just send it.

Disclaimer: Much of the information here is quoted from other sources. We try to keep things as up to date and accurate as possible. However, we are not responsible for the accuracy of the information contained herein, use the information here at your own risk. Also understand that there may be parts of this FAQ that you may not agree with, or may not feel are accurate. Feel free to point this out to us, but we reserve the right to leave it as it is.

Sexual & Reproductive Health

http://www.ppfa.org/ppfa/lev2-hlt.html

Sexual & Reproductive Health, from the Planned Parenthood Federation of America, provides sexual and reproductive health information on a variety of topics, including AIDS and HIV, herpes, pregnancy and prenatal health, a man's and a woman's guide to sexuality, and commonly asked questions about vaginitis. The site also offers breast cancer and adolescent information, excerpts from *The Planned Parenthood Women's Health Encyclopedia,* and current fact sheets on sexual and reproductive health.

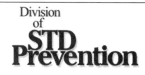

| Info | WhoWeAre | Action | Search | Links | Jobs |

Planned Parenthood®
Federation of America, Inc.

Sexual & Reproductive Health

For information about screening and treatment for sexually transmitted infections (including HIV), pregnancy-related care, or midlife services in your community -- or to make an appointment for counseling, services, or referral -- call toll-free 800/230-PLAN.

Breast Cancer
Be Aware – Learn the Risks –
Protect Yourself & Those You Love
(learn all about breast health on this site)

Topical Information Resources

STD Prevention

http://www.cdc.gov/nchstp/dstd/dstdp.html

STD Prevention, from the Centers for Disease Control and Prevention (CDC) Division of STD Prevention, includes telephone hotline listings to help prevent sexually transmitted diseases (STDs).

Division
of
STD
Prevention

What's New

Publications and Reports
What We Have Learned 1990 - 1995 – A collection of reports concerning research regarding STDs. Read the document on-line or download the Adobe Acrobat file for viewing and/or printing from your computer.

Software
STD*MIS 3.x – Program, report, and documentation files may be accessed and downloaded for current users or those wishing to evaluate **STD*MIS**, a CDC software application that

Tanqueray's American AIDS Rides

http://www.aidsride.org/

Tanqueray's American AIDS Rides provides information on bicycle rides planned to benefit AIDS. There are also highlights of rides from previous years.

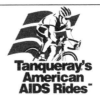

UNAIDS

http://www.unaids.org/highband/index.html

UNAIDS brings the AIDS activites of six United Nations organizations into a single synergistic effort. Services include press releases, fact sheets, epidemiologic data, women and AIDS, AIDS and human rights, World AIDS Day, and information about AIDS conferences.

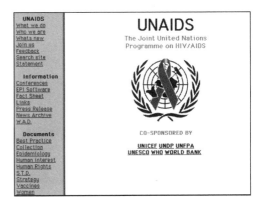

Unspeakable The Naked Truth About STDs

http://www.unspeakable.com/

Unspeakable The Naked Truth About STDs, sponsored by Pfizer, provides a variety of online resources for the prevention and treatment of sexually transmitted diseases (STDs). The site presents an interactive questionnaire, which enables the user to construct a risk profile for contracting an STD, offers a search tool for locating an STD clinic in your geographical area, and makes suggestions for more comfortably discussing the risk of STDs with your partner.

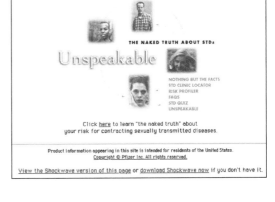

The Virtual Hospital
What You Need to Know About Sexually Transmitted Diseases, HIV Disease, and AIDS

http://www.vh.org/Patients/IHB/IntMed/Infectious/STDs/STDAIDS.html

What You Need to Know About Sexually Transmitted Diseases, HIV Disease, and AIDS provides topical information on the most common sexually transmitted diseases (STDs): how you get one, how it's transmitted, what it looks like and what the symptoms are, how you get tested, and what will happen to you if you don't get treatment. The site also includes articles on the proper use of a condom and HIV disease.

The Virtual Hospital®
the apprentice's assistant™

Iowa Health Book: Infectious Diseases

What You Need to Know About Sexually Transmitted Diseases, HIV Disease, and AIDS

Burroughs Wellcome Co.
Peer Review Status: Externally reviewed by Burroughs Wellcome Co.

Distributed at The American Medical Association Conference on Sexually Transmitted Diseases: Risk Assessment, Diagnosis, and Treatment

About STDs

"STDs" (sexually transmitted diseases) is a broad term that refers to as many as 20 different sicknesses, all of them transmitted by sex – usually through the exchange of body fluids such as semen, vaginal fluid, and blood. STDs can also be given by mothers to their babies. You can get some STDs, such as herpes, by kissing and caressing or close contact with infected areas – not just intercourse. Some STDs just make you feel uncomfortable. Some are more dangerous – if left untreated, they can cause permanent damage that leaves you blind, brain-damaged, or unable to have children. One, HIV (human immunodeficiency virus) disease, often leads to AIDS (acquired

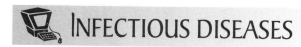

INFECTIOUS DISEASES

Café Herpé

http://www.cafeherpe.com/

Café Herpé, sponsored by SmithKline Beecham, provides a variety of resources about genital herpes. You can play an interactive Virus Trap quiz and answer the question of the week, read past answers to quizzes, learn about genital herpes and other related topics in the lounge, find information about virology in the buffet, take an awareness quiz, or join a newsgroup in the terrace.

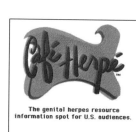

The genital herpes resource information spot for U.S. audiences.

※ Check out the <u>Virus Trap</u>– our new knowledge game.

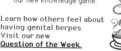
Learn how others feel about having genital herpes. Visit our new **Question of the Week.**

Reading Lounge

Everything you've wanted to know about <u>genital herpes</u> but were afraid to ask. Also, be sure to peruse our <u>gallery</u> of romantic art.

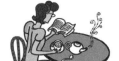
The Buffet

Get the Flu Shot, Not the Flu

http://fightflu.hcfa.gov/

Get the Flu Shot, Not the Flu, prepared in English and Spanish by U.S. Department of Health and Human Services, provides answers to questions about influenza (flu).

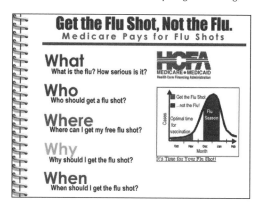

Hepatitis B Virus (HBV) Overview

http://www.hon.ch/Library/Theme/Hepatitis/

Hepatitis B Virus (HBV) Overview is an online version of Stuart Millinship's work on the hepatitis B virus. Click on the **Full Table of Contents** to view this Web version provided by Health On the Net Foundation.

Hepatitis Branch

http://www.cdc.gov/ncidod/diseases/hepatitis/hepatitis.htm

Hepatitis Branch, sponsored by the Centers for Disease Control and Prevention (CDC), contains fact sheets and an online slide set with a multimedia presentation of the epidemiology and prevention of viral hepatitis A through E.

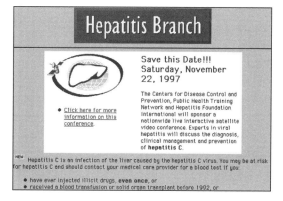

Hepatitis Zone

http://www.hep-help.com/

Hepatitis Zone, from Schering-Plough, provides basic information about hepatitis A, B, and C and understanding your liver.

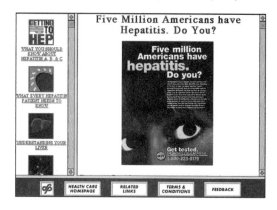

Herpes Advice Center

http://www.advicecenter.com/

Herpes Advice Center provides a wealth of information about herpes symptoms, treatment, transmission, and prevention, and management of herpes in pregnancy in the FAQ section. In addition, the site includes related resources and links.

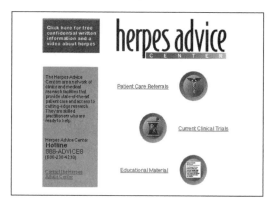

The Herpes Home Page

http://www.racoon.com/herpes/

The Herpes Home Page contains articles with information about this infectious disease, its treatment, the latest research about vaccines, and support groups.

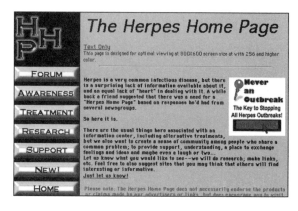

Herpes Zone

http://www.herpeszone.com/

Herpes Zone is a comprehensive resource that includes an introductory slide show, information about living and coping with herpes, questions and answers, a complete glossary, and related links to herpes sites.

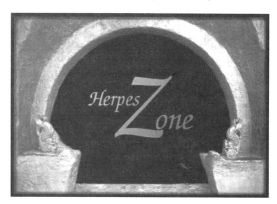

Infectious Disease WebLink

http://pages.prodigy.net/pdeziel/

Infectious Disease WebLink is a comprehensive listing of infectious diseases and related resources available on the Internet. Access to the page is free of charge and the site is updated regularly.

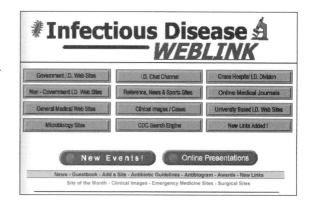

The National Center for Infectious Diseases

http://www.cdc.gov/ncidod/ncid.htm

The National Center for Infectious Diseases, a federal agency of the Centers for Disease Control and Prevention (CDC), contains extensive information on prevention, illness, disability, and death caused by infectious diseases in the United States and around the world. Topics include a list of diseases, travelers' health, emerging infectious diseases, electronic publications collection, and others.

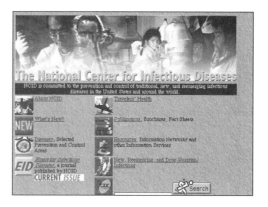

National Coalition for Adult Immunization

http://www.medscape.com/Affiliates/NCAI/

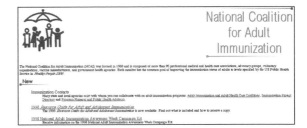

The National Coalition for Adult Immunization provides a variety of online immunization resources. The site includes the recommended adolescent and adult immunization schedules and a library of infectious disease fact sheets.

National Immunization Program

http://www.cdc.gov/nip/

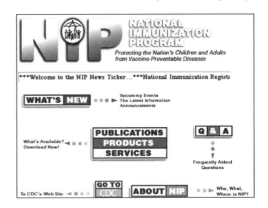

The National Immunization Program (NIP), from the Centers for Disease Control and Prevention (CDC), protects the nation's children and adults from vaccine-preventable diseases. For consumer immunization information for a variety of diseases, select **Frequently Asked Questions** and click on **General Q & A.**

Outbreak

http://www.outbreak.org/

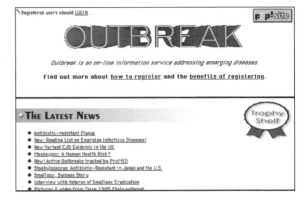

Outbreak is an online information service that keeps track of emerging infectious diseases. The site contains in-depth coverage of ebola, smallpox, malaria, and other diseases and also provides a worldwide collaborative database for collecting information about possible disease outbreaks.

The People's Plague Online

http://www.pbs.org/ppol/

The People's Plague Online, a companion to the public television program, presents an American chronicle of our history with tuberculosis and our ongoing fight against this deadly disease. For a list of quality tuberculosis sites, click on **Tuberculosis Resources.** The site also offers an interactive quiz about tuberculosis and audio and video excerpts from the program.

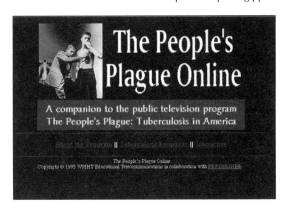

Tuberculosis Resources

http://www.cpmc.columbia.edu/tbcpp/

Tuberculosis Resources, from the Columbia University Department of Medical Informatics, contains online patient information pamphlets on detection, prevention, and cure of tuberculosis. The site also provides an extensive list of other tuberculosis sites.

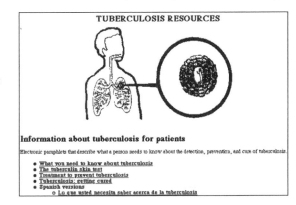

Yahoo! Directory of Infectious Diseases and Conditions

http://www.yahoo.com/Health/Diseases_and_Conditions/
Infectious_Diseases/

Yahoo! offers a comprehensive directory of infectious disease sites ranging from AIDS and HIV to yellow fever.

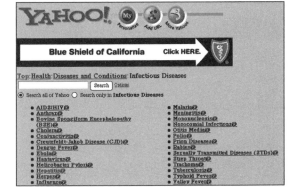

ORTHOPAEDIC PROBLEMS

American Academy of Orthopaedic Surgeons On-Line

http://www.aaos.org/

The American Academy of Orthopaedic Surgeons presents AAOS On-Line, a collection of patient education brochures in the public information section, assistance in finding a surgeon, and medical sites of interest to the consumer.

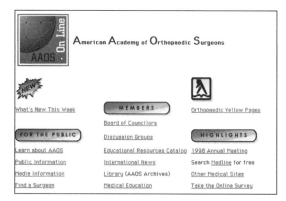

American College of Sports Medicine Online

http://www.a1.com/sportsmed/

The American College of Sports Medicine presents ACSM Online, the largest sports medicine and exercise science organization in the world. The site offers information and advice on sports-related injuries.

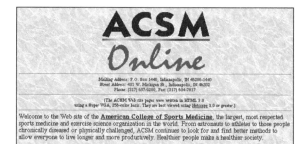

The American Orthopaedic Society for Sports Medicine

http://www.sportsmed.org/

The American Orthopaedic Society for Sports Medicine provides information on fitness and on the treatment, rehabilitation, and prevention of athletic injuries. The site includes a membership directory of 12,000 orthopaedic surgeons, sports medicine information, an ask the sports doctor feature, and links to related societies.

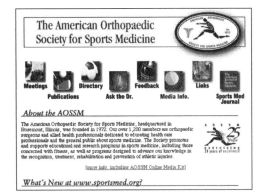

The Center for Orthopaedics and Sports Medicine

http://www.arthroscopy.com/

The Center for Orthopaedics and Sports Medicine provides information on the treatment of sports-related injuries for the upper and lower extremities. Injuries include ACL and meniscal injuries, rotator cuff disorders, and carpal tunnel syndrome.

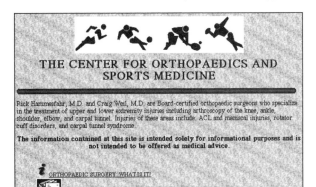

Hand Surgery

http://www.handsurgery.com/

Hand Surgery, from Southeastern Hand Center, provides treatment information on the hand and upper extremity conditions, including carpal tunnel syndrome, trigger fingers, ganglions, and arthritis.

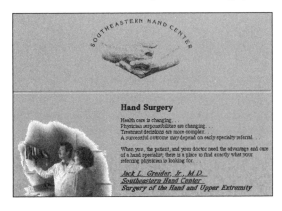

Health & Fitness

http://espnet.sportszone.com/editors/health/

Health & Fitness, from ESPN SportsZone and presented by Columbia Healthcare Corporation, provides sports medicine articles for health and fitness.

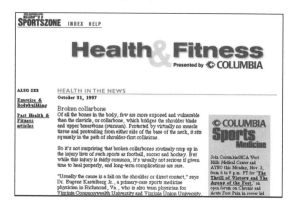

MMG Reference Library

http://www.sechrest.com/mmg/reflib.html

The Medical Multimedia Group (MMG) Reference Library contains a list of patients' guides to a variety of medical problems for carpal tunnel syndrome, low back pain, the knee, trauma disorders, the shoulder, and the foot and the ankle. Each medical problem includes an anatomical description.

Orthopaedic Links Patient Information Page

http://www.netshop.net/~cloughs/orthpat.html

The Orthopaedic Links Patient Information Page provides a variety of patient handouts ranging from amputations and back pain to rheumatoid arthritis.

Orthopaedic Resident's CyberLink LaunchPad

http://www.telusplanet.net/public/jasmith/

Orthopaedic Resident's CyberLink LaunchPad contains a comprehensive collection of orthopaedic resources, including online journals and articles, libraries, search engines, newsgroups, mailing lists, and related medical sites.

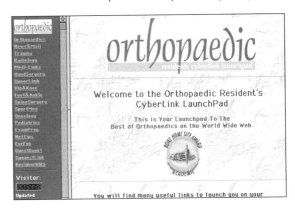

Osteoporosis and Related Bone Diseases

http://www.osteo.org

Osteoporosis and Related Bone Diseases, from the National Resource Center, provides a wealth of information about metabolic bone diseases, including clinical studies, news releases, and the latest research findings. The site offers prevention, early detection, and treatment information on Paget's disease, osteoporosis in men, osteogenesis imperfecta, and hyperparathyroidism.

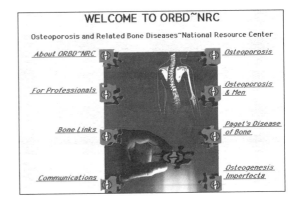

The Physician and SportsMedicine Personal Health

http://www.physsportsmed.com/personal.htm

The Physician and SportsMedicine Personal Health, a peer-reviewed monthly journal, provides a collection of personal health articles on exercise, nutrition, injury prevention, and rehabilitation for the active individual.

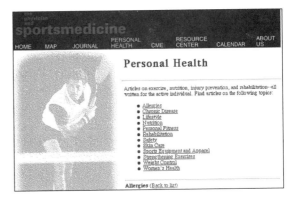

The Virtual Hospital
Patient Information

http://www.vh.org/Patients/IHB/Ortho/Ortho.html

Patient Information contains a collection of online orthopaedic resources ranging from Alcohol and Drugs Can Be Quite a Trip to Total Hip Replacement.

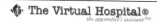

Wheeless' Textbook of Orthopaedics

http://www.medmedia.com/

The Wheeless' Textbook of Orthopaedics contains reliable and authoritative information on a variety of orthopaedic problems ranging from fractures to rickets. The articles are well written and illustrated. For an alphabetical index of topics, click on **Main Menu.**

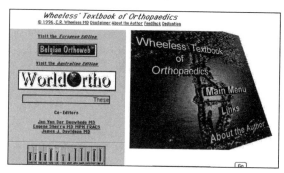

SKIN CARE AND SKIN CONDITIONS

AcneNet

http://www.derm-infonet.com/acnenet/

AcneNet, developed by Roche Laboratories and the American Academy of Dermatology, provides a comprehensive online acne resource with information on a variety of topics.

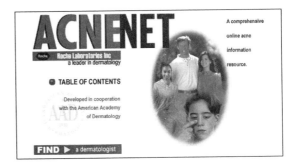

American Academy of Dermatology

http://www.aad.org/

The American Academy of Dermatology offers information for both the public and the medical community. The **Public Information** section includes nearly 45 educational and skin cancer articles that address a variety of skin conditions. In addition, the site supplies the names and addresses of patient advocacy groups and a search tool to help find a dermatologist near you.

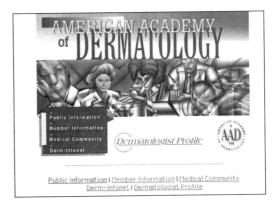

Clinique

http://www.clinique.com/

Clinique offers online skin care resources for both women and men. The **World of Clinique,** written for women, has an ask the expert feature, as well as a library with skin care tips. The **For Men Only** section features shaving and sports skin care tips and a variety of other men's health topics.

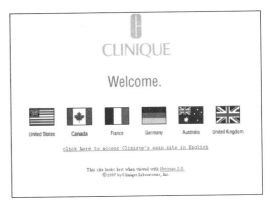

Cosmetic Connection

http://www.kleinman.com/cosmetic/

Cosmetic Connection, by Heather Kleinman, provides weekly tips, advice, and up-to-date information about cosmetic products. You can also ask Heather a question about skin care.

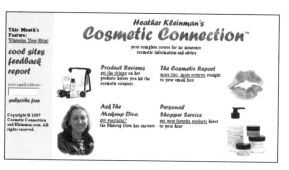

Dermatology & Aesthetic Health Focus.com

http://www.AestheticHealthFocus.com/

Dermatology & Aesthetic Health Focus.com provides a variety of resources about skin care and skin disorders, including skin cancer and habits for a healthy skin.

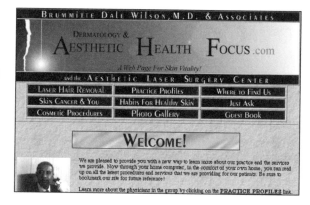

Dermatology Cinema

http://www.skinema.com/

Dermatology Cinema, created by dermatologist Vail Reese, explores the history of skin problems as seen in the movies. From the use of scars and unsightly blemishes in films to denote evil to Robert Redford's real-life skin transformation by overexposure to the sun, Dr. Reese covers the entire history of film.

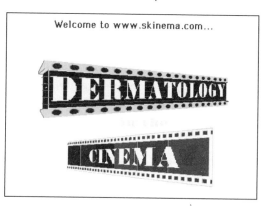

Dermatology Online Atlas

http://www.derma.med.uni-erlangen.de/bilddb/index_e.htm

Dermatology Online Atlas, from Germany, is an alphabetical index of color images and case studies.

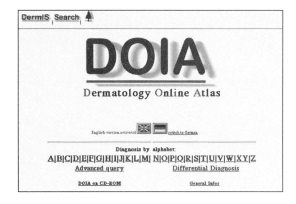

FaceFacts

http://www.facefacts.com/

FaceFacts, sponored by Roche Laboratories, contains an acne information library written in language for teenagers.

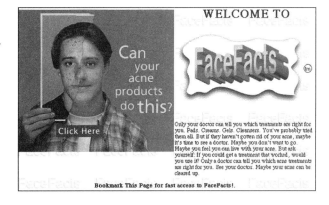

Living With Lupus

http://internet-plaza.net/lupus/

Living With Lupus, the home page of the Lupus Foundation of America, provides an assortment of resources for lupus disease, including commonly asked questions, up-to-date information, a health forum, a list of all local chapters, related links, and Dr. Robert G. Lahita's informative articles on causes, symptoms, testing, and treatment of lupus.

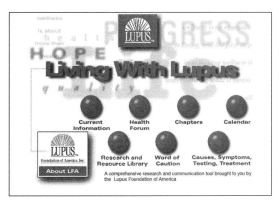

National Cancer Institute PDQ Patient Treatment for Melanoma

PDQ Patient Treatment for Melanoma, prepared by the National Cancer Institute, provides melanoma information. Topics include description, stages, treatment options, and recurrent melanoma.

http://wwwicic.nci.nih.gov/clinpdq/pif/Melanoma_Patient.html

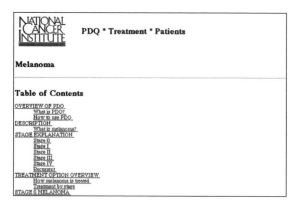

National Psoriasis Foundation

The National Psoriasis Foundation contains a wealth of information on psoriasis and its treatment. Click on the **Index** to find topics, including an ongoing NPF investigation, general psoriasis information and therapies, psoriasis research, NPF services and publications, and other related links.

http://www.psoriasis.org/

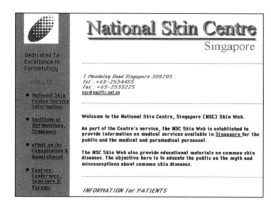

National Skin Centre

The National Skin Centre in Singapore provides information on common skin diseases, as well as the environment and your skin. To find these resources, scroll to Information for Patients and click on either resource on the left.

http://medweb.nus.sg/nsc/nsc.html

Skin Cancer Zone

http://www.skin-cancer.com/

Skin Cancer Zone, sponsored by Schering-Plough, provides a variety of online skin cancer resources. The site contains tips about protecting yourself from the sun's rays, treatment options, skin cancer and melanoma facts, games, related links, and support groups. For an overview of the site, click on **Site Map.**

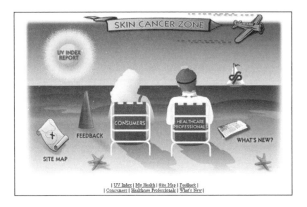

United Scleroderma Foundation

http://www.scleroderma.com/

United Scleroderma Foundation provides information about scleroderma (systemic sclerosis). Scroll to Features to find **Fact Sheet** and other resources.

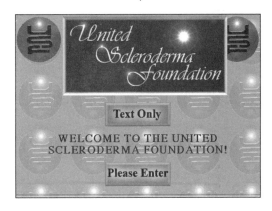

University of Iowa College of Medicine Department of Dermatology

http://tray.dermatology.uiowa.edu/

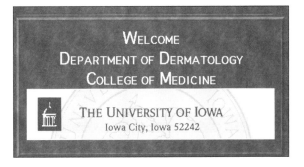

University of Iowa College of Medicine Department of Dermatology provides more than 25 patient information pamphlets on a wide variety of skin conditions. The Skin Cancer News section offers tips for protection against the sun and includes the latest news, research findings, and information about skin cancer. The site also contains a collection of professional and patient mailing lists and a list of patient support groups.

Vertigo Lounge

http://www.clearasil.com/home.html

Vertigo Lounge, from Clearasil and Proctor & Gamble, provides skin care information for teenagers. The site offers daily acne skin care tips, and the **Clearazine** section has a fact vs. fiction quiz, answers from the expert's file, and an online acne 101 course.

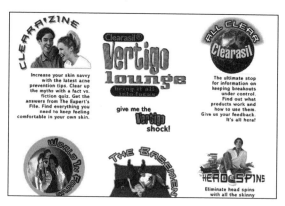

Vitiligo

http://biomed.nus.sg/nsc/vitiligo.html

Vitiligo, from the National Skin Centre in Singapore, contains treatment information and illustrations about this skin disorder. Vitiligo causes white spots on the skin, but is not contagious!

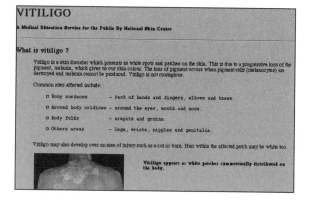

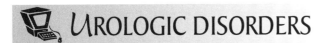

UROLOGIC DISORDERS

Fun With Urology

http://users.alphainfo.com/wlynes/

Fun With Urology, created by Dr. William Lynes, features a variety of genitourinary topics, including prostate cancer, cystitis, interstitial cystitis, urine infection, Peyronie's disease, and many others. The site also includes a section for female topics and a collection of related links.

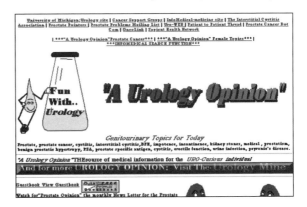

Kidney & Urologic Health

http://www.healthtouch.com/level1/leaflets/106107/106107.htm

Kidney & Urologic Health, from Healthtouch Online, provides a variety of resources on urologic disorders such as urinary tract infections and bladder control, benign prostatic hyperplasia (BPH), penis disorders, and other topics.

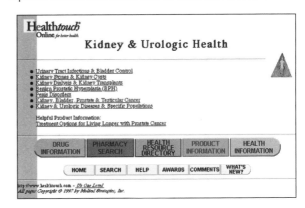

Patient Information on Urologic Diseases

http://www.niddk.nih.gov/UrologicDocs.html

Patient Information on Urologic Diseases, from the National Institute of Diabetes and Digestive and Kidney Diseases (NIDDK), contains a collection of patient information articles on urologic diseases. Topics include bladder control problems in women, impotence, kidney stones in adults, urinary tract infections, and others. The site also includes a list of organizations for referral information on urologic diseases.

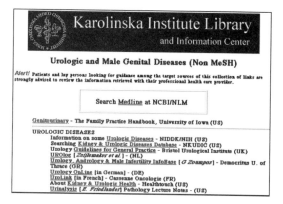

Urologic and Male Genital Diseases

http://www.mic.ki.se/Diseases/c12.html

Urologic and Male Genital Diseases, prepared by the Karolinska Institute Library and Information Center in Stockholm for its Medical Information Center, contains a comprehensive collection of links to infectious and noninfectious urologic and male genital diseases.

Urology Page

http://www.urolog.nl/uropage/uroeng.htm

The Urology Page provides patient information about urologic health problems of the kidneys, urinary bladder, urethra, prostate, penis, and testicles.

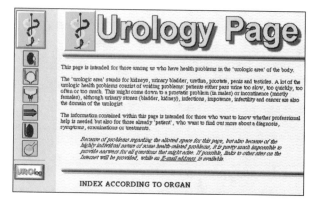

VISUAL DISORDERS AND EYE CARE

American Academy of Ophthalmology

http://www.eyenet.org/public/faqs/faqs.html

The American Academy of Ophthalmology provides detailed answers to FAQs about eye diseases, eye health, and safety. Among the reports are "Cataract Surgery," "Eye Safety for Children," and "AIDS, HIV, and the Eye." The site also offers an Ask the Doctor feature for answers to various eye conditions or users can ask via e-mail about a specific eye problem.

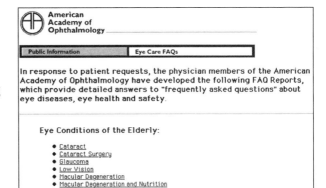

American Society of Cataract & Refractive Surgery, American Society of Ophthalmic Administrators Online

http://www.ascrs.org./

The American Society of Cataract & Refractive Surgery and the American Society of Ophthalmic Administrators provide patient information on cataract and refractive surgery, including the use of lasers.

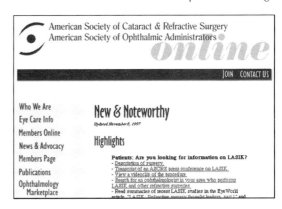

The Children's Hospital of Buffalo Department of Pediatric Ophthalmology

http://www.smbs.buffalo.edu/oph/ped/

The Children's Hospital of Buffalo Department of Pediatric Ophthalmology offers articles written in everyday language about a variety of topics related to ophthalmology and strabismus (misalignment of the eyes).

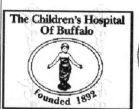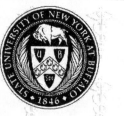

Welcome to The Department of Pediatric Ophthalmology at The Children's Hospital of Buffalo

Columbia Visual Health & Surgical Center

http://www.web-xpress.com/vhsc/

The Columbia Visual Health & Surgical Center provides comprehensive information about eye conditions and diseases, including retinal detachment, macular degeneration, floaters, flashing lights, glaucoma, and astigmatism.

◆ COLUMBIA
Visual Health & Surgical Center

- Columbia Healthcare Corporation
- About Visual Health & Surgical Center
- Professional Staff
- Our Facilities
- Medical Insurance Plans
- Free Community Outreach Programs
- Information About Eye Conditions and Diseases
- Eye Centers of Excellence

EyeNet

http://www.eyenet.org/

EyeNet, from the American Academy of Ophthalmology, provides a wealth of public information about eye care. The site includes a facts and myths quiz, tips for sunglass selection, eye anatomy, low vision resources, and an ask a doctor section. A search tool is also available.

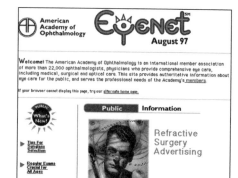

The Eyes Have It

http://www.aoanet.org/aoanet/

The Eyes Have It, presented by the American Optometric Association, includes a series of comprehensive, informative, and easy-to-read articles about eye care, vision conditions, lenses, and eye disease.

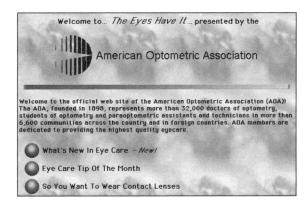

The Foundation Fighting Blindness

http://www.blindness.org/

The Foundation Fighting Blindness provides information about retinitis pigmentosa, age-related macular degeneration, Usher's syndrome, and other loss-of-vision diseases. Each disease includes a description, a treatment, and an inheritance factor.

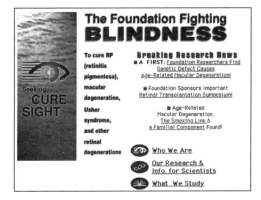

Glaucoma Research Foundation

http://www.glaucoma.org/

The Glaucoma Reasearch Foundation presents comprehensive glaucoma resources, including the online *Gleams Quarterly Newsletter,* with articles and interviews on glaucoma research, as well as an update and information about living with glaucoma. The **Understanding and Living with Glaucoma** resource offers a guide on treatments, therapies, and practical advice for people with glaucoma and their families. The site includes answers to FAQs about glaucoma and a telephone-based support network.

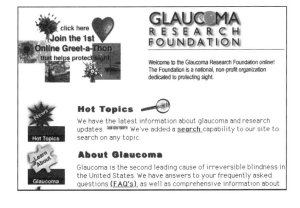

National Eye Institute

http://www.nei.nih.gov/

The National Eye Institute, from the National Institutes of Health, provides information about eye diseases and vision research in the section **Public and Patients.**

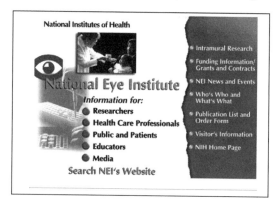

Steen-Hall Eye Institute

http://www.steen-hall.com/

Steen-Hall Eye Institute provides information on refractive surgery, cataract surgery, retinal conditions, plastic and reconstructive surgery, cornea, glaucoma, general eye care, and more.

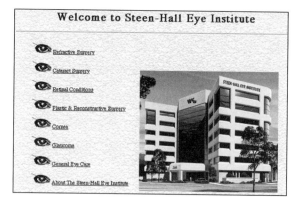

Tri-County Eye Physicians & Surgeons

http://www.med.upenn.edu/~ophth/

Tri-County Eye Physicians & Surgeons is a rich source of information about ophthalmology. The Vision section contains such topics as eye surgery, contact lenses, and permanent eyeliner, while the What's New section offers migraine headache sufferers an article that includes a definition, a discussion of precipitating factors, and a list of possible treatments. The site includes related links and a search tool.

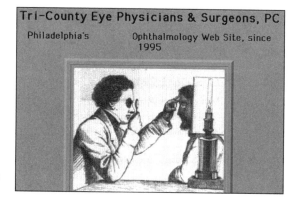

Vision and EyeCare FAQ

http://www.hon.ch/Library/Theme/VisionFaq/

Vision and EyeCare FAQ, compiled by the Health on the Net Foundation, provides a wide range of consumer health information relating to vision and eye care.

Your Medicine Cabinet

CHAPTER **13**

Abbott Laboratories Online

http://www.abbott.com/

Abbott Laboratories Online, a world-reknown pharmaceutical company, contains an **Abbott & Your Health** section with up-to-date information about disease research and medical products for HIV and AIDS, pediatric and adult nutrition, and kidney disease. To test your knowledge about HIV/AIDS, click on the **In the Community** section for an interactive quiz.

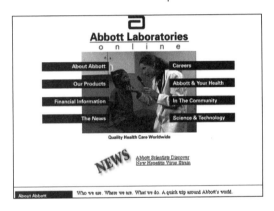

Antimicrobial Use Guidelines

http://www.biostat.wisc.edu/clinsci/amcg/amcg.html

Antimicrobial Use Guidelines, from the University of Wisconsin Hospital, provides treatment information on drugs for various diseases. You can search this guide alphabetically, by drug, by organism, by empiric therapy, by site, or by antimicrobial treatment of an HIV-infected patient.

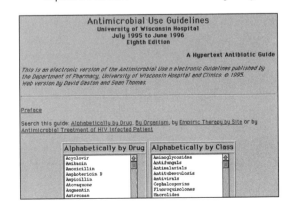

CenterWatch

http://www.centerwatch.com/

CenterWatch provides a collection of approximately 2000 clinical trials for a wide range of diseases, along with contact names for each trial. This service can be used to search for clinical findings, discover physicians and medical centers performing clinical research, and learn about drug therapies recently approved by the Food and Drug Administration (FDA).

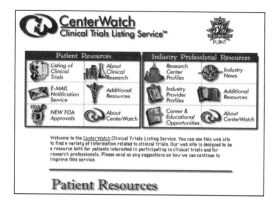

Cutaneous Drug Reaction Database

gopher://gopher.dartmouth.edu:70/11/Research/BioSci/CDRD

The Cutaneous Drug Reaction Database, from Dartmouth University, presents information on drug reactions that produce skin manifestations. It is updated yearly and a search tool is provided.

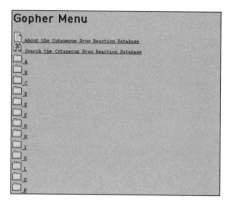

DARE-America.com

http://www.dare-america.com/

DARE-America.com is the Drug Abuse Resistance Education (D.A.R.E.) program designed to keep America's kids drug free. The site contains an online guide for parents and information for kids and teachers. To access this site, click on the lion **Daren.**

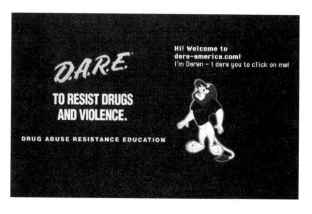

Drug InfoNet

http://www.druginfonet.com/

Drug InfoNet is one-stop shopping for drug information on the Internet. The site features sections on pharmaceuticals and drug interactions, drug manufacturers, health care news, and a "Medizine" about medicines and healthy living. Doctors and pharmacists answer questions regarding health care issues, and you can view the FAQs.

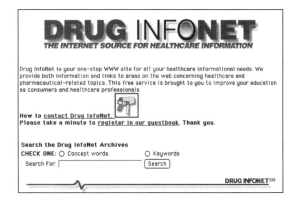

Drug Information

http://www.healthtouch.com/level1/p_dri.htm

Drug Information, from Healthtouch Online, enables you to find information on more than 7000 prescription and over-the-counter medications. Each description includes common uses, the proper ways to use it, its possible side effects, and other helpful information about the drug.

Drug Search from First DataBank

http://www.medscape.com/misc/formdrugs.html

Drug Search from First DataBank is provided by Medscape. Using the searchable drug database, you can find indications, dosing, precautions, and interactions for prescription and over-the-counter medications. In addition, you can search for drugs used to treat diseases. To access this site, click on the **cancel** button and select **register** at the top of the page. It's FREE!

Health A to Z Pharmaceuticals and Drugs

http://www.healthatoz.com/categories/PC.htm

Health A to Z Pharmaceuticals and Drugs is a searchable index of over 150 top-rated pharmaceutical-related sites for professionals and consumers. Categories include prescription drugs, over-the-counter drugs, drug research, and institutes and organizations. The site includes its own search tool.

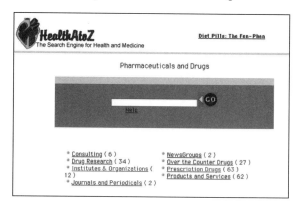

Health Centre Online

http://www.pharmasave.com/

Health Centre Online, from Pharmasave, provides a wealth of consumer health and drug information. The site includes an online bimonthly publication, *Healthnotes,* which answers some of the readers' questions (FAQ), a vitamin and mineral supplement guide, and a natural health supplement guide. In addition, the site updates its archive of related links monthly.

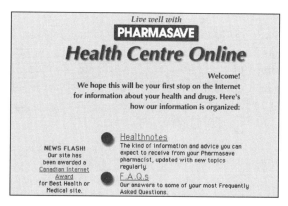

Infomed Drug Guide

http://www.infomed.org/100drugs/

The Infomed Drug Guide, based on a book published by Infomed-Verlags AG, provides online information on 100 commonly used drugs. To find information on the desired drug, click on the drug's name in an alphabetical index.

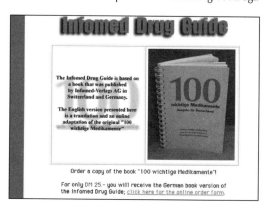

Internet FDA

http://www.fda.gov/

Internet FDA, maintained by the Food and Drug Administration (FDA), contains a variety of food and drug-related resources. Articles contain information about drugs, toxicology, cosmetics, children and tobacco, animal drugs, and other topics.

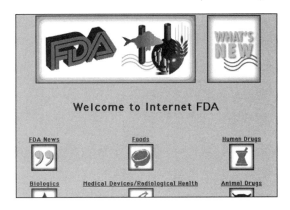

MCW & FMLH Drug Formulary

http://www.intmed.mcw.edu/drug.html

MCW & FMLH Drug Formulary, from the Medical College of Wisconsin (MCW) and Froedtert Memorial Hospital (FMLH), is a drug database in which you can enter a brand-name or generic drug name to make cost comparisons.

Medication Info Search

http://www.cheshire-med.com/services/pharm/med-form.cgi

Medication Info Search, from the Cheshire Medical Center in New Hampshire, lets you search for information on some of the more common prescription medications using keywords or by browsing the A to Z **Medication Index.**

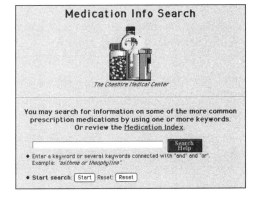

Medicine Box Remedy Corner

http://www.medicinebox.com/remedy.htm

Medicine Box Remedy Corner contains consumer-oriented information about medications, remedies, and other treatments. Medication categories include analgesics, antibiotics, muscle relaxants, and psychotropics.

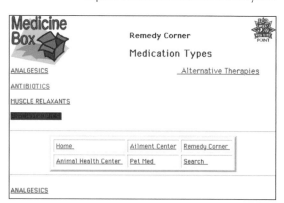

MedicineNet Pharmacy

http://www.MedicineNet.com/mni.asp?ag=Y&li=mni&ArticleKey=81

The MedicineNet Pharmacy provides a huge A to Z listing of major brand-name medications. Medications range from Accupril to Zyrtec.

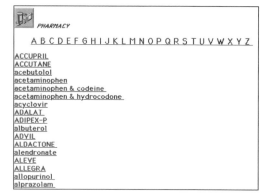

MedPharm

http://www.medfarm.unito.it/pharmaco/pharmaco.html

MedPharm provides a comprehensive collection of pharmaceutical sites on the Internet. Topics include pharmacology, drug industries, drug information, and much more.

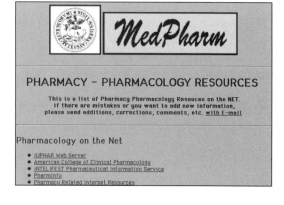

Medsite Navigator Drug Hub

http://www.medsitenavigator.com/searches/drugs.html

The Medsite Navigator Drug Hub is a searchable alphabetical index to clinical pharmacology. You can use the search tool or browse the index. Each drug entry includes its various brand names, a description, and a picture of its chemical composition.

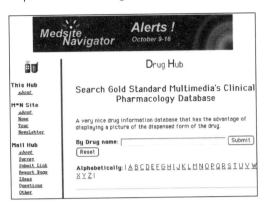

Onhealth Pharmacy

http://www.onhealth.com/onhealth/common/htm/hpphar.htm

Onhealth Pharmacy, from IVI Publishing, has nearly 8000 different types of drugs and drug information ranging from commonsense precautions to taking medicines. The site also includes what every conventional or alternative home medicine chest should contain, how to store various items, and for how long.

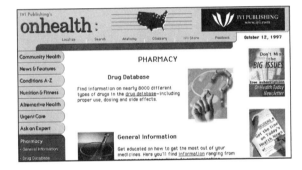

The People's Pharmacy

http://homearts.com/depts/health/kfpeopf1.htm

The People's Pharmacy, from HomeArts, contains hundreds of answers to readers' questions. Use the search engine or click on **Show me all People's Pharmacy columns** to browse a complete list of questions and answers about pharmacy issues. In addition, click on **More People's Pharmacy's** for more health-related information.

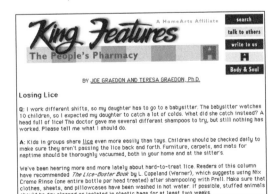

Pharmacology Departments World-Wide

http://www.kfunigraz.ac.at/ekpwww/linkinst.html

Pharmacology Departments World-Wide features a comprehensive list of university pharmacology departments around the world.

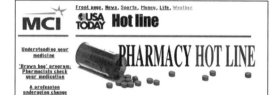

P HARMACOLOGY *D* EPARTMENTS
World-Wide
prepared by the Department of Experimental and Clinical Pharmacology of the University of Graz

North America (US)
United States of America
18.08.97

North America (non-US)
Canada, Mexico, Puerto Rico
01.08.97

South America
Argentina, Brazil, Chile, Venezuela
20.06.97

Europe (EU)
Austria, Belgium, Denmark, Finland, France, Germany, Greece, Ireland, Italy, Netherlands, Portugal, Spain, Sweden, United Kingdom
19.08.97

Europe (non-EU)
Bulgaria, Croatia, Czech Republic, Estonia, Hungary, Lithuania, Macedonia, Malta, Norway, Poland, Romania, Slovakia, Slovenia, Switzerland, Turkey, Yugoslavia
01.07.97

Middle East, Africa
Israel, Jordan, Kuwait, Lebanon, South Africa, United Arab Emirates
08.07.97

Asia
China (Hong Kong), Japan, Malaysia, Russia, Singapore, South Korea, Taiwan, Thailand
01.07.97

Australia and Oceania
Australia, New Zealand
01.08.97

You are welcome to include links to this page in your documents.
However, do not bookmark links to the partial lists since their URL may change.

Pharmacy Hot Line

http://www.usatoday.com/bestbets/bbthu/bbthu11.htm

Pharmacy Hot Line is a service of *USA Today* where you can ask pharmacists from across the country to answer your questions about prescription and over-the-counter drugs. You may call the toll-free number 1-800-422-8728 or use e-mail. In addition, the site provides information about drugs ranging from avoiding dangerous drug interactions to answers from readers' questions.

Front page, News, Sports, Money, Life, Weather

MCI   **USA TODAY Hot line**

PHARMACY HOT LINE

Understanding your medicine

'Brown bag' program: Pharmacists check your medication

A profession undergoing change

Defusing dangerous drug interactions

Some answers to readers' questions

Life front page

Previous hot lines

Avoiding dangerous drug interactions

Pharmacists from across the USA will answer your questions about prescription and over-the-counter drugs. Members of the National Association of Chain Drug Stores will answer phone calls at a toll-free number, 1-800-422-8728, beginning at 9 a.m. ET. You may also ask a question via email by clicking here.

Sample questions:

• I have prescriptions from two different doctors, could the two drugs cause a dangerous interaction?

PharmInfoNet Biotechnology Resources

http://pharminfo.com/

PharmInfoNet Biotechnology Resources features generic and brand-name pharmaceutical information for quick reference on drug interactions, side-effects, and dosage. The site also includes a searchable drug database in the **Drug Information** section, a **Disease Centers** section with links organized by medical specialty and specific medical conditions, a **PharmLinks** section with hundreds of pharmacy-related sites, a **Publication** section with clinical articles, and discussion groups. For an overview of the site, click on **Contents.**

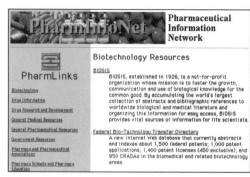

PharmInfoNet   **Pharmaceutical Information Network**

PharmLinks

Biotechnology
Drug Information
Drug Research and Development
General Medical Resources
General Pharmaceutical Resources
Government Resources
Pharmacy and Pharmaceutical Associations
Pharmacy Schools and Pharmacy Education

Biotechnology Resources

BIOSIS
    BIOSIS, established in 1926, is a not-for-profit organization whose mission is to foster the growth, communication and use of biological knowledge for the common good. By accumulating the world's largest collection of abstracts and bibliographic references to worldwide biological and medical literature and organizing this information for easy access, BIOSIS provides vital sources of information for life scientists.

Federal Bio-Technology Transfer Directory
    A new Internet Web database that currently abstracts and indexes about 1,500 federal patents; 1,000 patent applications; 1,400 patent licenses (450 exclusive); and 950 CRADAs in the biomedical and related biotechnology areas.

PharmInfoNet Drug InfoBase

http://pharminfo.com/drg_mnu.html

PharmInfoNet Drug InfoBase provides a browsable database of drug information, which can be searched by generic name or brand name. The site also includes a searchable database of information about new drugs and FAQs with answers about new drugs.

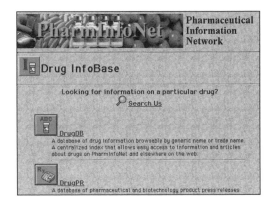

PharmWeb

http://www.pharmweb.net

PharmWeb, from the Department of Pharmacy at the University of Manchester, is a mega-directory of pharmacy information. The site lets you research your prescription, find newsgroups and mailing lists, participate in discussion forums, contact pharmacy societies worldwide, and much more. For an overview of the site, click on **PharmWeb Index.**

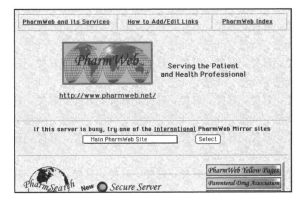

RxList

http://www.rxlist.com/

RxList is a searchable database on commonly prescribed and over-the-counter pharmaceuticals. This index identifies over 4000 drugs, the symptoms they are designed to treat, their interactions, and their side effects. In addition, you can search by imprint code, view **The Top 200,** and browse a huge collection of related links.

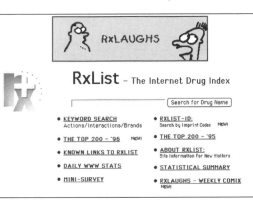

Taking Care of Your Health

http://www.Tylenol.com

Tylenol's Taking Care of Your Health provides general information on using drugs available at the supermarket (over-the-counter drugs), common illnesses, pain, and taking care of children.

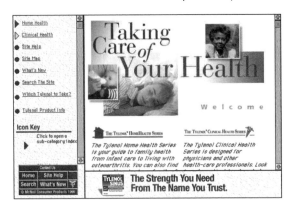

U.S. Pharmacopeia

http://www.usp.org/

The U.S. Pharmacopeia provides a collection of pharmaceutical resources for health care professionals and consumers. The **Drug Information** section includes a **Just Ask** feature that answers questions about the medicines that are used daily, and a **Standard Elements** database to enter the generic or brand-name drug or even an illness to learn more about the medications we take. You can also browse the **Standard Elements** database alphabetically.

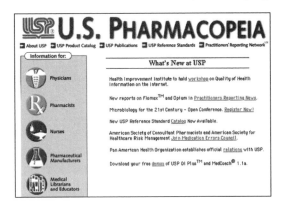

Virtual Library Pharmacy

http://157.142.72.77/pharmacy/pharmint.html

The Virtual Library Pharmacy contains a collection of pharmacy resources, including pharmacy schools on the Web, pharmacy databases, journals and books, and associations.

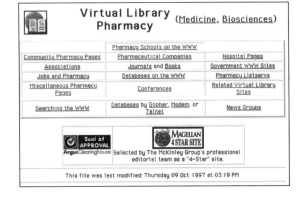

Vitamins Network

http://www.vitamins.net/

The Vitamins Network offers manufacturer-direct prices on thousands of vitamin, mineral, and herb products. The site also includes dozens of forums with message boards, chat rooms, and online guides for consumer briefs, for vitamins, and for herbs.

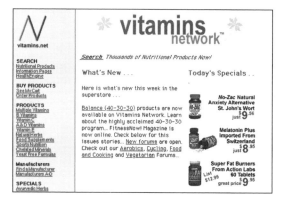

What Ails You?

http://www.nutrition-warehouse.com/What.Ails.You.html

What Ails You?, from the Nutrition Warehouse, contains a list of vitamins and supplements that may help health problems ranging from acne to yeast infections.

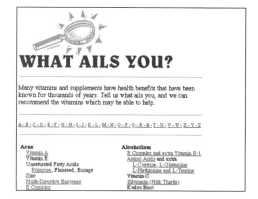

World Wide Pharmacy

http://www.ns.net/users/ryan/

World Wide Pharmacy provides the latest drug news in the New **Drug** section and a page of pharmaceutical sites in the **Reference** section.

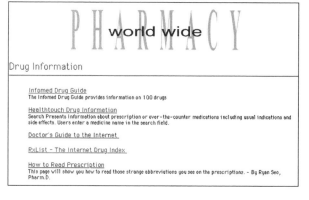

Selecting and Communicating With Your Doctors

CHAPTER **14**

1-800-Surgeon

http://www.SURGEON.org/

1-800-Surgeon is a surgeon referral service offering a free basic listing of surgeons' names and practices. You can search the database, browse an A to Z index, find a surgeon who performs a procedure you need, or click on a body part (male or female) to find a surgeon near you.

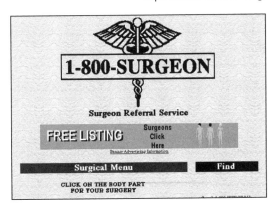

AMA Physician Select

http://www.ama-assn.org/iwcf/iwcfmgr206/aps?1798328487

AMA Physician Select provides information on virtually every licensed physician in the United States and its territories. Consumers can select a physician or verify the credentials of a known physician using a searchable database of more than 650,000 physicians. You can search for a physician by name or medical specialty. To access this service, click on **Accept** at the bottom of the page.

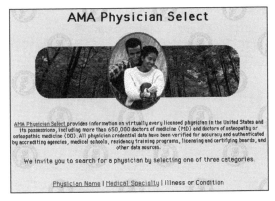

381

Ask An Expert: Health

http://www.askanexpert.com/askanexpert/cat/hea.html

Ask An Expert is a directory of health and medicine experts in over 40 different disciplines. An e-mail address and/or a link to the expert's Web site is provided for your query.

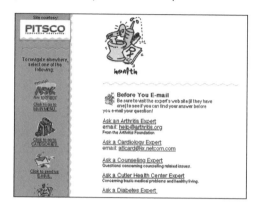

Ask the Anesthesiologist

http://www.csen.com/ask-the-anesthesiologist

Ask the Anesthesiologist is a directory of anesthesiologists from several countries, together with their e-mail addresses. You may e-mail them directly to receive responses to questions about anesthesia.

ASK THE ANESTHESIOLOGIST

Anesthesia is the first medical speciality. God "caused a deep sleep to fall upon Adam" for rib extraction (Genesis 2:21). Without anesthesia there are no operations. Even for minor operations the surgeons are using local anesthesia. Anesthesia changed the all natural history of medicine and it is still changing.

However, there is a widening gap between the anesthesia providers and the millions of patients.

Patients are afraid of the anesthesia more than they are afraid from the operations. Patients don't know exactly what are the options provided for their operations from the anesthesia point of view. Patients are signing the informed consent forms without being well informed regarding anesthesia.Patients don't know exactly how post-operative analgesia can make their post-operative pain disappear.

There is also a big difference in the state of anesthesia care among hospitals and countries.For the same operations patients are getting different kinds of anesthesia with different results.Many operations that could be done by regional anesthesia are still done by general anesthesia. For example, in a recent survey conducted in this website almost 80% of the anesthesiologists preferred regional anesthesia for their own operations.

Ask the Cardiologist

http://www.bev.net/health/cardiac/ask_cardio.html

Ask the Cardiologist, from the Cardiac HealthWeb, is an interactive site where Dr. J. Edwin Wilder answers questions related to the prevention and treatment of cardiovascular disease. You can also search the database of previous questions and answers or go to the **Topic List of Previous Questions.**

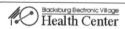

Blacksburg Electronic Village   **Cardiac**
Health Center   HealthWeb

CARDIAC HEALTHWEB HOMEPAGE
Ask the Cardiologist ‖ Health News ‖ Heart Disease ‖ Prevention ‖ Resources ‖ VT Cardiac Lab

 Ask The Cardiologist
Medical Advisor: J. Edwin Wilder, M.D.

About this Database

Ask the Cardiologist is an interactive question and answer database supported by educational grants from Merck & Company, Pfizer, Inc., and Novartis.

J. Edwin Wilder, M.D., will answer questions related to the prevention and treatment of cardiovascular disease. Dr. Wilder maintains a private practice in Cardiology in Blacksburg and is also an Adjunct Assistant Professor of Education in affiliation with the Virginia Tech Cardiovascular Rehabilitation Lab.

Selected questions will be answered anonymously online in the Cardiology Database.

Please Note: If you are having acute symptoms such as chest pain or breathing difficulties, please contact a health care professional immediately. Do not wait for an answer from *Ask the Cardiologist*.

Ask the Expert

http://www.mhsource.com/expert.html

Mental Health InfoSource provides an Ask the Expert feature where Dr. Ron Pies, an associate clinical professor of psychiatry at Tufts University and the popular *Psychiatric Times* columnist, will answer your mental health questions and post his responses the following Monday. To find an answer to a question, you can also read the current answered questions, browse the entire archive of previous answers dating back to 1996, search the archive, or go to the **consumer questions** section, which contains the entire archive arranged by topic ranging from attention deficit disorder/attention deficit hyperactivity disorder (ADD/ADHD) to women's issues.

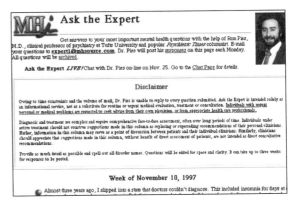

The Beth Israel Web Guide to Good Health

http://www.bimc.edu/

The Beth Israel Web Guide to Good Health, from Beth Israel Health Care System in New York, provides a wealth of consumer health resources, including an online **Physician & Referral Service** for the metropolitan New York City area and the **Ask the Doctor** feature with an extensive archive. In addition, the site offers **Health Information** on topics such as the heart and neurological disorders in children.

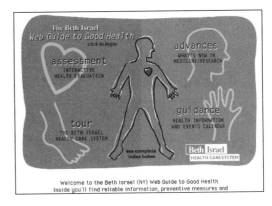

Docs Online

http://www.docsonline.com/

Docs Online is an online directory that enables you to locate dentists, physicians, health care providers, or hospitals in your geographic area. The parameters of the search tool include city, county, zip code, specialty, procedure, or insurance company.

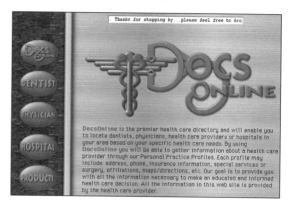

Doctorline

http://doctorline.com/

Doctorline is a nationwide resource for finding doctors, dentists, medical facilities, and health care plans. In addition, the site provides information about general health, diseases, and HMO care plans.

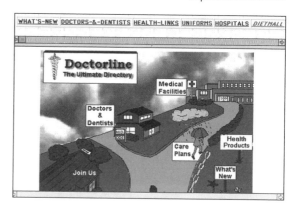

DoctorNet

http://www.doctornet.com/

DoctorNet offers the consumer numerous health/medical resources, including information from physicians about their specialties and their practices. Among the other resources are aids to finding a specialist, an online doctor's magazine, *DoctorNet Public Health Journal,* and an index of medical sites.

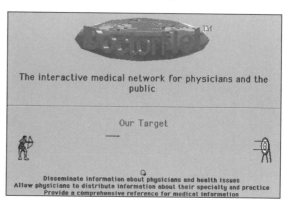

Doctors On-Line, Inc.

http://www.doli.com/

Doctors On-Line, Inc. provides medical advice from physicians licensed in the United States on ways to prevent heart disease, cancer, or diabetes, the three leading causes of death. The site offers a convenient and inexpensive way of consulting physicians by e-mail, toll-free telephone, or fax.

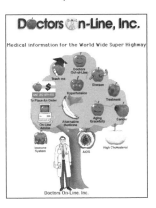

The Family Doctor

http://www.familydr.com/

The Family Doctor is divided into three main parts: (1) Ask the Doctor, (2) Doctor's Exam, and (3) Pharmacy. In Ask the Doctor, you may seek health information, which is categorized into 18 different sections. In Doctor's Exam, you may click on a body part, then seek a diagnosis, depending on a list of symptoms. In Pharmacy, you can find out what is in your new prescription via a search tool.

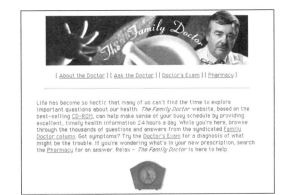

FindaDoc

http://findadoc.com/

FindaDoc provides an online directory of physicians, dentists, and health care professionals. Furthermore, in the Common Disease Symptoms section, a list of medical sites is provided.

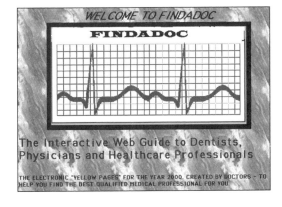

InteliHealth

http://www.intelihealth.com/

InteliHealth, home to Johns Hopkins Health Information, offers a treasure trove of health resources, including online quizzes, the top news headlines, fun interactive activities, and nearly one million pages of medical information. To have access to *all* the site's vast resources, you must register. It's free for the asking.

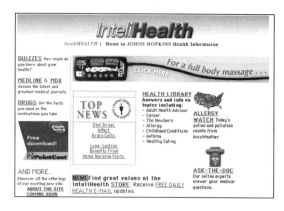

InteliHealth Ask the Doc

http://www.intelihealth.com/ih/ihtAskDocMain

InteliHealth Ask the Doc lets you submit your own medical questions to an online team of experts, or lets you review answers to the FAQs of doctors, nurses, and other health professionals.

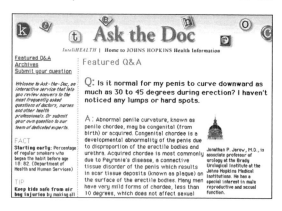

Medical Doctors Online

http://www.meddoctor.com/

Medical Doctors Online helps you locate the right medical doctor or health care services to meet your personal needs. The medical doctor locator searches the Internet and provides specific information on doctors and health care providers.

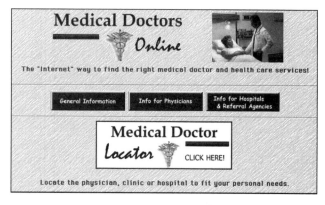

MedicineNet Ask The Experts

MedicineNet provides the Ask The Experts feature where consumers can ask all types of medical questions from the mundane to the technical. Consumers can submit questions to over 20 different specialty departments, including allergy, internal and family medicine, and cardiology, can view previous questions and answers in each specialty department, or can search the 1996 and 1997 databases.

http://www.medicinenet.com/ate.asp?ag=Y&li=MNI&x=l

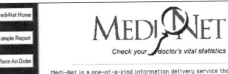

MediNet

http://www.askmedi.com/

MediNet, a commercial referral service, provides background information on every physician licensed to practice medicine in the United States. The service currently includes more than one million doctors.

Quackwatch

http://www.quackwatch.com/

Quackwatch, from Dr. Stephen Barrett, is a must-read for anyone seeking health advice online. The site can save you valuable time researching a questionable product or service on the Web. You can search previous answers and submit a question for Dr. Barrett to answer.

Questions to Ask Your Doctor Before You Have Surgery

http://www.pueblo.gsa.gov/cic_text/health/surgryqa.txt

Questions to Ask Your Doctor Before You Have Surgery, prepared by the Consumer Information Center of the U.S. General Services Administration, contains information that will help you make better decisions about your surgery.

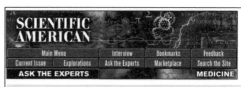

Scientific American Ask the Experts

http://www.sciam.com/askexpert/medicine/

Scientific American Ask the Experts allows you to ask a medical doctor a health question via e-mail. The site also contains a large archive of previous questions and answers.

Talk to our Doc

http://www.progest.com/Doctor.html

Talk to our Doc provides an online service where naturopathic doctors address your concerns about menopause and other female health issues. For a list of previous answers, scroll to Frequently Asked Questions of Our Doctors.

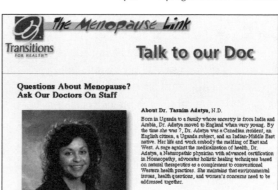

Insurance and Managed Care

CHAPTER 15

Aetna U.S. Healthcare

Aetna U.S. Healthcare is a national managed health care organization offering health information, and specialty health, and group insurance. For a goldmine of health information, click on **Health Topics.**

http://www.aetnaushc.com/

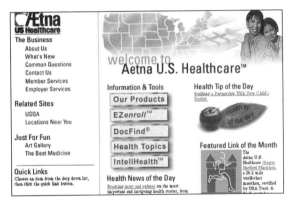

Art & Toons

Art & Toons is produced by Dr. John Capps, a health care consumer advocate. The site contains a collection of cartoons critical of HMOs and insurance companies.

http://users.aol.com/beetlebrox/jcapps.html

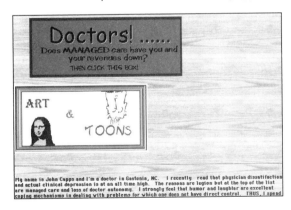

California Consumer HealthScope

http://www.healthscope.org/

California Consumer HealthScope, sponsored by the Pacific Business Group on Health, compares health plans, hospitals, nursing homes, and health care services on the quality features that are important to you.

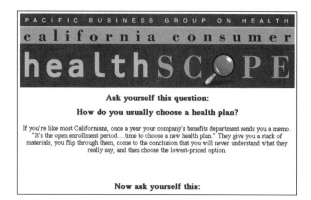

Cedars-Sinai Health System

http://www.csmc.edu/

The Cedars-Sinai Health System provides information for selecting health plans and insurance for yourself and your employees.

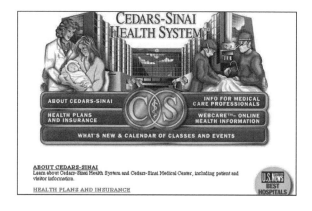

Center for Patient Advocacy

http://www.patientadvocacy.org/

Center for Patient Advocacy, a nationwide non-profit organization, offers advice on what to do when you have a complaint about your HMO and lists contact information for state insurance commissions.

Columbia/HCA Healthcare Corporation

http://www.columbia.net/

The Columbia/HCA Healthcare Corporation owns and operates more than 330 hospitals and other health care facilities with approximately 60,000 licensed beds in 36 states, England, and Switzerland. The site includes the HealthGate Wellness Center, the Columbia Virtual Hospital, a health manual, recipes, publications, an online facility and physician locator, and much more.

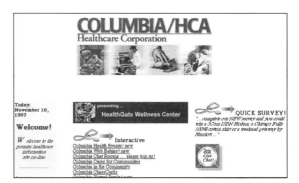

Empower!

http://www.comed.com/empower/

Empower!, the managed care patient advocate, is an evolving collection of online information designed primarily for managed care consumers and patients, and is intended to address issues relevant to the evolution of cost-efficient, high-quality managed health care services for consumers.

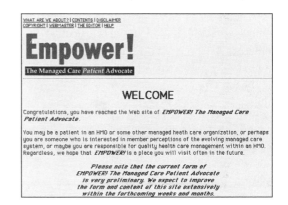

Harvard Pilgrim On-line

http://www.harvardpilgrim.org/

Harvard Pilgrim Health Care is New England's largest non-profit managed health care organization. Harvard Pilgrim On-line provides breast cancer awareness, the Wellesley Health Center, seasonal topics, featured articles, and a health library.

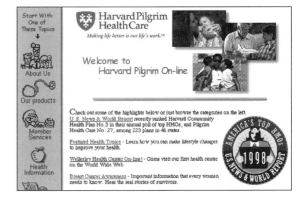

Health Care Financing Administration

http://www.hcfa.gov/

The Health Care Financing Administration (HCFA), a federal agency of the U.S. Department of Health and Human Services, administers two national health care programs, Medicare and Medicaid. These programs benefit more than 74 million people. The site includes statistics, an organizational telephone directory, and online publications.

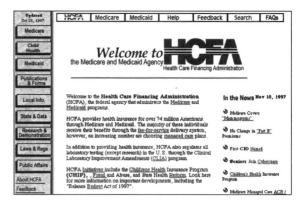

Health Hippo

http://www.winternet.com/~hippo/

Health Hippo is a collection of health policy and regulatory resources. Documents include congressional testimony, legislation, and recent supreme and appellate court decisions impacting managed care.

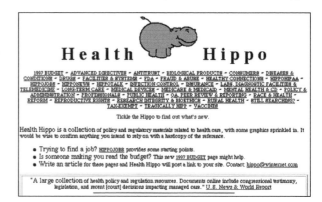

Health Net

http://www.healthnet.com/

Health Net offers health plan benefits and services throughout California. In addition, the site includes a collection of monthly health themes in the Wellness section with extensive consumer information on topics such as cholesterol, taking care of yourself, nutrition, and children's health issues. The site also presents a new health tip after each reloading.

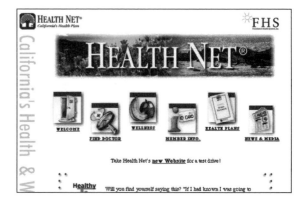

Health Policy Page

http://epn.org/idea/health.html

Health Policy Page, from Idea Central, contains articles about the current state of health care in the United States, including analyses of Medicare, Medicaid, and managed care.

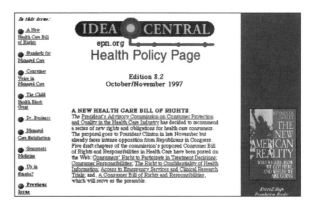

Humana

http://www.humana.com/

Humana is a network that contains information on medical-related news, products and services, a physician finder, local offices, and military health care services.

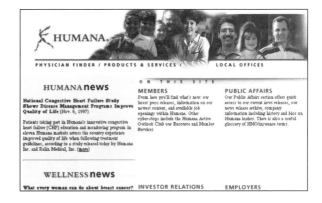

Kaiser Permanente

http://www.kaiperm.org/

Kaiser Permanente is a leading HMO. Its site includes the various health plans, employment opportunities, Permanente Medicine, and a list of locations. To learn about different health topics, click on **To Your Health.**

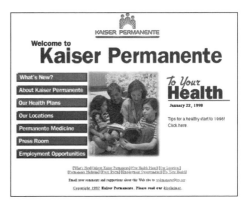

MedAccess Health Care Locator

http://www.medaccess.com/locator/hclocate.htm

MedAccess Health Care Locator provides information about all kinds of health care to help you make decisions about doctors, hospitals, or current types of health care insurance.

Murphy's Unofficial Medicaid Page

http://www.geocities.com/capitolhill/5974/

Murphy's Unofficial Medicaid Page is a guide to Medicaid-specific resources on the Internet. The site includes links to each state's Medicaid site and other related sites.

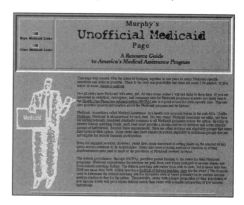

MVP Health Plan

http://www.mvphealthplan.com/

MVP Health Plan provides managed care for the state of Vermont and 30 counties in the state of New York. The site contains information on MVP and their doctors, health tips, games, and more!

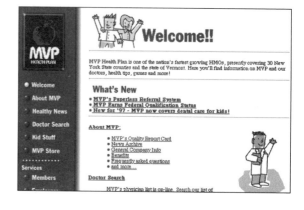

National Committee for Quality Assurance

http://www.ncqa.org

The National Committee for Quality Assurance serves as a watchdog group for managed care plans, provides information on accreditation, and issues report cards on quality. You can search for your HMO on their **Accreditation Status List** and see if your health plan has an Accreditation Summary Report.

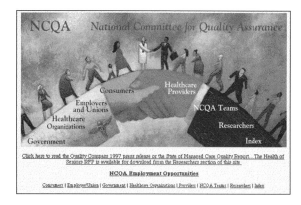

Prudential Health Care & Employee Benefits

http://www.prudential.com/healthcare/

Prudential Health Care & Employee Benefits provides benefits programs for employees and individuals. For an assortment of consumer health topics, click on **Staying Healthy.**

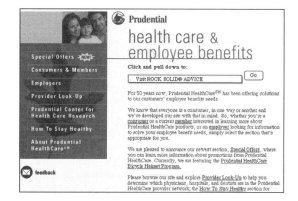

United HealthCare

http://www.uhc.com/

United HealthCare provides a **Resource Center** section with a guide to research on the effectiveness of managed health care plans. The **Living Smarter** section has general health information ranging from nutrition information to an ask a doctor checklist.

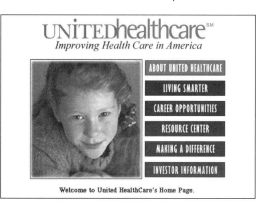

U.S. News Online

http://www4.usnews.com/usnews/nycu/hmoshigh.htm

U.S. News Online presents state-by-state rankings of America's top 223 managed care plans, including the 37 HMOs that earned the highest four-star rating. The site also provides an interactive quiz in the **Learning About HMOs** section.

What If You Didn't Have to Worry About Health Care?

http://www.bluecares.com/

What If You Didn't Have to Worry About Health Care?, the Blue Cross and Blue Shield Association Web site, is designed to serve your health care needs. You can connect to a huge network of locally operated Blue Cross and Blue Shield plans, find out what is new in the health care industry, or take a virtual tour of the human body. You can also browse through a list of sites for specific health care topics.

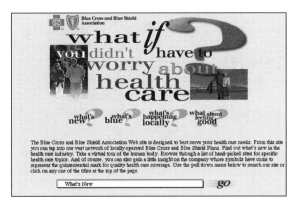

What You Need to Know About Surgery, Radiology, and Anesthesia

CHAPTER 16

1-800-Surgeon

http://www.SURGEON.org/

1-800-Surgeon is a surgeon referral service offering a free basic listing of surgeons' names and practices. You can search the database, browse an A to Z index, find a surgeon who performs a procedure you need, or click on a body part (male or female) to find a surgeon near you.

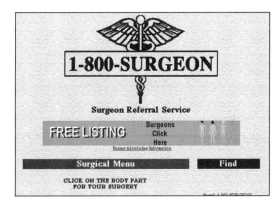

American College of Surgeons

http://www.facs.org/

The American College of Surgeons provides public information on patient choice, when you need an operation, and protecting your health. For an overview of the **Public Information** section, click on **Site Index** and go to that section.

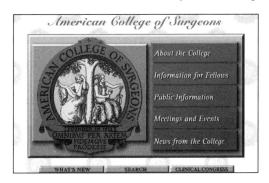

397

The Anaesthesia Server

http://www.medana.unibas.ch/

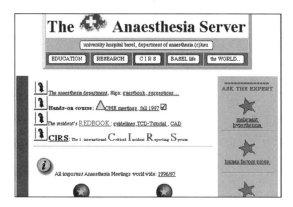

The Anaesthesia Server, from the University of Basel in Switzerland, provides the resident's *Redbook,* an online guide for anaesthesiologists. The site also includes an ask the expert feature where anesthesiology questions are answered via e-mail.

Anesthesia & Critical Care Educational Resources

http://dacc.uchicago.edu/education/

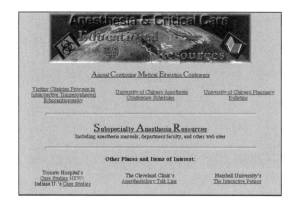

Anesthesia & Critical Care Educational Resources, from the University of Chicago, provides educational resources including anesthesia manuals and other Web sites. For a complete list of resources ranging from cardiac and pediatric anesthesia to pain and trauma treatment, click on **Subspecialty.**

Anesthesia.Net

http://anesthesia.net/

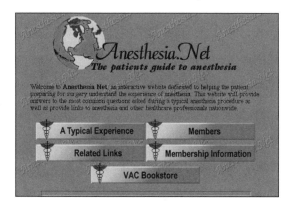

Anesthesia.Net is an interactive site to help a patient preparing for surgery understand the experience of anesthesia. The site provides answers to the most common questions asked about a typical anesthesia procedure and provides links to anesthesiologists and other health care professionals nationwide.

Ask the Anesthesiologist

http://www.csen.com/ask-the-anesthesiologist

Ask the Anesthesiologist is a directory of anesthesiologists from several countries, together with their e-mail addresses. You may e-mail them directly to receive responses to questions about anesthesia.

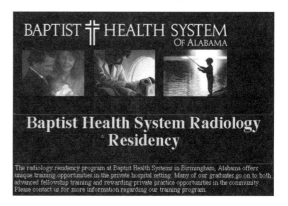

ASK THE ANESTHESIOLOGIST

Anesthesia is the first medical speciality. God "caused a deep sleep to fall upon Adam" for rib extraction (Genesis 2:21). Without anesthesia there are no operations. Even for minor operations the surgeons are using local anesthesia. Anesthesia changed the all natural history of medicine and it is still changing.

However, there is a widening gap between the anesthesia providers and the millions of patients.

Patients are afraid of the anesthesia more than they are afraid from the operations. Patients don't know exactly what are the options provided for their operations from the anesthesia point of view. Patients are signing the informed consent forms without being well informed regarding anesthesia.Patients don't know exactly how post-operative analgesia can make their post-operative pain disappear.

There is also a big difference in the state of anesthesia care among hospitals and countries.For the same operations patients are getting different kinds of anesthesia with different results.Many operations that could be done by regional anesthesia are still done by general anesthesia. For example, in a recent _survey_ conducted in this website almost 80% of the anesthesiologists preferred regional anesthesia for their own operations.

Baptist Health System Radiology Residency

http://www.wwisp.com/~bhsresidents/

The Baptist Health System Radiology Residency site, from The Baptist Health System of Alabama in Birmingham, has a **CyberRadiology** section with more than 165 links to teaching cases from the Internet organized by disease and body part. The teaching cases include the cervical spine, the hand and wrist, the pelvis, and the femur. Each case contains a description, a diagnosis, and an image.

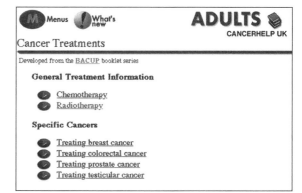

Cancer Treatments

http://medweb.bham.ac.uk/cancerhelp/public/treat/

Cancer Treatments, from CancerHelp UK, provides a free information service about cancer treatment developed from the *BACUP* booklet series. The site contains general information on chemotherapy and radiotherapy, along with specific information on treating breast cancer, colorectal cancer, prostate cancer, and testicular cancer.

Columbia Visual Health & Surgical Center

http://www.web-xpress.com/vhsc/

Columbia Visual Health & Surgical Center provides resources about diagnosis and treatment of ophthalmic abnormalities. The **Information About Eye Conditions and Diseases** section contains information on surgical tratment of astigmatism, cataracts, glaucoma, retinal detachment, and other eye disorders.

COLUMBIA
Visual Health & Surgical Center

- Columbia Healthcare Corporation
- About Visual Health & Surgical Center
- Professional Staff
- Our Facilities
- Medical Insurance Plans
- Free Community Outreach Programs
- Information About Eye Conditions and Diseases
- Eye Centers of Excellence

Laparoscopy.com

http://www.laparoscopy.com/

Laparoscopy.com provides information for the laparoscopic surgeon, including pictures, movies, and related links.

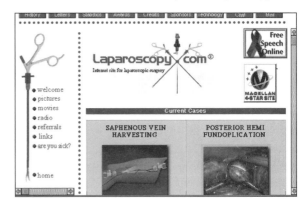

PRK Today Eye Site

http://www.prk.com/

PRK Today Eye Site provides information on excimer laser eye surgery, photorefractive keratectomy (PRK), and other corrective refractive surgical procedures, including RK, ALK, and laser-assisted in situ keratomileusis (LASIK). This site focuses on the facts about PRK, where to go for PRK and LASIK, and how to talk with the persons who are knowledgeable about laser eye surgery. The site also offers a comprehensive glossary of terms pertaining to vision correction procedures.

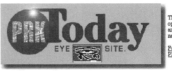

Laser Eye Surgery, PRK, LASIK

PRK**Today**
EYE   SITE.

This site has been optimized for Netscape 2.0 and Explorer 2.0 or newer.

For older versions, Please Click Here

PRK Today is dedicated to bringing you independent and unbiased information on excimer laser eye surgery, photorefractive keratectomy (prk) and other refractive eye surgery such as RK, ALK and LASIK. PRK laser eye treatments have made it possible for hundreds of thousands to see without depending on glasses or contacts. Find out the facts about PRK, where to go for PRK and LASIK, and how to talk with the people who know about laser eye surgery. Be sure to visit our PRK Guest Book before you leave.

Please read PRK Today Legal Disclaimer before proceeding.

Questions to Ask Your Doctor Before You Have Surgery

http://www.pueblo.gsa.gov/cic_text/health/surgryqa.txt

Questions to Ask Your Doctor Before You Have Surgery, prepared by the Consumer Information Center of the U.S. General Services Administration, contains information that will help you make better decisions about your surgery.

Radiation Therapy and You

http://rex.nci.nih.gov/NCI_Pub_Interface/
Radiation/radintro.html

Radiation Therapy and You is an online self-help guide prepared by the National Cancer Institute for persons undergoing radiation treatment for cancer. The guide provides information on what to expect and how to care for yourself during your treatment. It describes external radiation therapy and brachytherapy using radiation implants, the two most common types of radiation therapy. Information is included on radiation therapy methods and the general effects of treatment. There are also some self-help "pointers" for dealing with specific side effects.

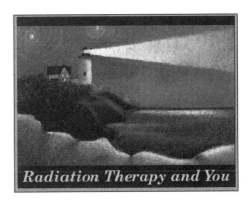

Radiologist.com

http://www.radiologist.com/

Radiologist.com is an Internet source for radiologists. Among its resources are a large collection of ultrasound sites, radiology sites, and educational sites.

RSNA Link

http://www.rsna.org/

RSNA Link is the Radiological Society of North America Web site that provides radiologists and allied health scientists with educational programs and materials. Among its varied resources are the Office of Research Development Database of Funding Opportunities, a database for researchers in the radiologic sciences, a collection of links to radiologic and other medical and scientific sites on the Internet, an online version of the monthly RSNA newsletter, and much more.

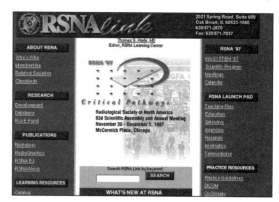

The Surgical Resource Network

http://www.ussurg.com/public/Home-Page.html

The Surgical Resource Network, sponsored by the United States Surgical Corporation, provides a variety of online resources for health professionals and patients. The **patient resources** section contains information about minimally invasive techniques and laparoscopic surgery.

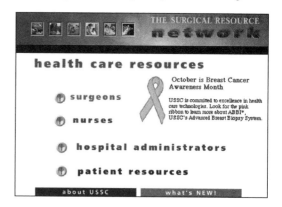

Vision Surgery & Laser Center

http://www.vslc.com

The Vision Surgery & Laser Center provides information on refractive surgery for correcting myopia (nearsightedness) and astigmatism using excimer laser procedures, including photorefractive keratectomy (PRK) and laser-assisted in situ keratomileusis (LASIK). The site also gives pointers on how to choose a qualified refractive eye surgeon.

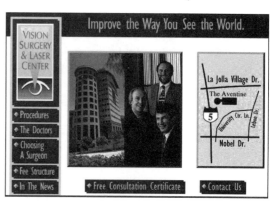

A Woman's Guide to Infertility & Gynecologic Surgery

A Woman's Guide to Infertility & Gynecologic Surgery, from the Atlanta Reproductive Health Centre WWW, has information on surgical procedures such as laparoscopy, microlaparoscopy, tubal sterilization reversal, endometrial ablation, and laparoscopic hysterectomy.

http://www.ivf.com/surgery.html

Atlanta Reproductive Health Centre WWW

A Woman's Guide To......

Infertility & Gynecologic Surgery

- Tubal Sterilization Reversal: A Patient Guide
- What's a Laparoscopy?
- Miracle Babies Chapter 16. Tubal Factor Infertility
- Microlaparoscopy A diagnostic surgical breakthrough.
- Endometrial Ablation offers a hysterectomy alternative
- Laparoscopic Hysterectomy speeds post-op recovery

Plastic Surgery

CHAPTER 17

Aesthetic Plastic Surgery

http://www.plasticsurgery-sf.com/

Aesthetic Plastic Surgery, Roger L. Greenberg's site, provides information on liposuction, breast augmentation surgery, facial plastic surgery, laser surgery, breast enlargement, eyelid surgery, and plastic surgery of the nose. The site contains a photo gallery of before and after photographs of surgical procedures.

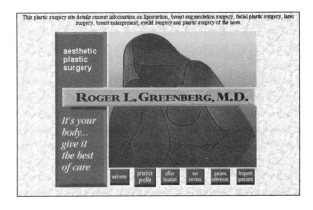

The Aesthetics Center

http://www.aesthetics.com/

The Aesthetics Center, the home page of the Banis-Derr Center, contains plastic surgery information for eyelids, rhinoplasty, breast lift, laser, face lift, and liposuction procedures. The **other** section provides information on plastic surgery for breast enlargement, breast reduction, breast reconstruction, and much more.

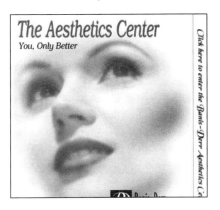

Beauty and the Beam

http://www.beautyandthebeam.com/

Beauty and the Beam is the online version of the book, *Beauty and the Beam: Your Complete Guide to Cosmetic Laser Surgery,* published by Quality Medical Publishing. To learn about the various laser procedures, click on **Cosmetic Laser Surgery Procedures.** To find more information about the book, scroll and click on **Frequently Asked Questions.**

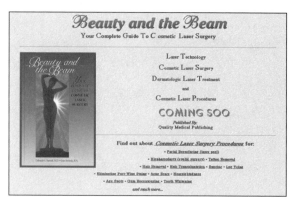

The Body Electric

http://www.surgery.com/

The Body Electric provides up-to-date information about plastic/cosmetic surgical procedures, including suction lipectomy (liposuction), face lifts, breast reconstruction, and more. The site includes a surgeon finder, as well as a **Body Area** feature, to explore the effects of plastic surgery on various parts of the body.

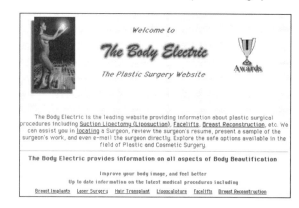

Center for Plastic Surgery

http://openseason.com/cps/

The Center for Plastic Surgery provides a variety of plastic surgery resources, including cosmetic, breast reconstruction, pediatric, and laser skin resurfacing procedures. For an overview of the site, click on **Index.**

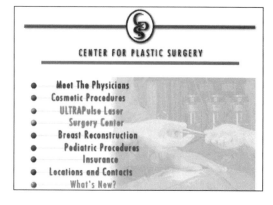

Cosmetic Plastic Surgery Online

http://www.surgery.org/enhanced/

Cosmetic Plastic Surgery Online, the American Society for Aesthetic Plastic Surgery (ASAPS) site, contains a variety of resources for aesthetic (cosmetic) plastic surgery. The site provides extensive information on procedures and finding an ASAPS surgeon. The **Media Center** features the latest news releases.

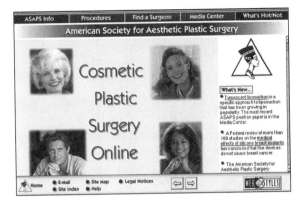

Dallas Plastic Surgery Institute

http://www.drhobar.com/

The Dallas Plastic Surgery Institute, maintained by Dr. Hobar, provides information on cosmetic and reconstructive plastic surgery. The site includes a list of procedures, before and after photographs, and FAQs.

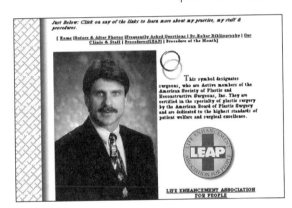

E-sthetics

http://phudson.com/

E-sthetics, maintained by Dr. Patrick Hudson, is the most comprehensive source of information about cosmetic surgery on the Web. Among the vast resources are plastic surgery after pregnancy, procedures for facial and body sculpturing, and related useful links. For an overview of the site, click on **Explore.**

Emory University School of Medicine Department of Surgery

http://www.emory.edu/WHSC/MED/SURGERY/plastic/

The Division of Plastic, Reconstructive, and Maxillofacial Surgery, from the Department of Surgery at Emory University School of Medicine, provides comprehensive services in reconstructive and aesthetic surgery. For inquiries, call the director, Dr. John Bostwick III, at 1-404-778-5761.

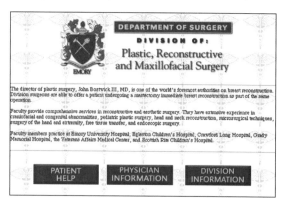

George H. Sanders, M.D.

http://www.drsanders.com/

George H. Sanders, M.D., a plastic surgeon, provides an online surgicenter in which he discusses why particular cosmetic and reconstructive procedures are done, what they achieve, and what the patient should expect following surgery.

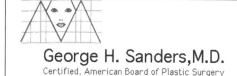

Lipoplasty

http://www.zilker.net/business/lsna/

Lipoplasty, from the Lipoplasty Society of North America, presents a patient guide to suction-assisted body contouring (liposuction). The site contains an explanation of what constitutes an appropriate candidate, the procedure itself, risk of complications, aftercare, and before and after pictures.

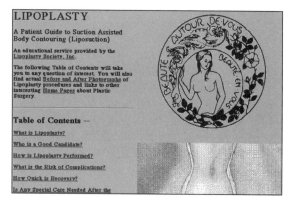

Mayo Rochester Aesthetic (Cosmetic) Surgery Center

The Mayo Rochester Aesthetic (Cosmetic) Surgery Center offers an online plastic surgery primer on physical dermabrasion, augmentation, and rejuvenation. Brief synopses are provided for the most common types of surgery, including fat removal, facial refinement, procedures for hair and teeth, and even tattoo eradication.

http://www.mayo.edu/staff/plastic/Cosmetic/CSOLMain.html

Mayo Rochester Aesthetic (Cosmetic) Surgery Center

Today, people of all ages take serious interest in nutrition and exercise as a way to enhance personal health and appearance. Aesthetic surgery offers another option for individuals to gain a better balance between the way they look and the way they feel. In most instances, the goal of aesthetic surgery is to improve the patient's sense of well-being while respecting and preserving the individual's unique attributes.

Contents

- Candidates for Cosmetic Surgery
- Preparation, Recovery, and Expense

MedMark Plastic Surgery

MedMark Plastic Surgery, maintained by Dr. Deok Hee Lee, contains a comprehensive list of the plastic surgery resources on the Internet, including general and consumer sites.

http://medmark.bit.co.kr/plastic.html

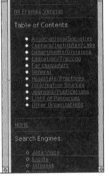

PLASTIC SURGERY

Associations/Societies

American Society for Aesthetic Plastic Surgery (ASAPS)
American Society for Surgery of the Hand
American Society of Ophthalmic Plastic and Reconstructive Surgery (ASOPRS)
Australian Society of Plastic Surgeons [ASPS]
Brazilian Society of Plastic Surgery
British Association of Plastic Surgeons
Dutch Society for Plastic Surgery
Societe Francaise Chirurgie Esthetique et Plastique
Spanish Society of Plastic, Reconstructive and Aesthetic Surgery [SECPRE]

Centers/Institutes/Labs

Garry Laboratory
Institute for Aesthetic and Reconstructive Surgery, Baptist Hospital
Institute of Craniofacial Plastic Surgery (SOBRAPAR)
Microsurgical Laboratories, Mcgill University
Restoration of Appearance and Function Trust (RAFT)
Institute for Reconstructive, Plastic & Burns Surgery Research

MedWeb Plastic Surgery

MedWeb, from Emory University Health Sciences Center Library, contains a list of plastic surgery sites on the Web.

http://www.gen.emory.edu/MEDWEB/keyword/plastic_surgery/plastic_surgery.html

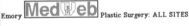

Emory   MedWeb   Plastic Surgery: ALL SITES

Other subcategories for plastic_surgery are listed at the bottom of this page

- Achieving Aesthetic Excellence - Dr. B. Scott Teunis (McLean, Virginia).
- Aesthetic Facial Surgery Center of Rockville (Rockville, Maryland).
- Aesthetic plastic surgery: official journal of the International Society of Aesthetic Plastic Surgery; official publication of the Lipoplasty Society of North America (tables of contents and abstracts; full text as Acrobat PDF files available to registered users).
- Aesthetic surgery journal: official publication of the American Society for Aesthetic Plastic Surgery (tables of contents and abstracts).
- American Society for Aesthetic Plastic Surgery (ASAPS).
- American Society of Plastic and Reconstructive Surgeons.
- Asociación Española de Microcirugía (A. E. M.) = Spanish Association of Microsurgery.
- Baylor College of Medicine Division of Plastic Surgery.
- Canadian journal of plastic surgery: official journal of the Canadian Society of Plastic Surgeons, Canadian Society for Aesthetic (Cosmetic) Plastic Surgery, Groupe pour l'Avancement de la Microchirurgie Canada (GAM).
- Case Western Reserve University Division of Plastic Surgery.
- Centro de Medicina Biológica y Estética (Alicante, Spain).
- Cirugía Plástica y Estética: Dr. J. Benito-Ruiz. (Barcelona, Spain).
- Clínica José Carlos Pallovez.
- Cosmetic-Trends.
- Craniofacial Surgery Discussion List operated by the Institute for Craniofacial Plastic Surgery (SOBRAPAR), in Campinas, Brazil.

Palm Beach Plastic Surgery Center

http://www.pbplasticsurgery.com

Palm Beach Plastic Surgery Center provides information about liposuction, the carbon dioxide (CO_2) laser, hair transplants, breast surgery, plastic and reconstructive surgery, face lifts, eye lifts, and male cosmetic surgery.

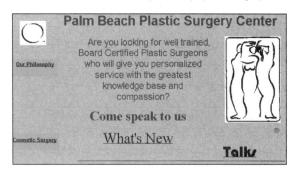

Plastic & Cosmetic Surgery

http://www.lookinggood.com/

Plastic & Cosmetic Surgery, from Dr. Alfonso Barrera, contains information about procedures and before and after photographs.

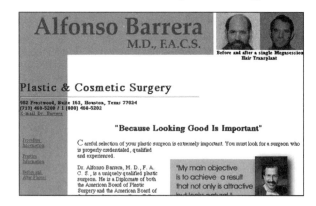

Plastic Surgery Information Service

http://www.plasticsurgery.org/

Plastic Surgery Information Service, the Web site of the American Society of Plastic and Reconstructive Surgeons (ASPRS), provides background information on the wide variety of cosmetic and reconstructive plastic surgery procedures and also offers a plastic surgeon referral service. The **FAQ** section contains answers to some of the questions most frequently asked about plastic surgery. The site also includes links to other medical associations and government organizations.

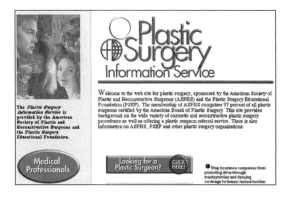

Plastic Surgery Lab

http://showbiz.starwave.com/showbiz/flash/surgery/

Plastic Surgery Lab, from ABCNews.com, is a fun, interactive site where you can mix and match facial features to create a new look for a male Hollyood celebrity.

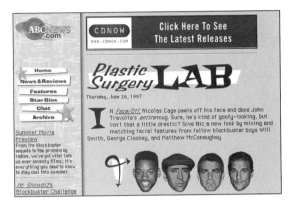

Plastic Surgery Network

http://www.plastic-surgery.net/

The Plastic Surgery Network provides a general overview of plastic/cosmetic surgery procedures ranging from face lifts to breast reconstruction. The site also offers advice on finding and choosing a qualified plastic surgeon, related links, and the plastic surgery site of the week.

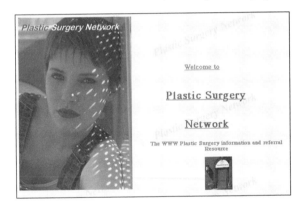

PLink

http://www.nvpc.nl/plink

PLink is a vast collection of plastic surgery resources organized by category. Categories include societies, university departments, doctors, private clinics, and many others.

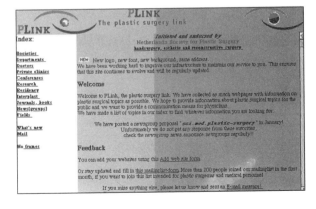

CHAPTER 18

Dental Care

http://www.agd.org/

Academy of General Dentistry

The Academy of General Dentistry is an invaluable dental care resource for consumers. **SmileLine Online** provides answers to your dental questions. You can ask an Academy dentist a question via e-mail or you can go to a list of dental FAQs with information on such items as children's oral health and infection control. The site also offers a **Consumer Information** category that provides online help for various dental concerns and links to dental organizations and academies.

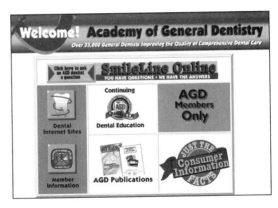

http://www.ada.org/

ADA Online

ADA Online, the American Dental Association Internet site, provides consumer information on dental care. The site's **consumer information** link is rich in resources and information on topics such as how to get the most out of a visit to the dentist, how to find a dentist, root canal treatment, and diet and dental health.

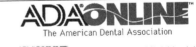

ADHA Online

http://www.adha.org/

ADHA Online, the American Dental Hygienists' Association Web site, provides a Consumer Center with oral health information and tips and a Kids' Stuff room with games, puzzles, and information on how kids can keep their teeth and mouths healthy.

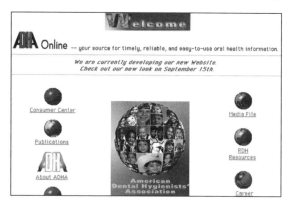

America's Finest Dentist Directory

http://www.afdd.com/

America's Finest Dentist Directory helps you locate a dentist near your home. The site includes useful dental links and the **dental miracles** section provides information on cosmetic dentistry.

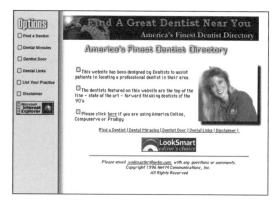

American Academy of Pediatric Dentistry

http://www.aapd.org/

The American Academy of Pediatric Dentistry covers a variety of topics, including parent information with 24 illustrated brochures addressing questions parents commonly ask, a directory of Internet links, and an online coloring book for kids.

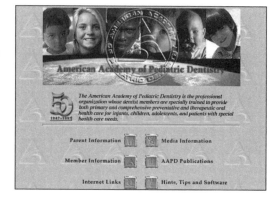

Ask an Oral Maxillofacial Surgeon

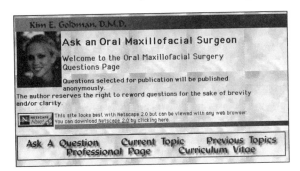

http://www.calweb.com/~goldman/

Ask an Oral Maxillofacial Surgeon, maintained by Dr. Kim E. Goldman, answers your oral surgery questions on such topics as wisdom teeth, orthognathic surgery, and chin augmentation.

Ask Dr. Tooth

http://www.dentistinfo.com/faska.htm

Ask Dr. Tooth contains **FAQs** with answers to previously asked questions. In addition, you can ask Dr. Tooth your own questions via e-mail.

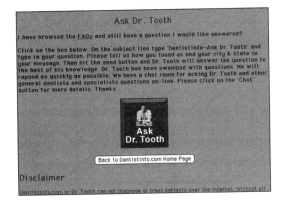

Basic Periodontology

http://www.odont.ku.dk/basic.periodontology/main.html

Basic Periodontology provides an overview of treatment of gum diseases such as gingivitis, periodontitis, and attachment loss. The site also includes related periodontal links.

CDA Online

http://www.cda.org/public/

CDA Online, the California Dental Association site, provides consumer resources, including dental health fact sheets and dental care articles.

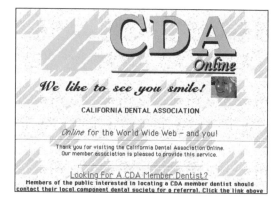

CDC's Oral Health Program

http://www.cdc.gov/nccdphp/oh/

The CDC's Oral Health Program, from the Centers for Disease Control and Prevention, provides information on oral health surveillance activities, prevention strategies such as fluoride and dental sealants, and recommendations for infection control.

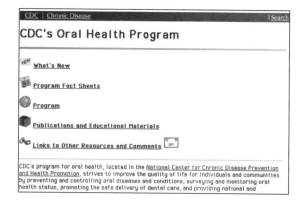

DDS4U Dentist Directory

http://www.DDS4U.com/

DDS4U Dentist Directory is a dentist referral service searchable by name, city, zip code, and specialty. At this site you can view a profile of your potential that includes education and services offered.

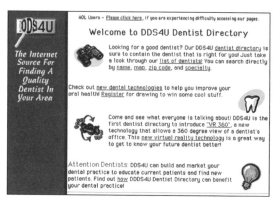

The Dental Consumer Advisor

http://www.toothinfo.com/

The Dental Consumer Advisor has a variety of
dental topics, including finding a dentist,
dental health fact sheets, an alphabetical list of
dental terms, and images and diagrams that
illustrate oral conditions.

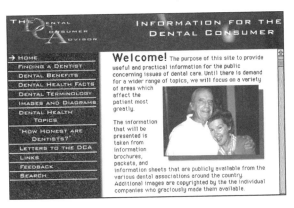

Dental Cyberweb

http://www.vv.com/dental-web/

Dental Cyberweb provides informative dental
articles for both patients and dentists. The site
also includes related dental links.

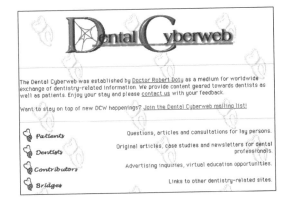

Dental Phobia & Anxiety

http://www.dentalfear.org/

Dental Phobia & Anxiety contains online help for
those suffering from dental phobia and anxiety. The
site also includes other dentistry links and a find a
dentist feature for Great Britain.

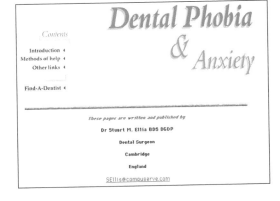

Dental Related Internet Resources

http://www.dental-resources.com/

The Dental Related Internet Resources provides a rich source of information for both dentists and consumers. Click on the **Dental Care** category to find a guide to dental products and general oral hygiene.

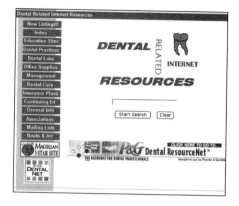

The Dental Site

http://www.dentalsite.com/

The Dental Site provides a variety of dental resources, including patient information, a discussion of dental benefit plans, articles on dental health, a feature describing treatments for dental anxiety and dental phobia, advice about how to choose a dentist, and links to related sites.

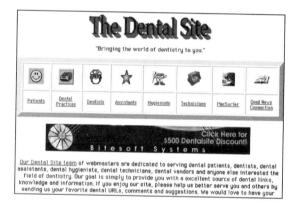

Dental Telecommunication Network

http://biz.onramp.net/Den-Tel-Net/

The Dental Telecommunication Network is an online monthly dental health journal with articles pertaining to various dental specialties. Topics include managed care, periodontics, and orthodontics with an archive of articles from 1994 to 1997.

Dental X Change

http://dentalxchange.com/

Dental X Change is an online service that contains a wealth of dental information. The site is directed toward general dentists, periodontists, pediatric dentists, students, and others interested in dentistry. Topics range from new dental products to getting your free home page and dentist directory posted.

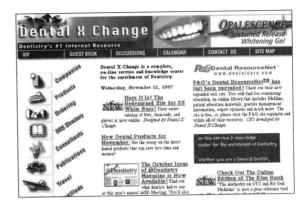

Dental-Find

http://www.dentalfind.com/

Dental-Find is a worldwide dental referral service.

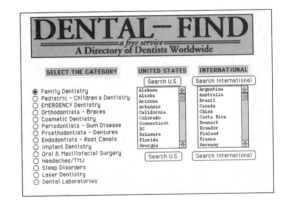

Dental-Related Internet List of Links

http://www.citizen.infi.net/~dmtrop/dental/dental3.html

Dental-Related Internet List of Links provides more than 2500 links related to the field of dentistry. Among those links are **dental societies, dental products for consumers, dental insurance companies, dental laboratories,** and others.

DentalBytes Mag-E-Zine

DentalBytes Mag-E-Zine is an online quarterly dentistry magazine with a wide array of charts, features, articles, and reports of interest to patients and dentists. The site also includes links to related sites on the Internet.

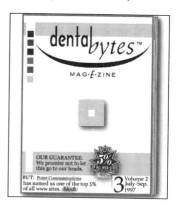

Dentist Directory

The Dentist Directory consists of three main parts: (1) Find A Dentist is a search tool that helps you find a dentist in your local area; (2) Patient Information Center answers FAQs about dental care and dentistry procedures; and (3) Ask A Dentist allows you to e-mail specific questions to a dentist who will reply within 24 hours.

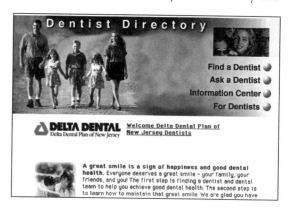

Dentist Guide to the Internet

Dentist Guide to the Internet is a dental directory providing a vast array of links categorized by resources, journals, and other areas of interest.

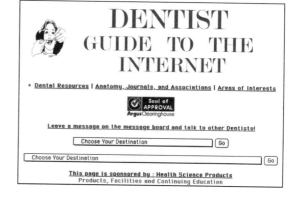

Dentist Hotline

http://www.dentisthotline.com/

Dentist Hotline is a comprehensive online resource for dental and oral care, including a database of qualified dentists.

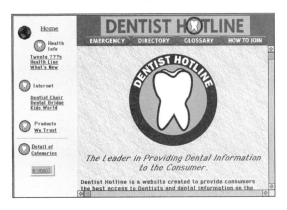

The Dentist Organization

http://www.dentist.org/

The Dentist Organization is a comprehensive dentistry site offering search services for a dentist ranging from general dentistry to periodontist. In addition, the site provides dental information on a variety of topics, including tooth development and wisdom teeth, an ask an expert feature, and live chat conferences on such topics as children's teeth and endodontics.

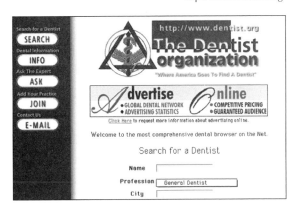

Dentistinfo.com

http://www.dentistinfo.com/

Dentistinfo.com offers a variety of dental health resources, including links to organizations and agencies. The site also provides answers to dental **FAQs** such as "Why should I replace a missing tooth?" and "How can I avoid getting cavities?"

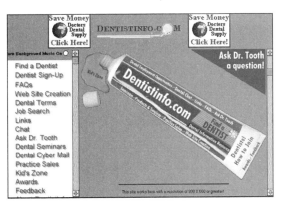

The Dentistry Homepage

http://www.pitt.edu/~cbw/dental.html

The Dentistry Homepage, from the Falk Library of the Health Sciences at the University of Pittsburgh, provides an enormous collection of dental resources, including those for diagnosis and treatment. The site includes everything you ever wanted to know about teeth, oral cavitities, associated structures, in addition to databases for additional inquiries.

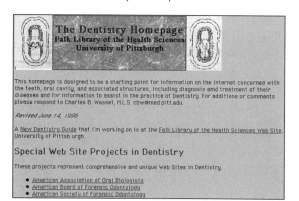

Dentistry Now

http://www.dentistrynow.com/Mainpage.htm

Dentistry Now provides dental information for the public and the health professional. The consumer resources include procedure information on a variety of dental topics and information and activities for children in the tooth fairy section. The site also features a list of dental schools worldwide.

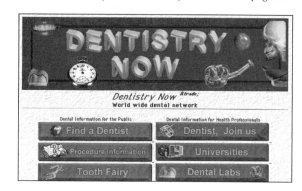

Dentistry On-Line

http://www.priory.co.uk/dent.htm

Dentistry On-Line has a variety of dentistry resources for both the consumer and the professional. The consumer topics include children's teeth, sealing teeth, oral hygiene problems, halitosis, and infections. The site also offers related dental links and a search tool.

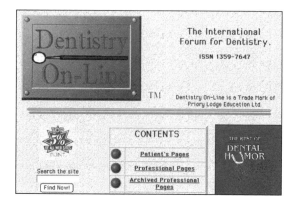

DHNet

http://jeffline.tju.edu/DHNet/

DHNet, from the National Center for Dental Hygiene Research, provides a variety of dental resources for the professional and the consumer. The **Consumer Information** page contains numerous informative articles on dental care.

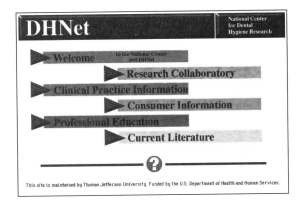

Dr. Dave's Dental Page

http://www.erols.com/dlucht/

Dr. Dave's Dental Page has patient information on such topics as the basics of tooth anatomy, implants, and HMOs and dentistry.

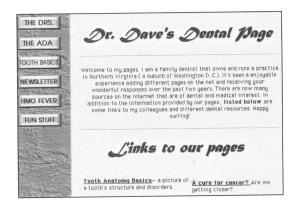

Dr. Spieler's Dental Zone

http://www.saveyoursmile.com/

Dr. Spieler's Dental Zone is an online dental resource with easy-to-read articles on various topics. The site also contains a **question-and-answer** section, a free newsletter, a health IQ quiz, and links to other medical resources.

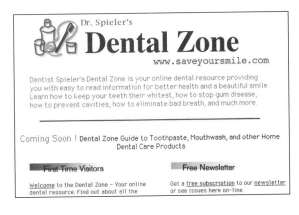

Einet Galaxy Dentistry

http://www.einet.net/galaxy/Medicine/Dentistry.html

Einet Galaxy Dentistry provides a compendium of dental resources, including articles, guides, periodicals, academic organizations, and much more.

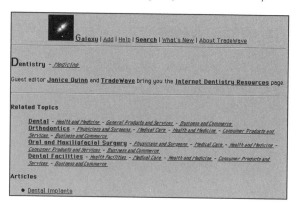

Family and Cosmetic Dentistry

http://www.familyinternet.com/dentist/

Family and Cosmetic Dentistry, home page of Dr. Kim Loos and Dr. R.K. Boyden, contains a plethora of dental resources. Among the resources are an ask the dentist feature with an archive of previous questions, what's new updates, online articles by dental experts, family tips for a better smile, and related dental links. The site can be viewed in eight different languages.

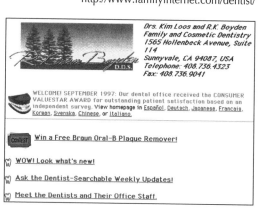

First Class Dentist Online

http://www.interpia.net/~dentist/

First Class Dentist Online contains a variety of dental resources, including Ask the Doc, Find a Doc, a newsletter, and dental sites.

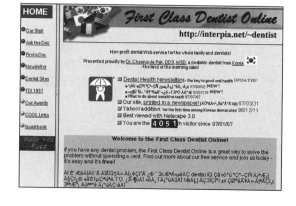

Gentle Dentistry

Gentle Dentistry is an online comprehensive guide to a variety of dental health topics, including dental diseases and treatments, replacement of teeth, cosmetic dentistry, long-lasting tooth whitening, prevention and oral hygiene, sealants/fluoride, drill-less fillings, children's dental health, and a quick guide to dental emergencies. The site also offers an online consultation service to get answers to dental care questions.

http://www.GentleDentistry.com/

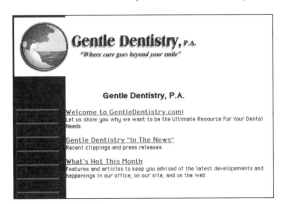

The Highlander Index of Dental Resources

The Highlander Index of Dental Resources is a large index to dental resources on the Internet. It contains more than 1000 links to dental sites, including a list of dental schools on the Web and searchable databases. The site also offers an interactive e-mail feature for analyzing your smile.

http://www.mindspring.com/~cmcleod/

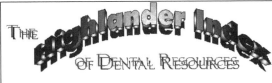

House Call

House Call, provided by Procter & Gamble's Dental ResourceNet, contains useful consumer information on dental problems and procedures, preventive oral care, and new directions.

http://www.dentalcare.com/soap/pg296/call.htm

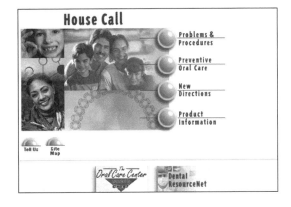

Internet Dentistry Resources

http://indy.radiology.uiowa.edu/Beyond/Dentistry/sites.html

Internet Dentistry Resources, from the University of Iowa College of Dentistry and The Virtual Hospital, is a comprehensive searchable index to a broad range of dental topics, including links to dental colleges, dental organizations and associations, dental education topics, dentist home pages, and much more.

©1994-1997 _The University of Iowa College of Dentistry_, in collaboration with the _Virtual Hospital_

Internet Dentistry Resources

Links found on this list are included for user's information only and are not endorsed by the University of Iowa College of Dentistry. If you wish to add or update an entry on this list, please contact _Janice Quinn_

Links to Dental Colleges

Dental Organizations and Associations

Dental Listservs, Dental Bulletin Boards and Newsgroups

List of Dental Journals

Dental Education Topics:

Kurt A. Butzin, D.D.S.

http://www.butzin.com/

Kurt A. Butzin, a general family dentist, provides information on a variety of dental topics ranging from children's teeth to root canals.

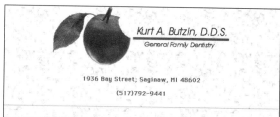

Kurt A. Butzin, D.D.S.
General Family Dentistry

1936 Bay Street; Saginaw, MI 48602

(517)792-9441

I graduated from Michigan State, _Go Spartans_, and the University of Detroit School of Dentistry and have been in private practice since 1981. I serve on the Michigan Dental Association Board of Trustees, the Saginaw Valley District Dental Society Executive Committee and I am member of the house of delegates of the American Dental Association. In 1994-95 I served as president of the Saginaw Valley District Dental Society. I'm an instrument rated private pilot and along with my colleague Dr. Gregory Rosecrans own and run Molarnet Technologies, Inc.

Ms. Flossy's Dental Hygiene News

http://www.geocities.com/HotSprings/7013/

Ms. Flossy's Dental Hygiene News provides information on dental hygiene, dentistry, and helpful hints for the consumer. The site includes links to other dental sites and dental newsgroups.

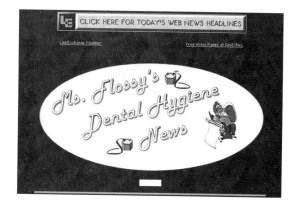

The Oral Care Center

http://www.pg.com/docYourhome/docCrest/

The Oral Care Center, produced by Crest, is loaded with helpful information on oral care. You can view a colorful animated flossing and brushing demonstration, take the Crest quizzes to find out how much you know about oral care, do a science experiment about tooth care, and much more.

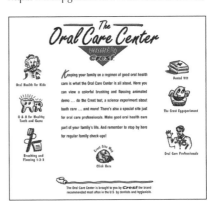

Oral Hygiene FAQ

http://www.colgate.com/Smiles/FAQ/

Oral Hygiene FAQ, from Colgate, provides answers to questions about oral health, dental care, and procedures.

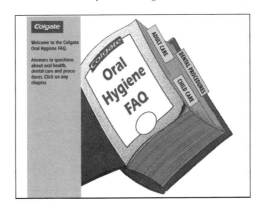

Oral B Convention of Ideas

http://www.oralb.com

Oral B Convention of Ideas provides a forum for exchanging information on oral care. Click on the **Oral Care at Home** section for a variety of family dental care resources. **I can do that too!** generates questions debunking common dental care myths, and the **Oral Care You Need to Know** category contains topics on oral care, answers to special dental problems, a glossary of terms, health links, and parent resources. In addition, the site provides a bulletin board to share ideas on dental care.

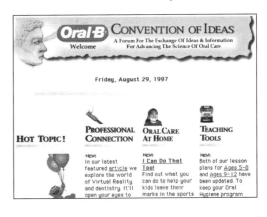

Orthodontic Centers of America

http://www.4braces.com/

Orthodontic Centers of America has patient information about orthodontics on the **FAQ Page.**

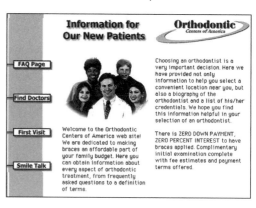

The Orthodontic Information Page

http://www.bracesinfo.com/

The Orthodontic Information Page contains a variety of consumer dental resources, including a discussion of why braces are necessary, kissing with braces, FAQs for adult orthodontic patients, teenage orthodontic patients, and parents of orthodontic patients, a dictionary of orthodontic terms, an orthodontic joke archive, fun facts about braces, new orthodontic products, helpful information for orthodontists, orthodontic links, and other information about orthodontics.

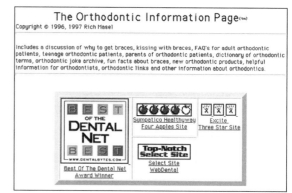

Patient Information

http://vhp.nus.sg/dentalweb/sdhf/sdhf/sdhf.html

Patient Information, from the Singapore Dental Health Foundation, provides online illustrated leaflets for patients on a variety of dental topics. Leaflets include "Braces Make You Beautiful," "Root Canal Treatment," and "Sealants Prevent Decay."

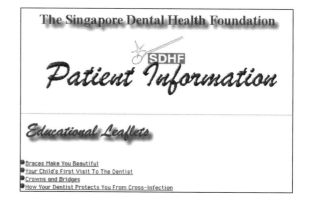

Pediatric Dentistry

http://www.flash.net/~dkennel/

Pediatric Dentistry furnishes information and links regarding pediatric dentistry. Among the topics are baby bottle tooth decay, natal and neonatal teeth, and athletic mouthguards.

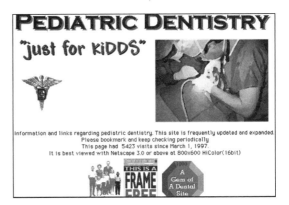

Practical Endodontics

http://www.endomagic.com/

Practical Endodontics provides information for dentists and non-dentists (consumers) on a variety of topics. You can also ask Dr. Kit Weathers questions via e-mail.

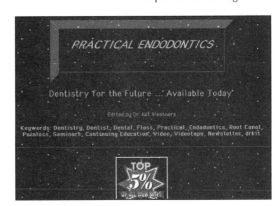

Pre-Dental Page

http://members.iglou.com/kale/Predental.HTM

Pre-Dental Page provides useful information for those considering the dental profession. The site includes information about dentistry, the basics of applying to a dental school, important publications, addresses, and phone numbers, dental schools in the United States on the Web, and links to related sites.

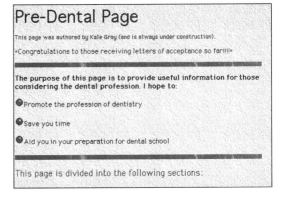

Quinline–Welcome to the World of Dentistry

http://www.quinline.com/

Quinline–Welcome to the World of Dentistry is a multimedia dental information resource on the Internet. The site includes a list of professional dental books, free dental software that can be downloaded, and related links.

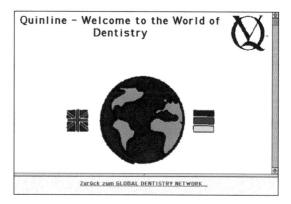

Smile Search

http://www.smilesearch.com

Smile Search is a cooperative network of licensed North American professionals dedicated to raising the profile and standards of dental care. The site contains dental information and links to dental associations and resources.

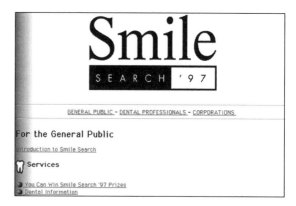

So, You Want To Be A Dentist?

http://www.vvm.com/~bond/home.html

So, You Want To Be A Dentist? provides consumer information on the different kinds of dentists, how to become a dentist, and how to take care of your teeth. The site also includes informative images of teeth.

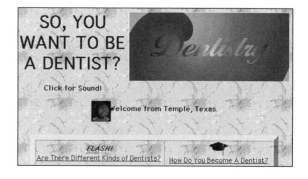

Sports Dentistry On Line

http://www.sportsdentistry.com/

Sports Dentistry On Line provides resources about dental/facial trauma prevention and treatment, what to do when a tooth is knocked out, athletic mouthguard types and designs, and general consumer information.

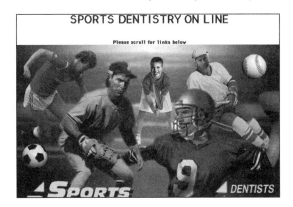

The Tooth Fairy Online

http://www.toothfairy.org/

The Tooth Fairy Online provides a variety of dental resources, including oral hygiene tips, FAQs, and information about baby teeth and flossing.

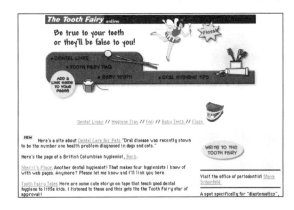

Tooth.net

http://www.tooth.net/

Tooth.net describes dental procedures and provides information on a variety of topics, including oral anatomy and plaque control.

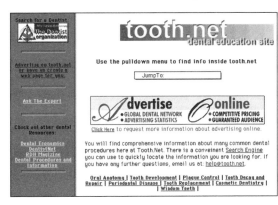

The "Virtual"–Dental Center

http://www-sci.lib.uci.edu/~martindale/Dental.html

The "Virtual"–Dental Center, Martindale's Health Science Guide, contains innumerable links to dental sites. The categories include dictionaries and glossaries, dental literature, online journals, dental anatomy browsers, and online courses and tutorials.

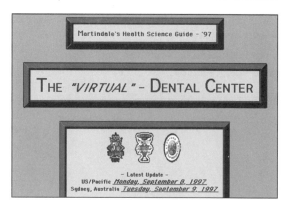

WebDental

http://www.webdental.com/

WebDental provides a variety of consumer resources, including patient information on the different dental specialties. The site also includes a directory of over 170,000 dentists and lists of professional associations and dental schools.

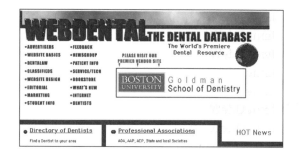

The Wisdom Tooth Home Page

http://www.umanitoba.ca/outreach/wisdomtooth/

The Wisdom Tooth Home Page addresses a wide variety of oral health issues and offers dental hygiene tips for adults, parents, and children. The site also includes related dental links.

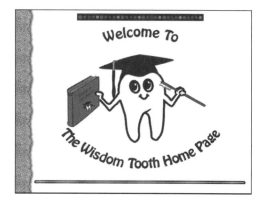

Alternative/ Complementary and Chiropractic Medicine

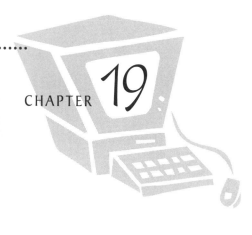

CHAPTER 19

Acupuncture.com

http://acupuncture.com/

Acupuncture.com discusses the benefits of traditional Oriental therapies: acupuncture, herbology, Qi Gong, Chinese nutrition, and Tui Na. The site also provides a list of practitioners around the world and a list of insurance companies that cover acupuncture. Finally, the site has many articles on the use of Oriental therapies in the treatment of medical conditions.

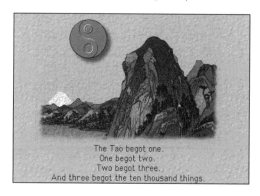

The Tao begot one.
One begot two.
Two begot three.
And three begot the ten thousand things.

Aesclepian Chronicles

http://www.forthrt.com/~chronicl/homepage.html

Aesclepian Chronicles is an online journal of the Synergistic Health Center of Chapel Hill, North Carolina. Synergistic medicine combines techniques of allopathic practice with holistic, alternative forms of healing.

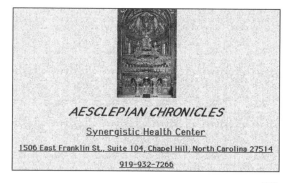

AESCLEPIAN CHRONICLES
Synergistic Health Center
1506 East Franklin St., Suite 104, Chapel Hill, North Carolina 27514
919-932-7266

The Alchemical Medicine Research and Teaching Association

http://www.teleport.com/~amrta/

The Alchemical Medicine Research and Teaching Association offers HealthWWWeb, a rich and broad resource to those interested in nontraditional approaches to health and medicine. Topics include acupuncture, herb dosing and prescribing, diet and nutrition, and homeopathy. Many links to related sites are available, as is a search tool.

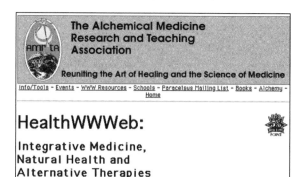

Alexandra Health Center

http://www.homeop.com/

Alexandra Health Center is an alternative medicine site that provides homeopathic cures and herbal formulas. Homeopathy is a holistic approach to medicine.

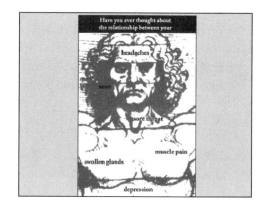

Algy's Herb Page

http://www.algy.com/herb/menu.shtml

Algy's Herb Page offers one-stop shopping for those interested in herbs for medicinal and cooking purposes. You can search a database for information on over 880 herbs, learn to grow and prepare your own herbs for remedies and cooking, and browse the site's library. In addition, there are news bites and articles exposing the false claims made by alternative health hucksters.

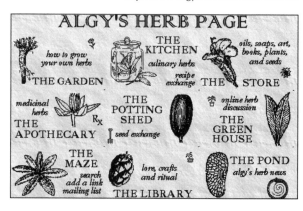

Alternative Health

http://members.aol.com/altamed/inter.htm

Alternative Health is a directory of alternative medicine sites on the Internet. General categories include Acupuncture, Aromatherapy, Ayurveda, Bach Flowers, Chiropractic, Gemstone & Crystal Healing, Herbs, Homeopathy, Nutrition & Orthomolecular, and Reiki. Access is also provided to search engines and to chat groups.

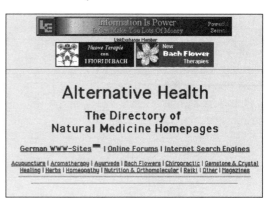

Alternative Medicine and Homeopathy

http://members.aol.com/bryonia

Alternative Medicine and Homeopathy offers information to those interested in alternative medicine. Many articles focus on topics such as AIDS, cancer, estrogen treatments, menopause, vaccinations, Nutrisweet, fluoride, and the Gulf War syndrome. Numerous links to related sites are available.

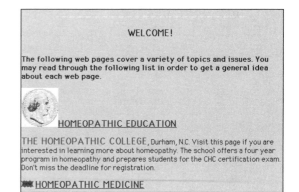

Alternative Medicine Connection

http://arxc.com/arxchome.htm

The Alternative Medicine Connection is an online information service for the holistic health community with interactive newsletters and patient resources. The site also includes a **MedSearch** feature for finding a holistic practitioner in your area.

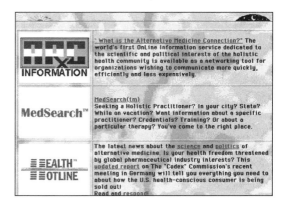

Alternative Medicine Digest

http://www.alternativemedicine.com/

The Alternative Medicine Digest presents summaries of alternative medicine articles found in journals, research, conferences, and newsletters. The site includes the current issue, an interactive index of back issues, and a search service for health practitioners.

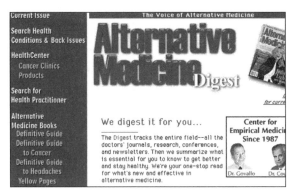

The Alternative Medicine Homepage

http://www.pitt.edu/~cbw/altm.html

The Alternative Medicine Homepage is a huge directory to sources of information about unconventional, unorthodox, unproven, or alternative medicine, as well as to complementary, innovative, or integrative therapy. Information comes in the form of search tools, consumer information, and related resources or links on the Internet.

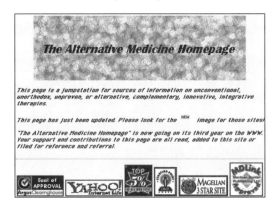

AltHealth Search

http://www.althealthsearch.com/

AltHealth Search is a resource center designed to help find alternative medical practitioners in your area. AltHealth Search has over 173,000 listings of alternative health care practitioners throughout the United States.

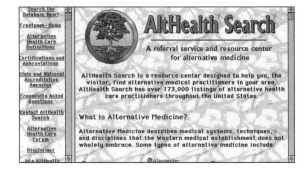

The American Association of Naturopathic Physicians

http://www.naturopathic.org/

The American Association of Naturopathic Physicians provides a variety of alternate health resources for naturopathic medicine. To find a collection of articles written by naturopathic doctors (NDs) for the public, click on **Library** in the Features section. You can also click on **Laughter As Medicine** for humorous articles on medicine.

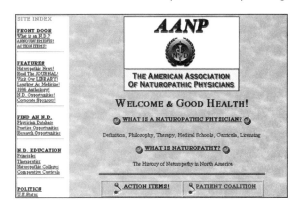

Ask Dr. Weil

http://cgi.pathfinder.com/drweil/

Ask Dr. Weil is an interactive site that provides answers to your health questions. The site contains an archive of past questions and answers, a top 10 list, healthy recipes, a bulletin board for posting questions, and a database to search for alternative health information on a disease, treatment, or remedy. Included in the database section is an alphabetical index of all Dr. Andrew Weil's questions and answers and material from his best-selling alternate medicine book, *Natural Health, Natural Medicine.*

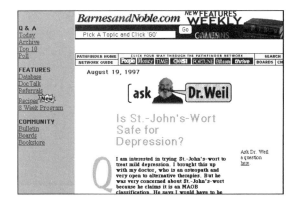

The Australian Alternative Health Directory

http://www.aahd.com.au/

The Australian Alternative Health Directory contains a list of resources for alternative health, including a directory of Australian health practitioners.

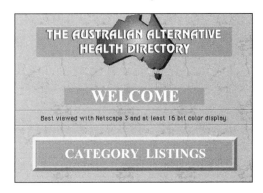

Australian Whole Health Home Page

http://aushealth.netconnect.com.au/

The Australian Whole Health Home Page provides information about herbs, meditation, hypnosis, dance therapy, an Australian practitioner directory, and much more.

Avicenna

http://www.avicenna.com/

Avicenna is a comprehensive alternative medicine resource free to all health care professionals and consumers. The site offers searchable databases, including free Medline access, reference materials, and tools for medical practice.

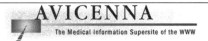

Ayurvedic Health Center

http://www.ayurvedic.org/

The Ayurvedic Health Center provides alternative medicine, home remedies for common diseases, based on basic principles of Ayurveda. The site includes a live chat room, where you can discuss your problems live with Ayurvedic experts, and newsletters, featuring tips and articles.

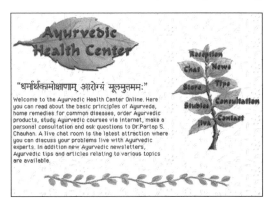

Botanical.com

http://www.botanical.com/botanical/mgmh/mgmh.html

Botanical.com features a searchable database of over 800 medicinal plants based on Mrs. M. Grieve's book, *A Modern Herbal,* published in 1931. You can search the database by the common name or by an ailment to find about a plant's actions, uses, or remedies. The site cautions that the information is meant for historical purposes only.

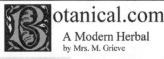

Chiro-Web

http://pages.prodigy.com/CT/doc/doc.html

Chiro-Web is an online connection to chiropractic resources on the Internet. The site provides up-to-date chiropractic information and includes links to other related health sites.

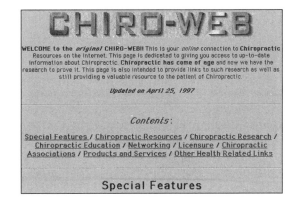

Chiropractic OnLine Today

http://www.panix.com/~tonto1/dc.html

Chiropractic OnLine Today provides a plethora of chiropractic resources for consumers. To find the resources, click on the **Main Menu,** scroll and select **Chiropractic** or **Education Corner.**

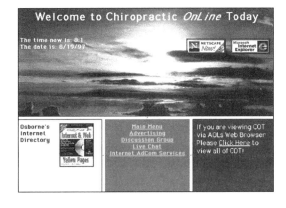

The Chiropractic Page

http://www.mbnet.mb.ca/~jwiens/chiro.html

The Chiropractic Page, maintained by John Wiens, from the Elmwood Chiropractic Centre in Winnipeg, provides a wealth of chiropractic resources, including a nutrition database that lets you determine the nutritional value of a particular food, software, research, organizations, health care and Internet resources, and colleges. You access these options by clicking on **The Full Chiropractic Page.**

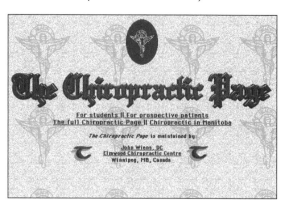

The Complimentary Health Network

http://www.cris.com/~prosch/biomed/index.shtml

The Complimentary Health Network, presented by Dr. Gus J. Prosch, Jr., provides comprehensive alternative medicine resources. The site includes a stop smoking page, information about dieting, chronic yeast infections and other diseases, online patient information for a variety of health-related topics, and related links to alternative medicine sites.

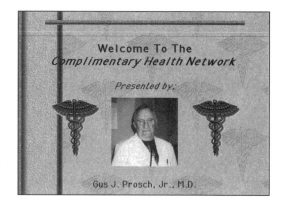

Delicious! Online

http://www.delicious-online.com/

Delicious! Online, based on the monthly *Delicious!* magazine of natural living, features articles on alternative medicine. Topics include nutritional supplements, diet, food preparation, organic foods, and homeopathy. The site also offers an archive of back issues, an index to conditions, diseases, and treatments, recipes for a variety of dishes, and related links.

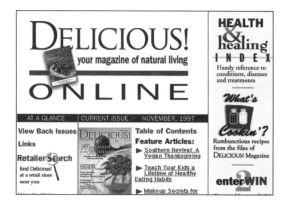

Directional Non-Force Technique

http://direct.nonforce.com/dnft/

Directional Non-Force Technique describes a unique chiropractic procedure in which the leg and/or the thumb are squeezed, as opposed to the snapping of the back. The site also includes links to other chiropractic sites.

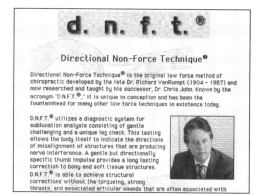

Dr. Bower's Complementary and Alternative Medicine Home Page

http://galen.med.virginia.edu/~pjb3s/
ComplementaryHomePage.html

Dr. Bower's Complementary and Alternative Medicine Home Page contains thousands of links for alternative and complementary medicine. Topics include complementary practices, treatment of specific diseases, and a list of related medicine links.

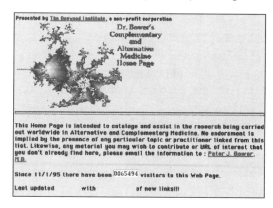

Environmental and Preventive Health Center of Atlanta

http://www.ephca.com/

Environmental and Preventive Health Center of Atlanta, from Dr. Stephen B. Edelson, reflects the alternative medicine point of view. It offers a great many articles, divided among five general categories: environmental and preventive medicine, diagnosis and treatment, chronic and autoimmune illnesses, women's medical challenges, and ADHA/autism/developmental delays.

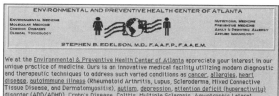

The Essential Garden

http://essentialgarden.com/

The Essential Garden presents alternative health news in the form of three magazines: *Well Being Journal, The Herb Blurb,* and *Richter's Herbletter.* The site also describes a number of alternative health products that employ aromatherapy.

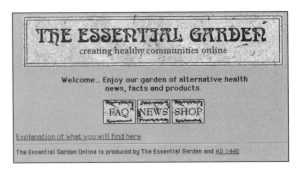

Gerson.org

http://www.gerson.org/

Gerson.org describes the Gerson Therapy, which is dedicated to the treatment of degenerative diseases (heart disease, diabetes, etc.) chiefly through a vegetarian diet, juices, and non-toxic medication. Articles from the *Gerson Healing Newsletter* are offered, as are links to other alternative medicine resources on the Internet.

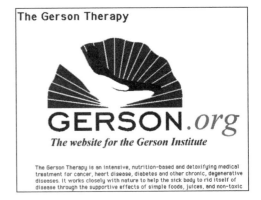

GroupWeb Directories

http://www.groupweb.com/health/alt_med.htm

GroupWeb Directories provides a directory of alternative medicine sites.

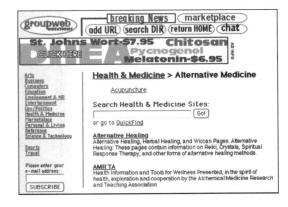

Healing-Arts Magazine

http://www.healing-arts.com/

Healing-Arts Magazine offers chiropractic health articles in the **Archives** under the Healthwatch section.

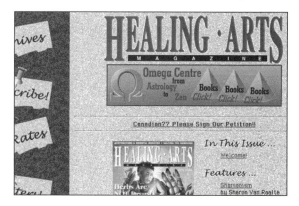

Health & Nutrition Breakthroughs

http://www.hnbreakthroughs.com/

Health & Nutrition Breakthroughs, an online version of the monthly magazine *Health & Nutrition Breakthroughs,* presents alternative medicine information and remedies based on food and supplement research. The site also features a nutrition question-and-answer service and back issues.

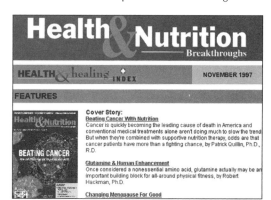

HealthWorld Online

http://www.healthy.net/

HealthWorld Online is a comprehensive collection of information on conventional, natural, and alternative health on the Internet. For an overview of this mega-site, click on **QuickN'Dex.**

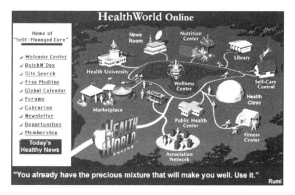

Henriette's Herbal Homepage

http://sunsite.unc.edu/herbmed/

Henriette's Herbal Homepage contains an online collection of annotated links to herbal matters.

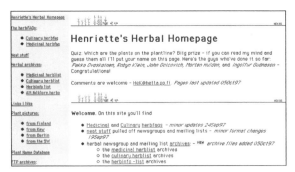

Herb Research Foundation

http://www.herbs.org/

The Herb Research Foundation is a research and educational organization focusing on herbs and medicinal plants. The site includes over 150,000 scientific articles with up-to-date information on thousands of herbs.

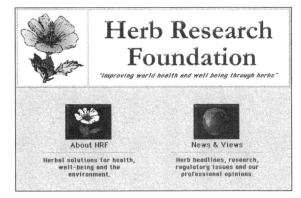

Herb Web

http://www.herbweb.com/

Herb Web contains an illustrated herb catalog that can serve as a handy reference to medicinal and botanical plants. The site also includes links to ethnobotanical resources.

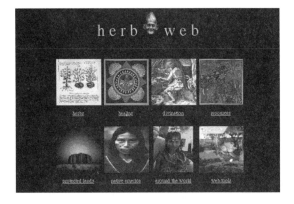

HerbNET

http://www.herbnet.com/

HerbNET is a comprehensive Web site devoted to those seeking information about herbs, herbal products and remedies, and publications on herbs. This site's magazine features the medicinal herb of the month, the edible flower of the month, and the essential oil of the month.

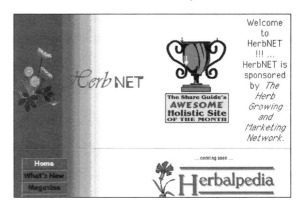

Holistic Healing Web Page

http://www.holisticmed.com/

The Holistic Healing Web Page contains articles on nutrition, yoga, breath work, toxic consumer products, and many other subjects. The site also offers more than 1000 links to other holistic healing sites, conference and retreat listings, case histories of healings and transformation, important news items, a holistic mailing list and newsgroups listings, practitioner directories, and much more.

Holistic Healing Web Page

Holistic healing and alternative medicine documentation, articles on nutrition, yoga, breathwork, toxic consumer products and many other subjects. 1000+ quality links to other holistic healing sites, conference and retreat listings, case histories of healings & transformation, important news items, holistic mailing list and USENET groups listings, practitioner directories, and much more!

The holistic medicine / alternative medicine -related information presented on this WWV page is not meant as medical advice. What is presented are IDEAS which can be discussed with your chosen healthcare practitioner.

Please send thoughts, comments, questions or design suggestions to mgold@holisticmed.com

Major Sections

- Articles and Documents Section
- Case Histories of Healing & Transformation
- Conferences, Retreats & Trade Show Listings
- News Bytes

- Web Page Links Index
- Internet Mailing List Index
- USENET Group Index
- Holistic Healing Bookstore in Association with Amazon.com

- What's New!
- Find a Holistic Practitioner!!!

- Humor

*** Creative Donation Web Page! ***

The Holistic Health Page

http://www.geocities.com/HotSprings/5940/

The Holistic Health Page is an alternative medicine site about homeopathy and herbs. The site, available in English, German, and French, includes holistic health directories and home pages.

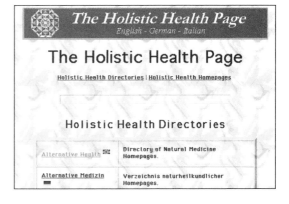

Holistic Internet Community

http://www.holistic.com/

The Holistic Internet Community provides a place to exchange information and resources to live a balanced life. The site contains articles, reviews, and essays written by leading holistic practitioners.

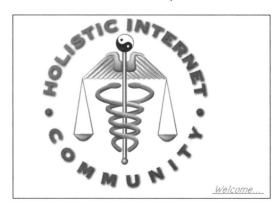

Homeopathy Home Page

http://www.dungeon.com/~cam/

The Homeopathy Home Page is a primer on treating illnesses with homeopathic medicine. The site contains a comprehensive collection of homeopathy sites, newsgroups, mailing lists, and links to other complementary resources.

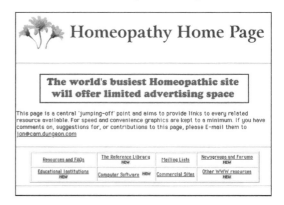

The Kahn Holistic pH Balance Evaluation

http://www.holistic.com/listings/zphbalance/drmjk.html

The Kahn Holistic pH Balance Evaluation provides information about the foods, minerals, vitamins, and herbs that can balance your body chemistry. The site offers an explanation of the Kahn pH Balance Theory and a list of holistic articles.

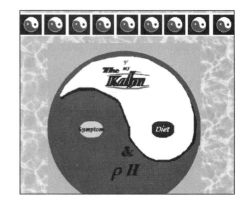

Maharishi Vedic Approach to Health

http://www.vedichealth.com/

Maharishi Vedic Approach to Health offers a holistic program for treating 32 chronic disorders, including asthma, arthritis, fatigue, and insomnia.

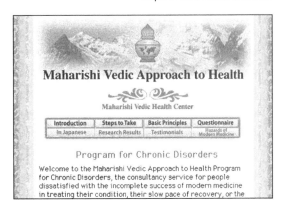

MedGuide

http://www.medguide.net/

MedGuide features a large database of selected Internet resources covering the spectrum of modern medicine and health care from A to Z. The site provides a search engine to find health information on subjects ranging from acupuncture to Zen and everything in between. In addition, the site offers lists of medical colleges and associations.

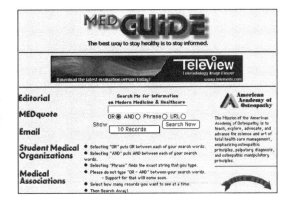

Meditopia!

http://www.meditopia.com/

Meditopia! is an Oriental medicine site with information about alternative medicine treatment of a variety of diseases using natural herbs.

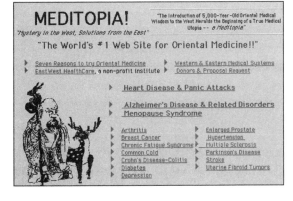

MedWeb Alternative Medicine

http://www.gen.emory.edu/MEDWEB/keyword/
alternative_medicine.html

MedWeb Alternative Medicine, from Emory University
Health Sciences Center Library, provides an extensive
alphabetical list of alternative medicine sites categorized
by topic. The index covers everything from acupuncture
to wellness.

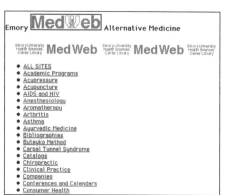

The Menopause Link

http://www.progest.com/

The Menopause Link contains online holistic medicine
resources for women in menopause. Women can read
humorous stories about their menopause experiences,
sample articles in the newsletter, *Natural Solutions,* or
review previously answered menopause questions.
Women can also e-mail their own stories with the
possibility of publication, and even get answers to a
menopause question from a homeopathic doctor.

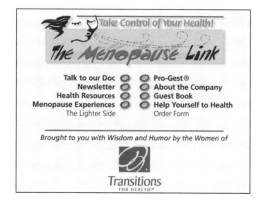

Mother Nature's General Store

http://www.mothernature.com

Mother Nature's General Store provides a
menu of choices, including chat rooms and a
recipe exchange. There is also general information on various health-related topics such
as aromatherapy, herbology, and vitamins and
a library to search for alternative health
articles.

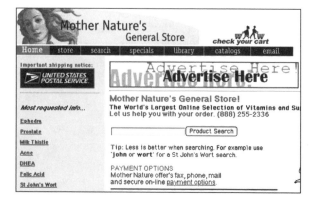

The Natural Connection

http://www.natural-connection.com/

The Natural Connection contains a rich storehouse of resources, including a directory for holistic practitioners, online publications such as *Yoga Journal* and *Macrobiotics Today,* a kitchen full of recipes, health, healing, and fitness discussion groups, and tips from famous natural foods chefs.

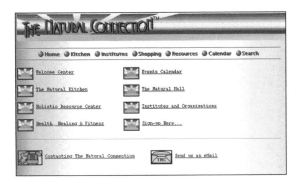

Natural Health Village

http://www.naturalhealthvillage.com/

Natural Health Village contains legislation, legal information, and debates about natural health issues, along with a list of congressional e-mail addresses in the **Town Hall** section. The **Learning** section features an extensive collection of alternative sites. The site invites you to subscribe to its free weekly electronic newsletter, *Natural HealthLine.*

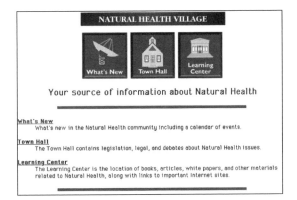

Nutrition Guide

http://www.nutrition-warehouse.com/NWGuideMain.html

Nutrition Guide, from the Nutrition Warehouse, provides an A to Z remedies guide to alternative medicines ranging from acidophilus to wild Mexican yam.

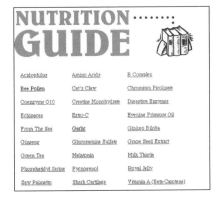

Nutrition Science News

http://www.nutritionsciencenews.com/

Nutrition Science News, an online version of the monthly magazine *Nutrition Science News*, features comprehensive information on vitamins, minerals, herbs, homeopathy, nutraceuticals, and other supplements. The site also contains an archive of issues dating back to 1995.

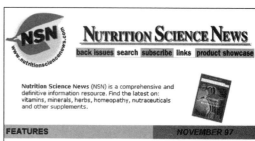

Office of Alternative Medicine

http://altmed.od.nih.gov/

The Office of Alternative Medicine, part of the National Institutes of Health, provides information about complementary alternative medicine (CAM) therapies, treatments, and practitioners. Click on **What is CAM?** to find this information. To find a list of alternative medicine government reports, select **Information Resources** and click on **OAM Clearinghouse** for the online publications.

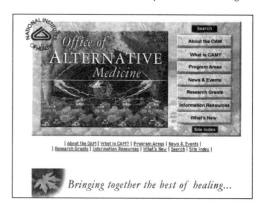

Physical Therapy and Chiropractic

http://www.batnet.com/nopain/

Dr. Gale McIntosh offers long-lasting healing to her patients by combining chiropractic treatment with physical therapy. The site also includes related links.

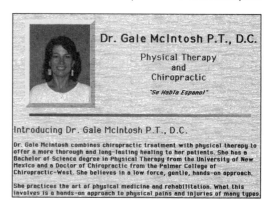

The Richard and Hinda Rosenthal Center for Complementary & Alternative Medicine

http://cpmcnet.columbia.edu/dept/rosenthal/

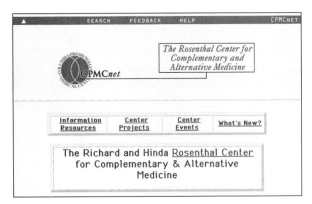

The Richard and Hinda Rosenthal Center for Complementary & Alternative Medicine contains a collection of alternative and complementary medicine sites. Click on **Information Resources** to find these sites.

The Road Back Foundation

http://roadback.org

The Road Back Foundation discusses an alternative treatment for various arthritic conditions, which involves the use of antibiotics in combination with an anti-inflammatory drug.

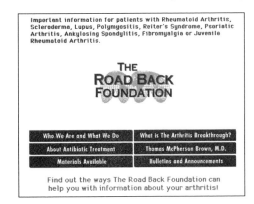

The Share Guide

http://www.shareguide.com/

The Share Guide is an online magazine focusing on holistic health, personal growth, and environmental awareness. The magazine features articles on a variety of topics and has related links to holistic health resources.

THE SHARE GUIDE

Holistic Health Zine & Resource Guide

Welcome to *The Share Guide*, a magazine focusing on holistic health, personal growth and environmental awareness. Our goal is to make information available for people actively working to improve themselves and the planet. We feature thought-provoking articles on a variety of subjects, and resources that support conscious change and harmony with the earth. We are constantly expanding and updating this site; our network of holistic health businesses & conscious web sites is growing daily – **bookmark this site and visit us often!**

Solutions to Health Problems

http://www.nutramed.com/zeno/

Solutions to Health Problems reflects the point of view of alternative medicine. It contains many articles describing health problems that may be related to diet, allergy, nutrition, or environmental factors. The areas of nutrition and the environment are given special emphasis at this site.

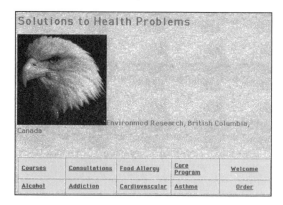

University of Washington Medicinal Herb Garden

http://www.nnlm.nlm.nih.gov/pnr/uwmhg/

The University of Washington Medicinal Herb Garden is an online resource for herbalists, medics, and botanists of all levels. Click on an **index** of common names to find information along with a photograph about a specific herb.

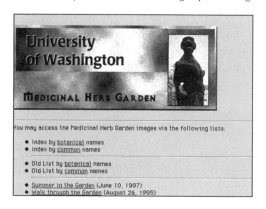

Vads Corner

http://www.geocities.com/HotSprings/2188/

Vads Corner, Dr. M. Vadivale's home page, is an index to hundreds of medical and health-related sites, including many search tools. In addition, there are links to many medical journals and to search engines.

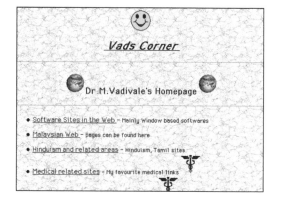

Vegetarian Pages

http://www.veg.org/veg/

Vegetarian Pages is an index to links of interest to vegetarians and vegans. FAQs are answered and links to another major index are offered. The site contains readers' recipes, articles about nutrition and health, and a worldwide list of vegetarian and vegetarian friendly restaurants.

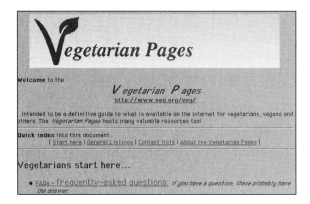

Vegetarian Resource Center

http://www.tiac.net/users/vrc/

Vegetarian Resource Center contains links to vegetarian discussion groups, sites, and various information in the areas of vegetarian diet and lifestyle.

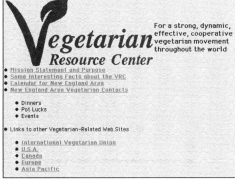

The Vegetarian Resource Group

http://www.vrg.org

The Vegetarian Resource Group is a mega-site with basic facts on vegetarianism and how to become a vegetarian. The site includes lists of vegetarian literature and teaching materials, recipes and vegetarian food replacements, a vegetarian search engine, feeding vegan kids, a guide to non-leather goods, and vegetarian online links to finding vegetarian stuff on AOL, CompuServe, MSN, and other commercial services.

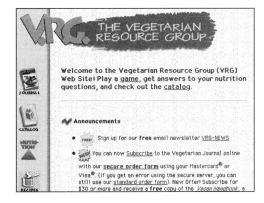

The Vegetarian Society of the United Kingdom

http://www.veg.org/veg/Orgs/VegSocUK/

The Vegetarian Society of the United Kingdom, established in 1847, provides a collection of online resources for healthy living. The site includes an index with hundreds of vegetarian recipes for every occasion, information sheets, a health and nutrition section, and youth pages.

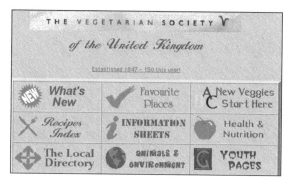

Veggie Heaven

http://www.webserve.co.uk/Veggie/

Veggie Heaven, created by Rosamond Richardson, furnishes over 160 vegetarian recipes, amazing facts and figures, and much more. There are tasty recipes for main dishes, salads, desserts, and other things.

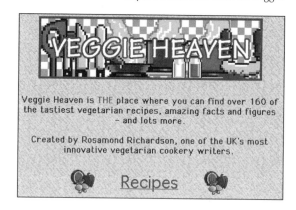

Veggie Life Magazine

http://www.egw.com/vlm.htm

Veggie Life Magazine is a complete healthier lifestyle reference with more than 100 full-color pages of tips, techniques, recipes, and remedies covering organic gardening, optimum nutrition, herbal health, and plant-based well-being for health conscious consumers.

Veggies Unite!

http://www.vegweb.com/

Veggies Unite!, an online guide to vegetarian living, contains a directory of over 2000 vegan recipes. In addition, the site offers a grocery list maker, a weekly meal planner, and a monthly e-mail *VegWeb* newsletter.

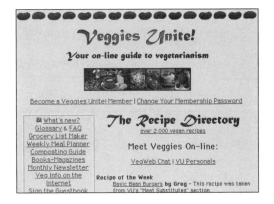

VegSource

http://www.vegsource.com/

VegSource offers news, recipes, information, and discussion boards related to vegetarianism and other topics. Two featured participants, Charles Atwood, M.D., and Ruth Heidrich, Ph.D., provide answers to health questions as well as fitness and nutrition information.

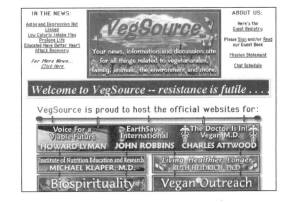

The Virtual Vegetarian

http://www.vegetariantimes.com/

The Virtual Vegetarian, created by *Vegetarian Times*, contains veggie recipes, information about natural remedies, discussion boards, and other vegetarian resources.

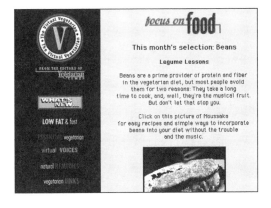

Wellspring Media

http://www.wellmedia.com/

Wellspring Media provides online information promoting a holistic approach to health. The *Wellness* newsletter features brief articles on topics such as nutrition, aging, fitness, and women's health, as well as advice on medication and maintaining healthy relationships. The site also includes links to other holistic resources.

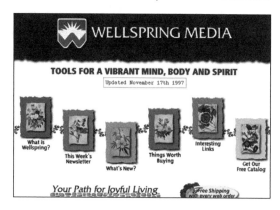

The World Source

http://www.intelligent-health.com/

The World Source provides a variety of health topics for alternative medicine, including daily health headlines and an Eye On Medicine page with an A to Z directory of garden herbs from around the world. To find these resources, scroll to the **Health Related** section.

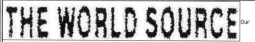

Physical and Developmental Disabilities

CHAPTER 20

Access-Able Travel Source

http://www.access-able.com/

Access-Able Travel Source, organized by a disabled person, provides information on wheelchair-accessible trips.

Accommodations Resources

http://pursuit.rehab.uiuc.edu/pursuit/dis-resources/
accommodations/accommodations.html

Accommodations Resources contains an extensive list of disabilities such as attention deficit disorder (ADD), vision impairments, Tourette's syndrome, and learning disabilities. Each disability is defined, with characteristics and classroom accommodations.

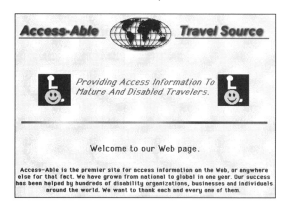

American Hyperlexia Association

http://www.hyperlexia.org/

The American Hyperlexia Association home page provides information on the condition of hyperlexia, differential diagnosis among hyperlexia, autism, pervasive developmental delay, and Asperger's syndrome, and on speech and language disorders. The site also includes articles on inclusion and remediation techniques.

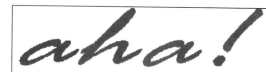

A MERICAN H YPERLEXIA A SSOCIATION H OME P AGE

Please sign our guestbook

☞ NEW CSLD Sponsored Conference on Fast ForWord ☜

The Center for Speech and Language Disorders is Sponsoring a one-day conference on exciting new brain research and the Fast ForWord therapy for language disordered children. Click the above link for detailed information.

☞ NEW The Hyperlexia Parents' Page ! ☜

Americans with Disabilities Act Document Center

http://janweb.icdi.wvu.edu/kinder/

The Americans with Disabilities Act Document Center contains copies of the Americans with Disabilities Act of 1990. The site also provides links to other Internet sources with disability information and sources concerning occupational health and safety.

Americans with Disabilities Act Document Center

ADA Statute, Regulations, ADAAG (Americans with Disabilities Act Accessibility Guidelines), Federally Reviewed Tech Sheets, and Other Assistance Documents

[Home | Documents | Links | Kinder]

This site has been cited as a 3-Sept-96 *Times Pick* by the Los Angeles Times, rated among the top 5% of all sites on the Internet by Point Survey, and rated as a Three Star *** site by both Magellan and Mental Health Net.

To view this page without tables, click here

Created by Duncan C. Kinder

with the assistance of the Job Accommodation Network, the

Great Lakes Disability and Business Technical Assistance Center, and

The Arc Home Page

http://thearc.org/

The Arc Home Page describes the nation's largest voluntary organization commited to the welfare of children and adults with mental retardation and their families. The site offers many articles, especially with regard to advocacy, and related links.

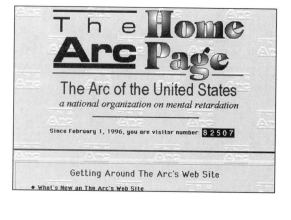

The Arc Home Page

The Arc of the United States
a national organization on mental retardation

Since February 1, 1996, you are visitor number: 8 2 5 0 7

Getting Around The Arc's Web Site

• What's New on The Arc's Web Site

The Arc's Q&As and Other Fact Sheets

http://thearc.org/qaindex.html

The Arc's Q&As and Other Fact Sheets provides information about mental retardation and other developmental disabilities in the following categories: services/support, Social Security, the Americans with Disabilities Act, mental retardation, community living/employment, health promotion and prevention, and education. Almost all information is offered in a question-and-answer format.

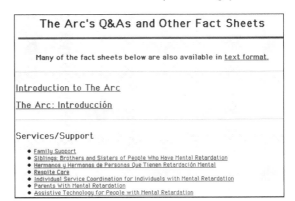

Attention Deficit Disorder

http://add.miningco.com/

Attention Deficit Disorder (ADD), part of the Mining Company Web site, contains a collection of articles and links to ADD sites.

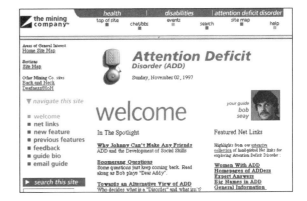

Attention Deficit Disorder and Related Issues

http://www.ns.net/users/BrandiV/

Attention Deficit Disorder and Related Issues, created by Brandi Valentine, offers a vast collection of online resources for ADD/ADHD.

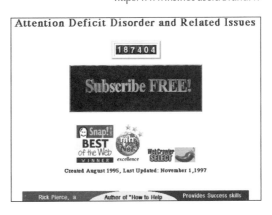

Attention Deficit Disorder WWW Archive

http://www.realtime.net/cyanosis/add

Attention Deficit Disorder WWW Archive, started by Meng Meng Wong from the University of Pennsylvania, contains resources ranging from diagnostic criteria to tips for living with attention deficit disorder.

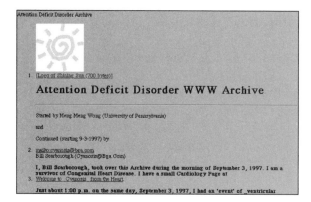

Autism Resources

http://web.syr.edu/~jmwobus/autism/

Autism Resources, maintained by John Wobus, is a comprehensive collection of online autism resources organized by topic. The site includes general disabilities, general information on autism, mailing lists, news sources, methods and treatments, related links, and other topics.

Blindness Resource Center

http://www.nyise.org/blind.htm

The Blindness Resource Center contains hundreds of links related to access technology, eye diseases and visual conditions, organizations, braille, and computer technology for persons with visual impairments. The site is adapted for special access perspectives for persons with visual impairments.

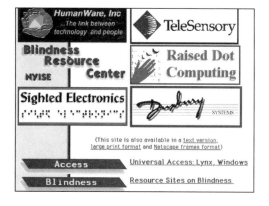

Center for the Study of Autism

http://www.autism.org/

The Center for the Study of Autism provides information and resources on various topics related to or about autism.

Center for the Study of Autism

Jump to Table of Contents

The Center for the Study of Autism (CSA) is located in the Salem/Portland, Oregon area. The Center was established in 1991 and was first located in Newberg. In 1994, the Center moved to Beaverton; and in 1996, the Center moved to Salem. The Center provides information about autism to parents and professionals, and conducts research on the efficacy of various therapeutic interventions. Most of the research is in collaboration with the Autism Research Institute in San Diego, California. If you would like to write to us, our mailing address is: Center for the Study of Autism, P.O. Box 4538, Salem, OR 97302, U.S.A.

This Web page was developed to provide information on various topics related to or about autism. **This Virtual Web Site was made possible by the generosity of Khera Communications, Inc.**

We hope you find this information helpful.

Table of Contents

Overview of Autism
[Chinese version] [English version] [Korean version] [Spanish version]

Children and Adults with Attention Deficit Disorders

http://www.chadd.org

Children and Adults with Attention Deficit Disorders discusses attention deficit disorder (ADD) as it affects both children and adults, but ADD in children is clearly the emphasis at this site. There is information about both conventional and controversial treatment, about parenting a child with ADD, about ADD in the classroom, and about legal rights and services. A link to government resources is offered, as are links to other sources of information on the Internet.

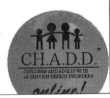

Hear our Public Service Announcement

Special Offer! Join C.H.A.D.D. Now and receive a free gift.

Meet the Board of Directors / 1996 Annual Report

CH.A.D.D.
CHILDREN AND ADULTS WITH
ATTENTION DEFICIT DISORDERS

DISCLAIMER

What is CH.A.D.D.®?

Children and Adults with Attention Deficit Disorders (CH.A.D.D.) is a nonprofit parent-based organization formed to better the lives of individuals with attention deficit disorders and those who care for them.

Through family support and advocacy, public and professional education and encouragement of scientific research, CH.A.D.D. works to ensure that

CH.A.D.D.
CHILDREN AND ADULTS WITH
ATTENTION DEFICIT DISORDERS

online!

Clinician's View

http://chili.rt66.com/cview/

Clinician's View provides therapists and parents with resources for helping people with special needs. The site includes a monthly journal article, a parent therapist forum for exchanging information, an ask the experts service for posting questions, a clinician's corner, an information line, and related links.

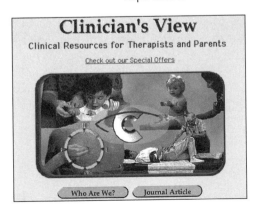

Clinician's View

Clinical Resources for Therapists and Parents

Check out our Special Offers

Who Are We?   Journal Article

Deaf World Web

http://dww.deafworldweb.org/

Deaf World Web is the largest and leading multipurpose deaf Web site and provides deaf-related resources from around the world.

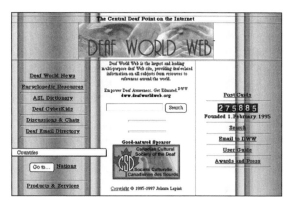

Deafness

http://deafness.miningco.com/

Deafness, from the Mining Company, provides online information and links to related sites about deafness.

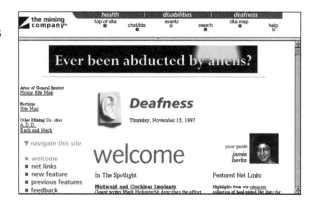

Disability Net

http://www.disabilitynet.co.uk/

Disability Net is a worldwide information and news service for all disabled people and people with an interest in disability issues. Among its vast resources are links to useful disability information and a soapbox so you can share your opinions.

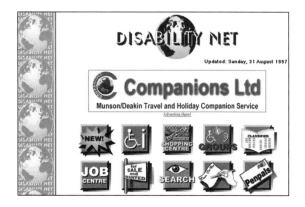

Disability Resources, Inc.

http://www.geocities.com/~drm

Disability Resources, Inc. is a non-profit organization that publishes online *Disability Resources Monthly*. The site includes the **DRM WebWatcher,** an easy-to-use guide to Web resources, and **Librarians' Connections,** with information about listservs, professional associations, and assistive technology to librarians who serve people with disabilities.

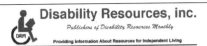

Discover Technology Web Site

http://discovertechnology.com/

The purpose of the Discover Technology Web Site is to share information that is pertinent to people with disabilities and those professionals who provide services. The site includes a comprehensive list of related links, adaptive software by category and the location so you can download their demos, and a list of pen pals who only use voice communication.

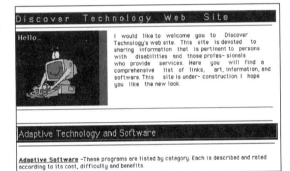

Down Syndrome WWW Page

http://www.nas.com/downsyn/

The Down Syndrome WWW Page has links to every aspect of this congenital disease. Among the resources are articles, FAQs, organizations, and support groups.

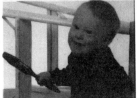

Dwarfism

http://www-bfs.ucsd.edu/dwarfism/

The Dwarfism site provides resources about restricted growth, including a mailing list, medical information, and other related organizations.

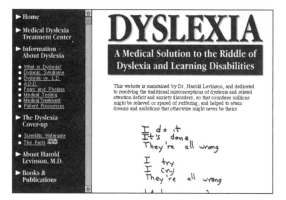

Dyslexia

http://www.dyslexiaonline.com/

Dyslexia, maintained by Dr. Harold Levinson, presents information about the misconceptions of dyslexia and related attention deficit and anxiety disorders.

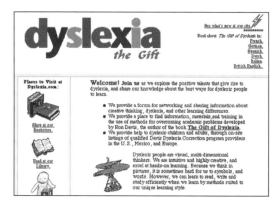

Dyslexia The Gift

http://www.dyslexia.com/

Dyslexia The Gift, based on the Ron Davis book, provides a forum for sharing information about dyslexia and other learning difficulties. The site contains information and articles on materials and methods for overcoming academic dyslexic problems.

Health & Disability Index Page

http://www.ability.org.uk/health.html

The Health & Disability Index Page provides a huge collection of indexes on many topics, including anorexia, autism, blindness, and epilepsy. For an alphabetical list of all the indexes, scroll to the bottom of the page and click on **Full A-Z Index.** Each index contains articles, reports, and fact sheets. The site also includes a chat room, a bulletin board, and related links.

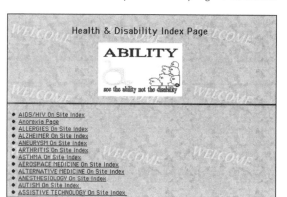

Hearing Help-On-Line

http://www.betterhearing.org/

Hearing Help-On-Line, from the Better Hearing Institute, informs persons with impaired hearing and the general public about hearing loss and the help that is available through medicine, surgery, amplification, and other rehabilitation. The site provides comprehensive information on hearing loss, tinnitus, and hearing aids, as well as a directory of hearing care providers and famous people with hearing loss.

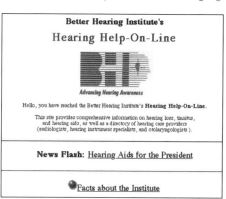

How to Guide the Blind

http://biomed.nus.sg/access/guideblind.html

How to Guide the Blind provides illustrated information on how sighted people can guide the blind.

National Information Center for Children and Youth with Disabilities

http://www.kidsource.com/NICHCY/

The National Information Center for Children and Youth with Disabilities, part of KidSource Online, contains a collection of articles, fact sheets, and information for parenting children with a range of disabilities and developmental disorders.

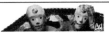

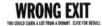

WRONG EXIT
YOU COULD LEARN A LOT FROM A DUMMY. CLICK FOR DETAILS.

National Information Center for Children and Youth with Disabilities

P.O. Box 1492
Washington, DC 20013-1492
1-800-695-0285 (Voice/TT)
(202) 884-8200 (Voice/TT)

NICHCY Articles and Information

- NICHCY: Parenting A Child With Special Needs ***NEW***
- A Guide to Children's Literature and Disability (1989-1994)
- Questions Often Asked About Special Education Services
- Having a Daughter With a Disability: Is it Different For Girls?

National Institute on Life Planning for Persons With Disabilities

http://www.sonic.net/nilp/

The National Institute on Life Planning for Persons With Disabilities, affiliated with Sonoma State University, is a national clearinghouse dedicated to helping persons with disabilities and their families plan for the future. This site includes a life planner database, life planning listserv, publications, questions and answers, and national training programs.

IF YOU HAVE A DISABILITY OR A LOVED ONE WITH A DISABILITY, THIS IS THE MOST IMPORTANT SITE YOU WILL EVER VISIT. IT WILL HELP YOU PLAN FOR THE FUTURE.

NATIONAL INSTITUTE ON LIFE PLANNING
FOR
PERSONS WITH DISABILITIES

Administrative Office, P.O. Box 5093, Twin Falls, ID, 83303-5093
Fax 208-735-8562 E-Mail: rlee@sonic.net

NILP is a national organization dedicated to promoting transition, life and person centered planning for all persons with disabilities and their families. Because it is a diverse and the only professional membership association made up of teachers, lawyers, planners, social workers, advocates, etc., it provides this special Web page to help families obtain the latest information on transition, life and person centered planning, government benefits, advocacy, guardianship, aging, housing, supported employment, etc.

If you have a disability or if you have responsibility for a person with a disability,

One A.D.D. Place

http://www.greatconnect.com/oneaddplace/

One A.D.D. Place has a wealth of information about attention deficit disorder/attention deficit hyperactivity disorder (ADD/ADHD), including an adult checklist, famous people with ADD, an online library with newsletters, articles, and references, and related links to ADD/ADHD sites.

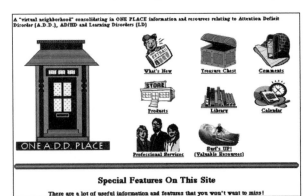

A "virtual neighborhood" consolidating in ONE PLACE information and resources relating to Attention Deficit Disorder (A.D.D.), AD/HD and Learning Disorders (LD)

What's New   Treasure Chest   Comments

Products   Library   Calendar

ONE A.D.D. PLACE

Professional Services   Surf's UP! (Valuable Resources)

Special Features On This Site

There are a lot of useful information and features that you won't want to miss!

Our-Kids

http://rdz.stjohns.edu/library/support/our-kids/

Our-Kids is an excellent source of information for parents and caregivers of children with various disabilities. The site also contains links to disability-related sites and listservs.

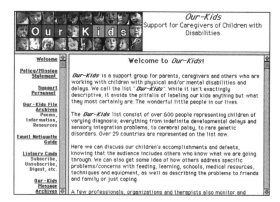

Rehabilitation Medicine

http://weber.u.washington.edu/~rehab/

Rehabilitation Medicine, from the University of Washington School of Medicine in Seattle, offers online illustrated patient pamphlets for spinal cord injury and polio. Titles include "The Late Effects of Polio," "Bowel Care," "Maintaining Healthy Skin," and "Pressure Sores." The site also provides a collection of rehabilitation links.

Solutions

http://disability.com/

Solutions, sponsored by Evan Kemp Associates, links people with disabilities and chronic health conditions to resources, products, and services that promote active, healthy independent living. Among its online features are **Sound Off** where you can post your opinions on selected health care topics, 1995 and 1996 back issues of the *One Step Ahead* (OSA) magazine, **Solution Center,** an exchange for OSA readers, and an extensive collection of disability sites.

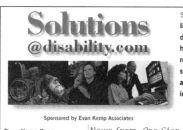

Spinal Cord Injury Resources

http://www.eskimo.com/~jlubin/disabled/sci.htm

Spinal Cord Injury Resources, compiled by Jim Lubin, provides a comprehensive list of sites organized by topic.

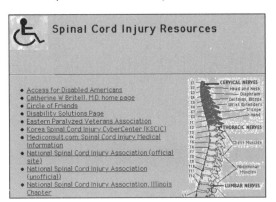

Western New York Disabilities Forum

http://freenet.buffalo.edu/~wnydf/

The Western New York Disabilities Forum provides a disabilities library, Social Security information, links to newsletters, information on strokes, the Americans with Disabilities Act, other disability-related sites, and a searchable index.

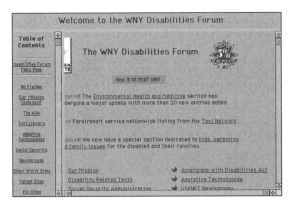

Death and Dying

CHAPTER 21

Bereavement Resources

http://www.funeral.net/info/brvres.html

Bereavement Resources contains a variety of bereavement categories, including FAQ—alt.support.grief, What is grief?, The Grieving Process, Children and Grief, and Grief Tips.

Bereavement Resources

Mourning Light Webring

This Mourning Light Grief Support WebRing site is owned by allen@funeral.net.
Click for the [Next Page | Skip It | Next 5 | Random site]
Want to join the ring? Click here for info.

Mourning Light Webring   next

Resources Directory

FAQ - alt.support.grief	Sharing With Others' ("news:alt.support.grief")	Grief Shared Is Grief Diminished With Bill Chadwick
What is Grief?' Some Helpful Information	Grief Briefs'	Suicide-' Frequently Asked Questions
About Bevreavement	Children And Grief	Thanatolinks
Source Music	Compassionate Friends	Pen Parents

DeathNET

http://www.islandnet.com/~deathnet

DeathNET provides a wide range of materials related to the legal, moral, medical, historical, and cultural aspects of human mortality.

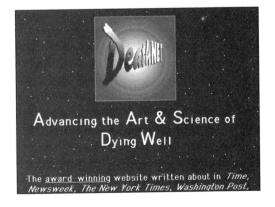

Advancing the Art & Science of Dying Well

The award-winning website written about in *Time, Newsweek, The New York Times, Washington Post,*

Emotional Support Guide

http://asa.ugl.lib.umich.edu/chdocs/support/emotion.html

The Emotional Support Guide has resources for people who are experiencing chronic illness, physical loss, and bereavement, their friends and families, and caregivers. The site includes discussion groups, directories to various non-Internet support groups nationwide, and documents in which people share their advice or experiences.

> **❧ Emotional Support Guide ❧**
>
> **Internet Resources for
> Physical Loss, Chronic Illness, and Bereavement**
>
> This is a guide to emotional support resources on the Internet for people who are experiencing physical loss, chronic illness, and bereavement; their friends and families; and caregivers. Some of the support resources you will be able to find through this guide are electronic discussion groups, directories to various non-Internet support groups nationwide, and documents in which people share their advice or experiences. We have not included resources that are primarily directed at professionals, medical resources without an emotional support component, or advertisements for fee-based services.
>
> We hope that the listings in this guide will be helpful to you, whatever situation of chronic illness, physical loss, or bereavement you may be facing.
>
> Joanne Juhnke and Chris Powell
> University of Michigan, School of Information and Library Studies
> July 1995, Version 2.1
> URL: http://asa.ugl.lib.umich.edu/chdocs/support/emotion.html

Grief Support Resources on the Internet

http://www.transweb.org/fordonorfamilies/grief_support_net.html

Grief Support Resources on the Internet provides a list of grief-related Web sites and a list of grief support newsgroups.

> **Grief Support Resources on the Internet**
>
> Grief-Related Web Sites
>
> - GriefNet, a comprehensive resource
> - WidowNet
> - Frequently Asked Questions about Grief
> - Children and Grief, an article
> - Bereavement Resources in the Emotional Support Guide
> - Growth House's grief and bereavement page
>
> Grief Support Groups
>
> - alt.support.grief (see the group's FAQ file for more information about the group, and about grief in general)
> - The Compassionate Friends
> - Pen Parents, which matches bereaved parents in similar situations for correspondence via the mails.
>
> If you are interested in contributing information to this page or have ideas as to how to improve it, please let us know.
>
> Return to "A Home Page for Donor Families"

GriefNet

http://rivendell.org/

GriefNet is a collection of resources for those experiencing loss and grief. The site includes bereavement, death, dying, and resources.

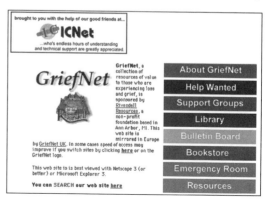

Growth House, Inc.

http://www.growthhouse.org

Growth House, Inc. has a comprehensive index of Internet and local resources related to death and dying, hospice care, bereavement, grief, and AIDS and HIV disease. For an overview of the site, click on **Topic Index.**

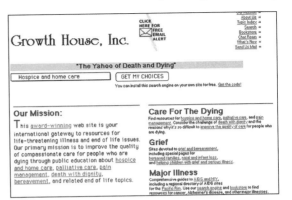

Hospice Foundation of America

http://www.hospicefoundation.org/

The Hospice Foundation of America provides information on how to select a hospice and publications and videos.

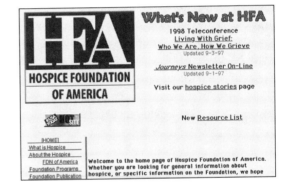

Hospice Hands

http://hospice-cares.com/

Hospice Hands contains a variety of long-term health care resources, including a library of patient/family handouts, a chat room, related links, and a question-and-answer forum to ask specific questions or read the questions of others.

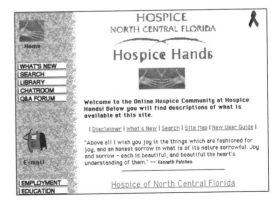

Hospice Web

http://www.teleport.com/~hospice/

Hospice Web is a comprehensive resource of hospice care. The site includes a list of hospices, an electronic bulletin board for questions and answers, an excellent FAQs section, and links to other hospice information on the Web.

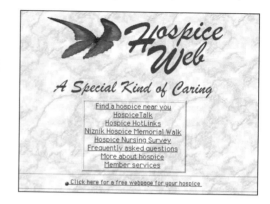

The Kevorkian Verdict

http://www.pbs.org/wgbh/pages/frontline/kevorkian/

The Kevorkian Verdict is a "Frontline" special on the life and legacy of the "suicide doctor." The site includes death interviews with four patients and their families that can be heard on RealAudio, background information on Dr. Kevorkian, legal issues, and the views and practices of doctors.

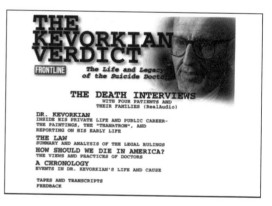

Pen-Parents Home

http://pages.prodigy.com/NV/fgck08a/PenParents.html

Pen-Parents Home is an organization for grieving parents and grandparents. Pen-Parents matches bereaved parents in similar situations so they can correspond by e-mail or regular mail.

Webster's Death, Dying & Grief Guide

http://www.katsden.com/death/

Webster's Death, Dying & Grief Guide, created by Kathi Webster, a nurse, contains links to a wide variety of information on end-of-life issues, including hospice care.

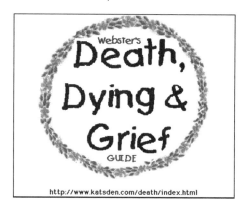

WidowNet

http://www.fortnet.org/~goshorn/

WidowNet is a resource for widows by widows and widowers. The topics include grief, bereavement, recovery, and other beneficial information for people of all ages, backgrounds, and situations who have suffered the death of a loved one.

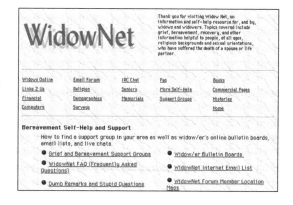

Electronic Newsstand

CHAPTER 22

American Medical Association Publications Home Page

The American Medical Association Publications Home Page contains online editions of the *American Medical News* and links to condition-specific sites on the Internet.

http://www.ama-assn.org/public/journals/

American Medical Association
Physicians dedicated to the health of America

Welcome to the AMA Publications Home Page

This is where you'll find the Web editions of the AMA's Scientific Publications and *American Medical News*, plus physician recruitment advertising, Science News press releases on the latest reports in the AMA journals, links to our condition-specific Web sites, and more.

This site is provided as a public service by the AMA. You can access the full range of features on our site, including abstracts, letters to the editor, selected full-text, a searchable archive and more, with no charge or obligation. We do ask that you complete a brief, one-time visitor form to help us know better who is visting our site, but filling out this form is not required to access our content.

The Boston Globe

The Boston Globe, in its online edition, covers the current and previous weeks' health news. In addition, the online edition contains health/science stories, health articles by its featured columnists, the latest health news from the AP, and links to health-related sites.

http://www.boston.com/globe/healthscience/

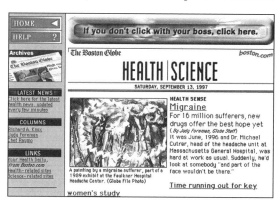

CHID Online

http://chid.nih.gov/

CHID Online, a combined health information database, provides titles, abstracts, and citations for health information and health education resources from the National Institutes of Health (NIH) and the Centers for Disease Control and Prevention (CDC).

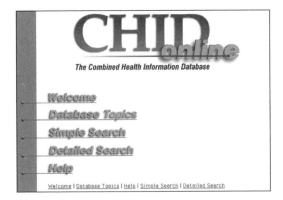

CNN Interactive Health

http://cnn.com/HEALTH/

CNN Interactive Health, updated daily, features current news stories on important health issues. For previous topics, use the search tool or scroll to the **More Stories** section.

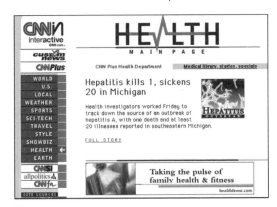

CNN Interactive Year in Review

http://cnn.com/EVENTS/1996/year.in.review/health/

CNN Interactive Year in Review presents the Top 10 Health Stories of 1996. The site includes an online quiz to test your knowledge.

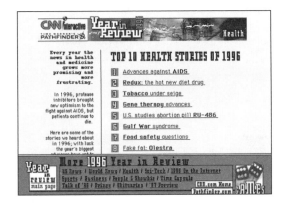

Consumer Health Information

http://www.nih.gov/health/consumer/conicd.htm

Consumer Health Information, from the National Institutes of Health, has a comprehensive list of online consumer health resources of the most requested NIH publications.

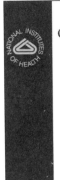

Consumer Information Center

http://www.pueblo.gsa.gov/

The Consumer Information Center of the U.S. General Services Administration has full-text versions of hundreds of the best federal consumer publications. To find health-related publications, click on **Special Stuff, Food & Nutrition,** or **Health.** The Center also includes a search engine.

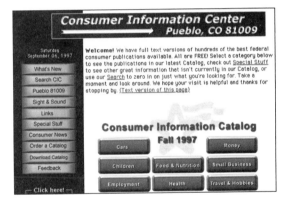

Current Medical News

http://www.healer-inc.com/

Current Medical News, a bimonthly magazine, provides the general reader with summaries of the most recent clinical studies and medical research selected from original articles published in scientific journals. The online edition contains articles on topics ranging from Alzheimer's disease to the causes of hay fever.

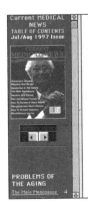

Daedalus

http://www.brooks.af.mil/AL/SD/DAEDALUS/

Daedalus, the Aeromedical Library Online, provides access to thousands of online medical resources, including journals, United States and international libraries, search engines, and databases.

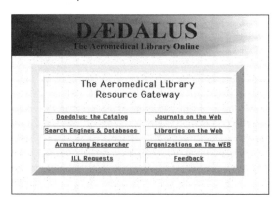

Ecola Newsstand Health

http://www.ecola.com/news/magazine/health/

The Ecola Newsstand contains shelves of health, fitness, holistic, and medical magazines. In addition, the site offers online newspapers from around the world.

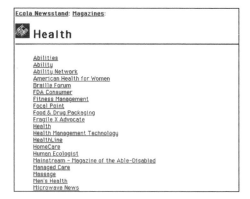

Electronic Newsstand

http://www.enews.com/channel/0,1026,11,00.html

The Electronic Newsstand contains a huge collection of health and medical magazines with information on alternative medicine, disability and rehabilitation, nutrition, fitness, mental health, and the health needs of seniors. Within the nutrition category, for example, there are over 30 magazines with sample articles from past and recent editions.

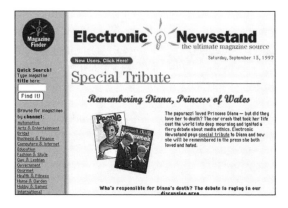

FDA Consumer

http://www.fda.gov/fdac/496_toc.html

The FDA Consumer contains all the articles published online by the U.S. Food and Drug Administration (FDA). The site covers all issues from 1985 to the present. Scroll to bottom of the page and click on **Back Issues** to find an archive of health-related topics.

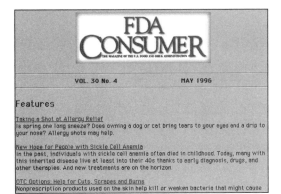

Fox News

http://www.foxnews.com/health/

Fox News presents daily featured health stories and news. For a list of the week's health headlines, click on **Health Wires.**

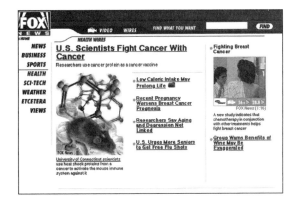

Harvard Health Publications

http://www.med.harvard.edu/publications/Health_Publications/

Harvard Health Publications, from Harvard Medical School, provides timely and reliable health news and information for both the consumer and the health care professional. To view selected articles from the five current monthly newsletters, click on **Newsletter Features.** The site also includes the **By the Way, Doctor** section where experts answer your health and medical questions and the A to Z **Glossary** with definitions of common medical terms from Harvard Health Publications.

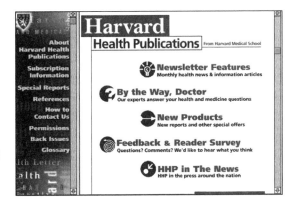

Health A to Z News

http://www.healthatoz.com/news.htm

Health A to Z News, updated bimonthly, presents the latest news in health and medicine. The service also includes archives of previous issues from 1996. To receive more information regarding current headlines in Health A to Z News and the monthly Health Alert, complete the free online registration form.

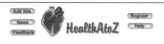

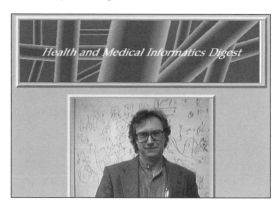

Health and Medical Informatics Digest

http://maddog.fammed.wisc.edu/hmid/hmid.html

Health and Medical Informatics Digest, from the School of Medicine and Nursing at the University of Wisconsin, provides reviews of Internet health care sites.

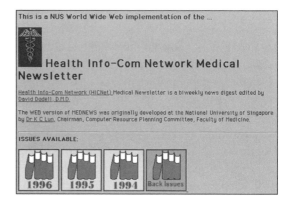

Health Info-Com Network Medical Newsletter

http://ch.nus.sg/MEDNEWS/

Health Info-Com Network Medical Newsletter is an online biweekly digest of health-related news, with issues dating back to 1994.

HealthBeat Articles

http://healthlinks.washington.edu/your_health/hbeat

HealthBeat is a newsletter published by the University of Washington Health Sciences Center. The site currently features brief articles on common health issues such as "Understanding Hepatitis," "Avoid the Rash," and "Dental X-rays." The site also includes past articles dating back to 1994.

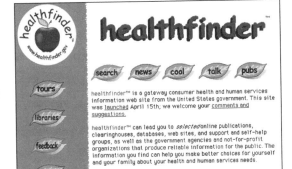

HealthFinder

http://www.healthfinder.gov/

HealthFinder, sponsored by the U.S. government, provides the public with reliable health information from a variety of sources. You can access selected online publications, clearinghouses, databases, Web sites, and support and self-help groups, as well as government agencies and non-profit organizations. To find a list of health topics and information about different age groups, click on **Tours.** The site includes a powerful search tool.

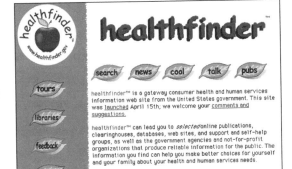

Healthy Kids

http://www.enews.com/magazines/healthykids/

Healthy Kids is a bimonthly magazine providing parents with medical advice for their kids from infancy to young adolescence. The site has the approval of the American Academy of Pediatrics.

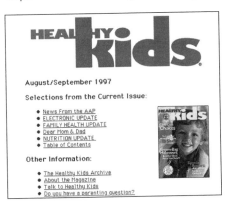

HELIOS

http://www.helios.org/bio.html

HELIOS presents daily medical and health science news.

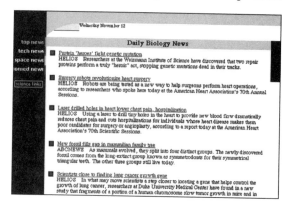

HMS Beagle

http://biomednet.com/hmsbeagle/

The HMS Beagle is a biweekly magazine offering articles, debates, reviews, and editorials about biomedical research. The categories include biological science, medicine/health, and biotech pharmaceutical. To view over 90 journals and newsletters, you can browse headlines and brief summaries of stories.

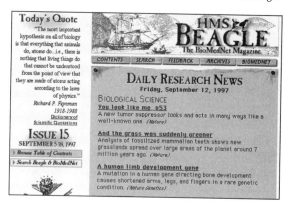

Information Television Network

http://www.itvisus.com

The Information Television Network offers a wealth of online medical information, links to other health-related sites, and upcoming program schedules and summaries of its award-winning "Cutting Edge Medical Reports" and "Healthy Women 2000" programs.

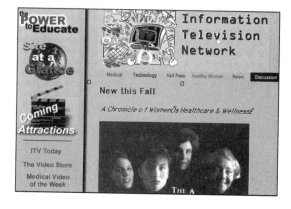

InfoSeek News Channel

http://www.infoseek.com/
Topic?tid=1486&sv=IS&nh=10&CAT=Health

InfoSeek News Channel features the top
headlines daily, including health care news.
The site also provides an interactive tool to
personalize your searches in seeking the health
care information you want.

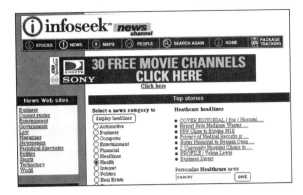

Integrated Newswire

http://www.artigen.com/newswire/health.html

The Integrated Newswire provides daily links to
articles from the leading online news sources
for health. For an archive of older stories, scroll
to the bottom of the page.

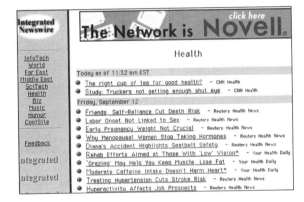

Internet Medical News Channel

http://www.primenet.com/~xerit

The Internet Medical News Channel provides
complete health and medical news from participating
government and private organizations.

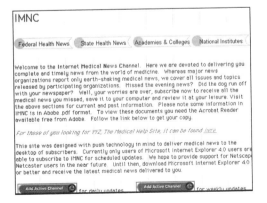

IVI Online

http://infoventures.microserve.com/

IVI Online, a service of Information Ventures, Inc., provides online summaries of the latest research and journal news for electric and magnetic fields, herbicides and pesticides, chemicals and other hazards in the workplace, pharmaceuticals, and cancer.

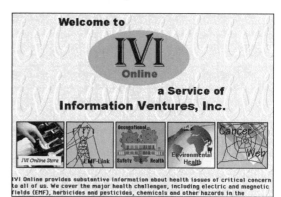

John Labovitz's E-Zine-List

http://www.meer.net/~johnl/e-zine-list/

John Labovitz's E-Zine-List, updated monthly, is a directory of electronic magazines around the world, accessible via the Web, Gopher, FTP, e-mail, and other services. Scroll to "Here are the 80 most popular keywords" and click on **health** to find magazines covering a variety of topics.

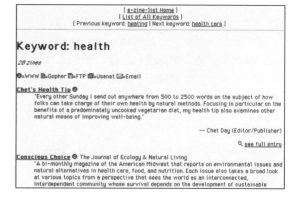

Kaiser Permanente California Web Site

http://webzine.ca.kaiserpermanente.org/

Kaiser Permanente California Web site provides an online magazine, *Partners in Health,* with articles about health maintenance and personal wellness. The site is updated regularly with topics such as stress and your health and cold and flu.

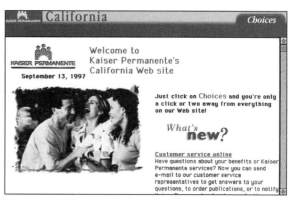

Los Angeles Times

http://www.latimes.com/HOME/NEWS/HEALTH/

The Los Angeles Times presents online articles from the Monday's health section in the *Los Angeles Times* newspaper. The articles usually focus on a health theme and cover a variety of topics. In the medicine section, the site posts daily articles ranging from personal stories to children's health issues.

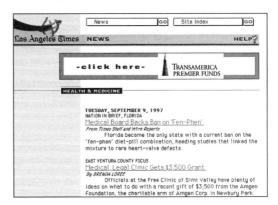

The MedAccess Newsletter

http://www.medaccess.com/newsletter/current/news.htm

The MedAccess Newsletter is an online bimonthly newsletter featuring general health articles, a health quiz, and healthy recipes. The site also includes past issues dating back to January 15, 1996.

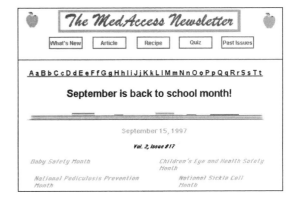

Medical Breakthroughs

http://www.ivanhoe.com/

Medical Breakthroughs, reported by Ivanhoe Broadcast News, provides the latest weekly reports and medical news on a variety of health topics, including tooth care, fighting cavities, Alzheimer's disease, and children's and women's health concerns. You can also search an archive of back issues by key word or browse one of the 13 categories. For a free e-mail subscription, click on **First-To-Know Bulletin.**

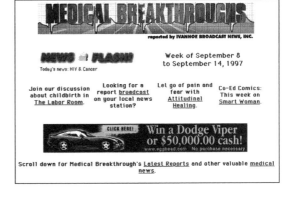

The Medical Reporter

http://www.dash.com/tmr/

The Medical Reporter, created by medical journalist Joel R. Cooper, is an online monthly health magazine that contains hundreds of medical articles written for the savvy consumer. For a list of articles, click on **TMR Subject Index.**

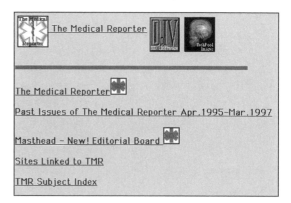

Medical Tribune

http://www.medtrib.com/

Medical Tribune, sponored by *The New York Times Syndicate,* is an online bimonthly news service that provides up-to-date health care information. The site includes archives to past issues, a debate feature where physicians face-off, and a cyberguide to top-regarded medical sites.

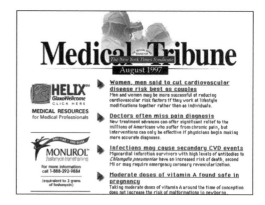

Medical World Search

http://www.mwsearch.com/

Medical World Search indexes the full content of the major medical sites on the Web, assisted by a thesaurus of 540,000 medical terms. The site can search PubMed, Alta Vista, Hotbot, Infoseek, or WebCrawler separately or altogether.

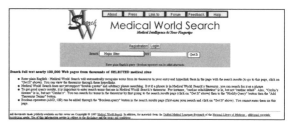

MedPulse—What's New at Medscape

MedPulse is Medscape's free weekly e-mail newsletter. Its featured articles include depression in the elderly, jail fever, and who will fund pharmaceutical research on breast, ovarian, and cervical carcinoma. For a subscription to a newsletter, you must complete a free registration form.

http://www.medscape.com/Home/MedPulse/MedPulse.html

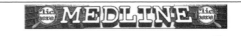

Medsite Navigator Medical Journals

Medsite Navigator contains an A to Z listing of online medical journals on the Web. It includes a brief description of journals and direct links to their Web sites.

http://www.medsitenavigator.com/med/Journals_pr.html

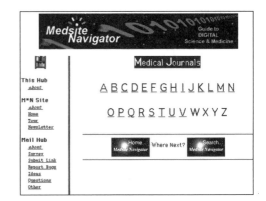

MigraineZine

MigraineZine is a bimonthly online magazine that claims that all migraines are caused by caffeine withdrawal.

http://www.batnet.com/spencer/

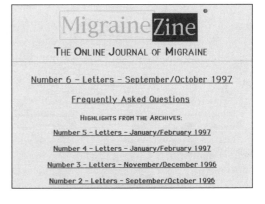

Nando Health/Science

http://www.nando.net/nt/health/

Nando Health/Science provides a daily collection of health and science articles gathered from various news and print sources. Titles include "Heart Transplant Patient Climbs Mountains," "Enzyme May Be Key to Emphysema," "Diet Alternatives May Also Have Risks, Doctors Caution," and "Sun Is Heating Up, Researchers Say." You can also search the Health/Science database for previous articles.

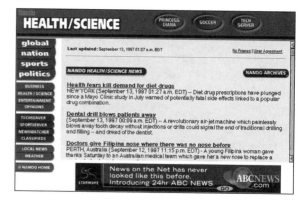

The New England Journal of Medicine

http://www.nejm.org/

The New England Journal of Medicine, owned by the Massachusettes Medical Society, is a weekly journal that reports the results of important medical research around the world. The site includes collections of full-text articles for asthma, breast cancer, molecular medicine, and kidney disease and summaries of articles from the the current week's journal. Journal articles from 1990 can also be searched by topic or by author.

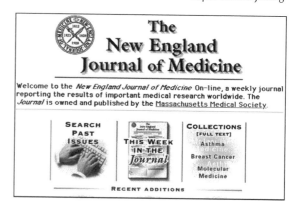

NewsFile

http://www.newsfile.com/

NewsFile contains more than 26,000 summaries of disease-related articles from CW Henderson weekly publications. The site also includes full-text articles of the top news stories.

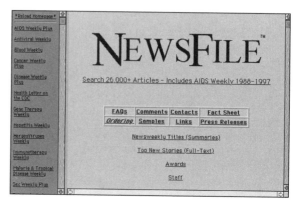

NewsPage Healthcare

http://www.newspage.com/

NewsPage Healthcare presents today's headlines for a variety of healthcare industries.

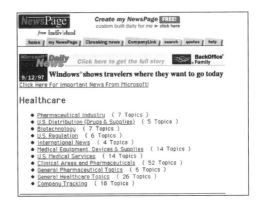

OncoLink Cancer News

http://cancer.med.upenn.edu/cancer_news/

OncoLink Cancer News, updated monthly from the University of Pennsylvania Cancer Center, provides cancer news from various media sources. The site includes previous cancer news from 1994 to 1997.

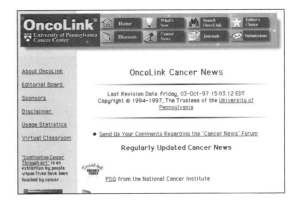

OSH-Link: An Occupational Safety and Health Electronic Resource

http://infoventures.com/osh/

OSH-Link: An Occupational Safety and Health Electronic Resource features the *Cancer Web Report,* a monthly publication summarizing the latest cancer news from research and medical journals. The site also includes health reports from various hazardous materials encountered in everyday life.

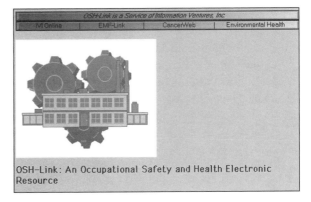

Parenting in Arkansas

http://ach.uams.edu/parenting/

Parenting in Arkansas, published twice a year by the Arkansas Children's Hospital, offers sample issues containing helpful parenting and medical information. You can request a free subscription to *Parenting in Arkansas* mailed directly to your home.

Spring 1997
Volume 6, No. 1

Fall 1996
Volume 5, No. 2

Spring 1996
Volume 5, No. 1

Request a free subscription to Parenting in Arkansas mailed directly to your home.

Return to Arkansas Children's Hospital

The Philadelphia Inquirer Health & Science Magazine

http://sln.fi.edu/inquirer/inquirer.html

The Philadelphia Inquirer Health & Science Magazine presents online the articles from the Monday's health/science section in the The *Philadelphia Inquirer* newspaper. Articles are easy to read and cover a wide variety of topics.

The Philadelphia Inquirer

Health & Science
M A G A Z I N E

Each Monday, *The Philadelphia Inquirer* publishes a section devoted to covering current topics in science and medicine. The Franklin Institute Science Museum offers enhanced re-prints of feature stories from that section. Background information, teacher resources, multimedia, and interactivity are added to the articles, providing a continually changing source of science news for classroom use.

Extra!!!

Mystery of the mummies

Physician's Weekly

http://www.physweekly.com/

Physician's Weekly, an online medical magazine, provides highlights and analysis of medical news. The current and recent issues can be accessed and medical information can be searched in the archives. Each issue contains In the News, Point/Counterpoint, Clinical Updates, This Week's Lead Story, and This Week's Chart.

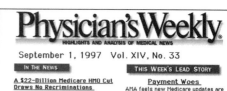

Physician's Weekly
HIGHLIGHTS AND ANALYSIS OF MEDICAL NEWS

September 1, 1997   Vol. XIV, No. 33

IN THE NEWS

A $22-Billion Medicare HMO Cut Draws No Recriminations

Lipase Inhibitor Aids Weighty Diabetics and Nondiabetics

Old Drug Shrinks Meningioma

POINT/COUNTERPOINT

Should physicians participate in discussions on the Net?

CLINICAL UPDATES

STROKE: Black and white diabetics: similar rates

THIS WEEK'S LEAD STORY

Payment Woes
AMA feels new Medicare updates are worse than a freeze

PR NewsWire Health/Biotech

http://www.prnewswire.com/health/newshealthcare.html

PR NewsWire presents daily online the latest
health/biotech news from a wide range of
companies, institutions, and government
agencies. The site includes a news archive
of pharmaceutical, biotechnology, and
health care companies.

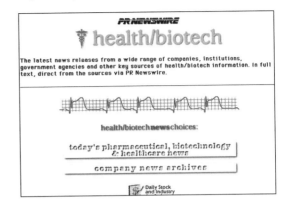

Priory Lodge Education

http://www.priory.co.uk/

Priory Lodge Education publishes a series of
online journals for a variety of medical
specialties, including anesthesia, dentistry,
general practice, psychiatry, medicine, chest
medicine, family medicine, and pharmacy. Each
journal offers extensive patient health
information.

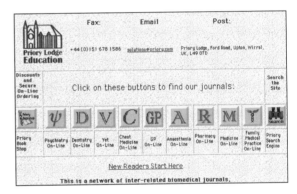

PubMed

http://www.ncbi.nlm.nih.gov/PubMed/

PubMed, a powerful consumer search tool of the
U.S. National Library of Medicine, offers free access
to over 9 million documents in Medline, including
links to related articles. A parent, for example, can
enter the words "ear infections" or "cold remedies"
to search for information about treating these
common kids' ailments.

ReutersHealth

http://www.reutershealth.com/

ReutersHealth, a comprehensive medical news service for both consumers (**Health eLine**) and professionals (**Medical News),** covers the most important news in health and medicine each business day. The site delivers in-depth medical information from over 300 medical journals and other sources. There is health information on men, women, and children's health, diet, exercise, treatment advances, and disease management. The site offers a search tool.

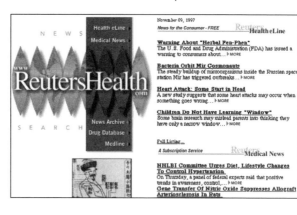

ScienceDaily

http://www.sciencedaily.com/topic_health_medicine.htm

ScienceDaily, an online magazine, provides daily the breaking news about the latest discoveries and hottest research projects in health and medicine. For more news summaries, scroll to the bottom of the page.

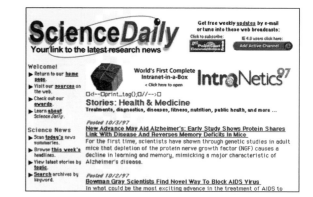

The Six Senses Review

http://www.sixsenses.com/

The Six Senses Review contains health care and medical sites indexed by category and evaluated by a panel of health care experts. For a list of the top-rated sites, click on **Seal Winners.**

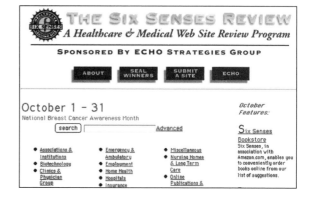

UC Berkeley Library Web Electronic Journals

UC Berkeley Library Web contains an alphabetical index of electronic public health journals, including *AIDS Information Newsletter* and *Pediatrics*.

http://www.lib.berkeley.edu/PUBL/ejournals.html

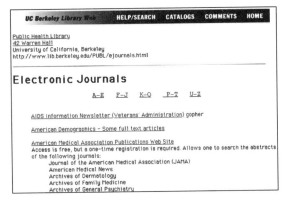

University of California at Berkeley Wellness Letter

The University of California at Berkeley Wellness Letter, brought by Electronic Newsstand, provides online monthly articles for a variety of healthy living topics. The topics include nutrition and weight control, self-care, prevention of cancer and heart disease, buying guides to foods and health-related products, and safe driving. The site also includes archives of previous articles.

http://www.enews.com/magazines/ucbwl/

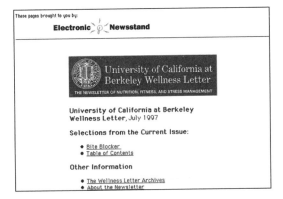

University of Washington HealthLinks

University of Washington HealthLinks provides an alphabetical list of electronic journals and newsletters for health and medicine.

http://healthlinks.washington.edu/journals/

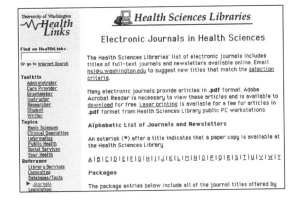

U.S. National Library of Medicine Health Services/ Technology Assessment Text

http://text.nlm.nih.gov/

U.S. National Library of Medicine includes Health Services/Technology Assessment Text (HSTAT), an online health library containing thousands of government publications. You can use the site's powerful search tool to find information about innumerable medical topics. The abstracts and citations found in the database are based on government research findings and are written with the consumer in mind.

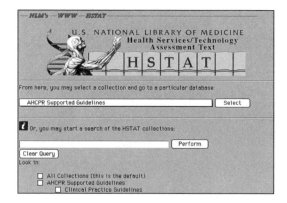

USA Today Health

http://www.usatoday.com/life/health/lhd1.htm

USA Today provides daily health-related news stories. The site includes a topic index to previous health stories and hot lines to find answers to diet, foot, and sports injury problems.

The Virtual Medical Center

http://www.mediconsult.com/

The Virtual Medical Center, provided by Mediconsult.com, offers an immense amount of health information from leading medical journals, medical institutions, government agencies, and non-profit organizations. The site includes over 50 topics and a search tool to help find the information you want.

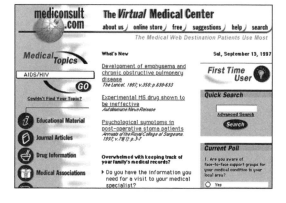

Washingtonpost.com

http://www.washingtonpost.com/wp-srv/WPlate/m-health.html

Washingtonpost.com, from *The Washington Post,* has online every Tuesday health articles from the newspaper's print edition. You can also consult experts and read answers to readers' questions in the site's **health issues.**

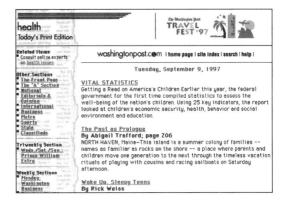

WebMedLit

http://www.webmedlit.com/

WebMedLit tracks over 23 medical journals to view the latest medical literature on the Web by topic. The site also provides a search tool for more specific research.

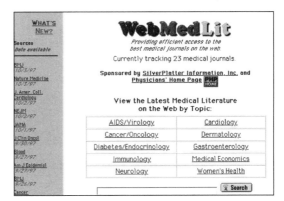

Wellness Wise Electronic Journal

http://fermi.jhuapl.edu/wej/

Wellness Wise Electronic Journal is an online biweekly newsletter consisting of transcripts from the Dr. David J. DeRose's daily syndicated radio program, *WellnessWise,* and selections from Phylis Autin's *Science/Health Abstracts.* Topics cover traditional and alternative therapies for prostate cancer, women's health, elderly health care, heart disease, lung cancer, and other medical problems. You can subscribe to the free newsletter via e-mail.

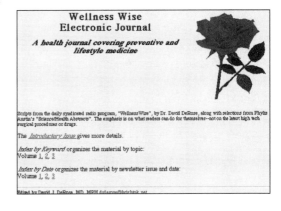

What's News

http://www.gene.com/ae/WN/

What's News, from Access Excellence, provides weekly news reports on biomedical topics from a variety of sources, including journals, conferences, and the Internet. To browse a collection of previous updates with hundreds of science and medical articles, click on **Archive.** Access Excellence also offers its own key word search engine.

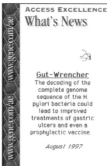

Yahoo! News

http://www.yahoo.com/headlines/health/

Yahoo! News, from the Reuters News Service, has ten health/medicine news stories daily. You can read descriptions of the stories by clicking on **Health Summary.** The site also includes archives of the previous week's stories and a search tool.

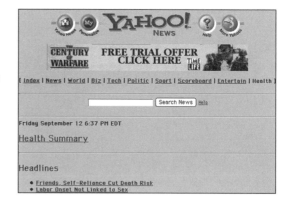

Your Health Daily

http://yourhealthdaily.com/

Your Health Daily offers in-depth articles on a variety of health news topics. Click on **More News** for an archive of past articles or click on **Health Topics** to view articles organized by topics. In addition, the site has a search tool and discussion groups.

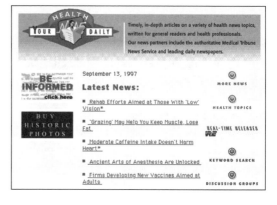

CHAPTER 23

Health Directories

Achoo

http://www.achoo.com

Achoo is one of the most comprehensive health care databases on the Internet with over 7000 indexed and searchable health care sites. The site is organized by categories that include Human Life, Practice of Medicine, Business of Health, and What's New.

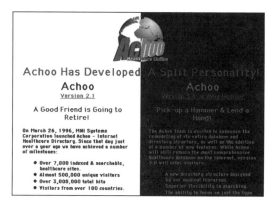

AOL NetFind

http://netfind.aol.com/aol/Reviews/Health_and_Medicine

AOL NetFind contains reviews of health and medicine sites sorted into 16 categories. The categories include Children's Health and Disabilities, Fitness, Geriatrics, Nutrition, Substance Abuse, and Veterinary Medicine.

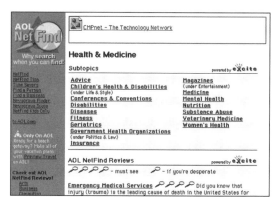

Best of the Web

http://www.luckman.com/yp/

Best of the Web, from Luckman Interactive, contains an extensive collection of reviewed health and medical sites. Categories include addictions and recovery, geriatrics, hospitals and medical centers, medical schools, sports medicine, and much more.

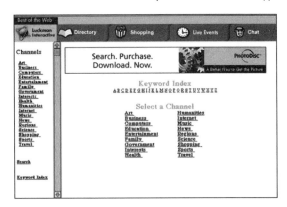

Britannica Internet Guide

http://www.ebig.com/

Britannica Internet Guide, by the Encyclopedia Britannica, is a collection of reviewed sites that are organized by category. The **Health and Medicine** category includes topics ranging from general medicine to specialties and related fields. To find the health and medicine contents, click on **Expanded Outline.**

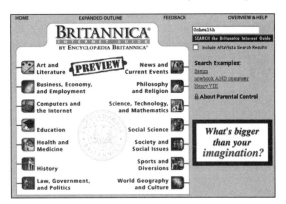

Combined Internal Medicine & Pediatrics

http://ourworld.compuserve.com/homepages/anduril/medicine.htm

Combined Internal Medicine & Pediatrics is an extensive directory of internal medicine and pediatric sites on the Internet. Categories include general information, medical links, specific pediatric sites, medical associations, doctors' home pages, and others.

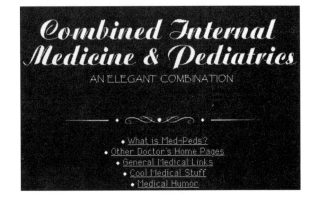

Doctor's Guide to the Internet

http://www.pslgroup.com/docguide.htm

Doctor's Guide to the Internet contains a variety of online resources. Scroll to **Of Interest to your Patients** to find a wealth of information and resources on topics such as AIDS/HIV, diabetes, insomnia, menopause, migraine headaches, and schizophrenia. In addition, the site offers the latest medical news from conferences, the literature, newswires, and the Internet.

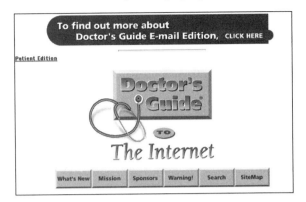

Dr. MEDMarket

http://dr.medmarket.com/indexes/indexmfr.html

Dr. MEDMarket features an A to Z health services index to medical resources ranging from Accredited Allergy Associates to Wellness on the Web. To find this index, click on **Medical Resources.** You can also use a search tool to find medical information in this index.

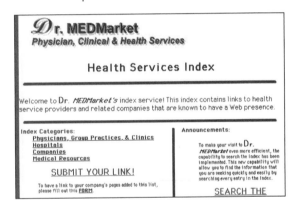

Edmund's Home Page

http://www.li.net/~edhayes/ed.html

Edmund's Home Page provides a large catalog of links to medical professions, including pharmacy, nursing, and dentistry. The site is updated weekly.

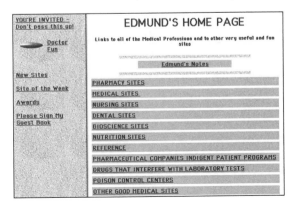

Einet Galaxy

http://galaxy.einet.net/galaxy/Community/Health.html

Einet Galaxy is a powerful resource to a wide range of health and medical information. Among the topics are aging, disabilities, environmental medicine, diseases and disorders, exercise, surgery, and travel. Scroll to the bottom of the page to find other Einet Galaxy directories for **Medicine, Health and Medicine,** and **Public Health.**

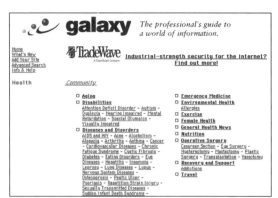

Essential Links to Medicine

http://www.el.com/elinks/medicine/

Essential Links to Medicine provides online resources to medical directories, newsletters, libraries, and facilities, as well as an index of diseases, medicine, and other health-related information.

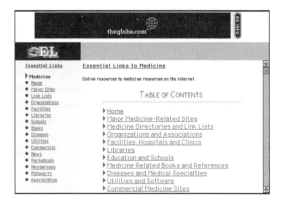

Excite

http://www.excite.com/channel/health/

Excite, an Internet search engine, offers a directory of health topics ranging from alternative medicine to women's health. The Health & Science News section has the latest news on AIDS, the environment, and other health topics.

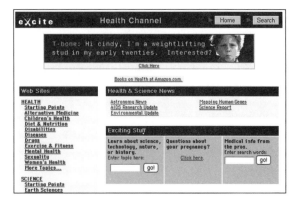

HandiLinks to Health

http://www.ahandyguide.com/cat1/health.htm

HandiLinks to Health contains thousands of health sites sorted into categories ranging from abortion alternatives to weight loss.

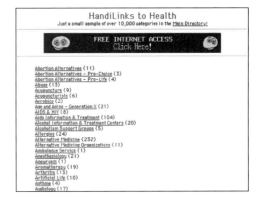

Hardin Meta Directory of Internet Health Sources

http://www.arcade.uiowa.edu/hardin-www/md.html

Hardin Meta Directory of Internet Health Sources offers a vast collection of informative health-related sites. Topics include allergy, anesthesiology, psychiatry/mental health, toxicology, and much more.

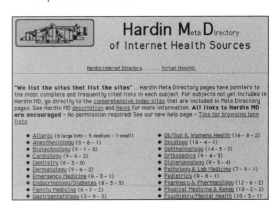

Health

http://www.useekufind.com/health.htm

Health contains a rich assortment of resources for a variety of topics, including health and medical issues, patient education, nutrition, health problems and illness, mental health, kid's health and safety, women's health, and men's health. Furthermore, the site offers four search engines for access to thousands of other health and medicine links.

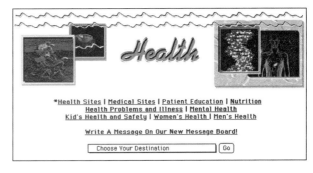

Health

http://home.miningco.com/health/

Health, from the Mining Company, provides a wide variety of health resources for alternative medicine, diseases, disabilities, fitness, health care, women's health, and mental health. The site is updated daily.

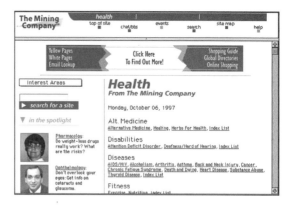

Health A to Z

http://www.healthatoz.com/

Health A to Z contains thousands of health and medical sites sorted into categories. Categories range from allied health to women's health. The site also includes a search tool.

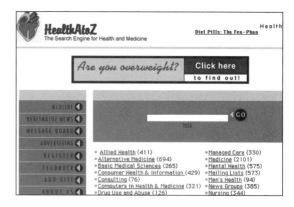

Health and Fitness Information

http://www.silcom.com/~dwsmith/

Health and Fitness Information is a giant supermarket of resources compiled by Douglas W. Smith and Sheelah R. Smith of the Santa Barbara Health Center. Categories include WWW search tools, general health-related sites, health news, chiropractic, fitness, nutrition, and specific disease-related sites.

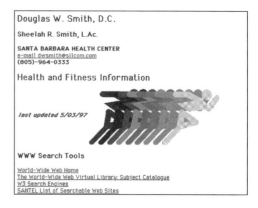

The Health Atlas of Long Beach Community Medical Center

http://www.lbcommunity.com/atlas/

The Health Atlas of Long Beach Community Medical Center allows quick and easy access to health-related information on the Internet. Each site in the Health Atlas has been categorized and rated for content and technical merit. You can search by category or by key word, or you can browse an alphabetical index.

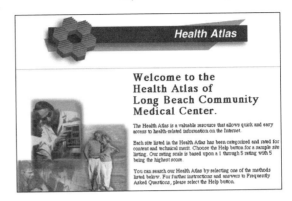

Health Care Information Resources

http://www-hsl.mcmaster.ca/tomflem/top.html

Health Care Information Resources is a comprehensive directory of annotated health-related sites organized by categories, including Health Sites, Wellness, Alternative Medicine, and Illness. There is also a listing of medical societies and university departments.

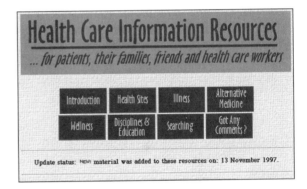

Health Information Highway

http://www.stayhealthy.com/

The Health Information Highway, from the Wellness Interactive Network, provides thousands of health information resources on the Internet, including a directory of sites, a drug information database, disease management and prevention information, medical usegroups and databases, and health risk assessment and self-assessment tools.

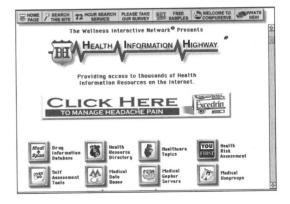

Health On the Net Foundation

http://www.hon.ch

The Health On the Net Foundation offers the excellent MedHunt search engine for locating health and medicine information from its own database of selected sites and from the entire Internet.

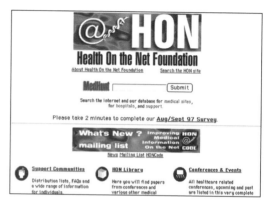

Health Resources

http://alabanza.com/kabacoff/Inter-Links/medicine.html

Health Resources, from Inter-Links, has a catalog of Internet health resources with health/medical information, meta-lists, daily news sources, and online libraries of health articles and references.

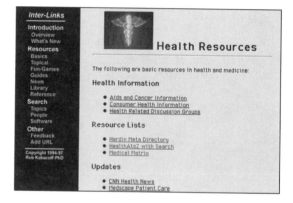

Health Sciences Library System Internet Resources

http://www.hsls.pitt.edu/intres/alphi.html

Health Sciences Library System Internet Resources, from the University of Pittsburgh, provides an A to Z index to Internet resources ranging from AIDS and HIV to virology.

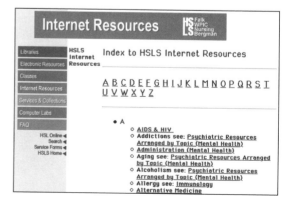

HealthCity

http://www.healthcity.com/

HealthCity is just a click away from expert information about health, medicine, and medical issues from all over the world. Enter **HealthCity** to find an alternative care clinic, library, health club, newspapers, whole family park, and valuable resources.

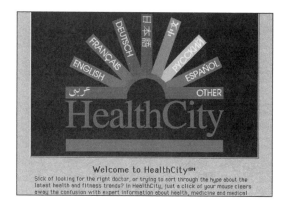

HealthGate

http://www.healthgate.com/

HealthGate offers numerous databases for health, wellness, and biomedical information. The site includes a wide range of topics for adult and children's illnesses, surgical procedures, medical tests, prescription and non-prescription drugs, sports injuries, and pregnancy.

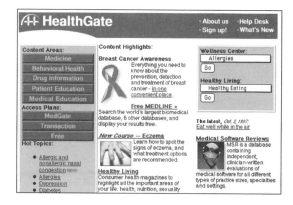

HealthSeek

http://www.healthseek.com/

HealthSeek provides a wealth of health information for health care professionals and consumers alike. The site includes a message board to present your views, medical resources, a catalog of online journals and newsletters, a list of professional health organizations, and a collection of consumer health sites.

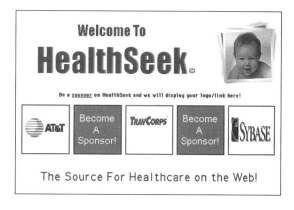

Healthtouch Online

http://www.healthtouch.com/

Healthtouch Online provides a wide variety of health resources, including drug information, a health resource directory, and medical topics ranging from allergies to sexually transmitted diseases (STDs).

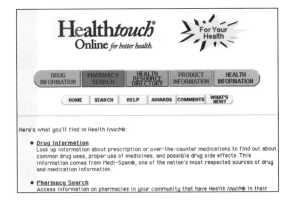

HealthWeb

http://healthweb.org/

HealthWeb, created by a dozen of the leading academic medical centers in the Midwest, provides a library of health-related sites for consumers and health care professionals. To find an alphabetical list of topics, click on **Subjects.** The **Consumer Health** topic in the list contains an A to Z index of Internet resources, online publications, and professional organizations.

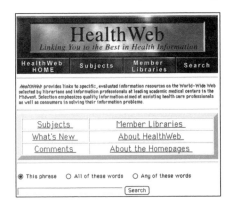

HealthyWay

http://www1.sympatico.ca/healthyway/

HealthyWay features health communities with topics ranging from active living to women's health. At the top of the page, click on **Health Links Index** to find an A to Z list of topics.

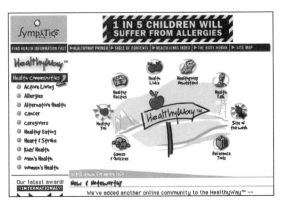

i-Explorer

i-Explorer contains 100 Internet directories, including **Health and Medicine.** This directory offers health, fitness, and medical articles. Each area includes its own search engine.

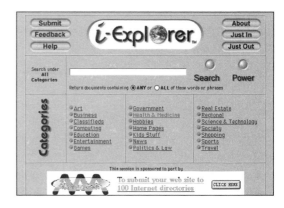

Internet Health Resources

The Internet Health Resources provides access to a broad range of health resources, as well as articles on over 50 general topics ranging from allergies to women's health. Links to cancer and diabetes are extensive. A searchable database of over 4000 prescription and over-the-counter medications is also included.

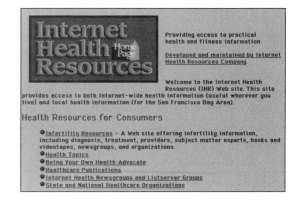

Internet Sleuth

Internet Sleuth provides information on a variety of health topics ranging from alternative medicine to pharmacology. The site also includes search engines from major health sites to help access information quickly.

Librarians' Index to the Internet

http://sunsite.berkeley.edu/InternetIndex/

The Librarians' Index to the Internet is a searchable, annotated, subject directory of close to 3000 Internet resources chosen for their usefulness. Click on **Health, Medicine** for over 65 authoritative sites on health-related topics.

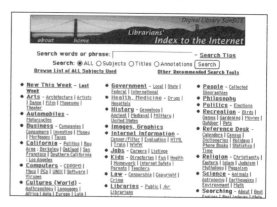

LookSmart

http://www.looksmart.com/r?lvp&e53940

LookSmart, from *Reader's Digest,* provides a health and fitness directory of medical sites. The directory includes Best of the Web, Ask a Professional, Family Health, Diet/Nutrition, and other categories.

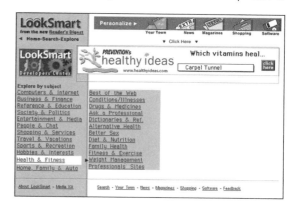

Lycos Health

http://www.lycos.com/health/

Lycos, an Internet search engine, selects the top 5% health sites on the Internet. To browse the top 5% health sites, click on **Top 5%** at the top of the page. Select **Health** in the topic directory and click on **Alphabetic.** The health categories of interest to consumers are alternative medicine, conditions, fitness, and nutition and diet. The site also presents daily health headlines.

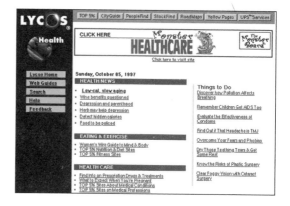

Magellan Internet Guide

http://mckinley.com/magellan/Reviews/
Health_and_Medicine/index.mag

Magellan Internet Guide provides reviews of health and science sites covering topics such as advice, children's health, diseases, sexuality, and women's health.

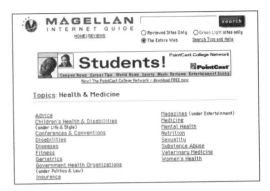

Martindale's Health Science Guide

http://www.sci.lib.uci.edu/HSG/HSGuide.html

Martindale's Health Science Guide contains a virtual medical center with departments ranging from anatomy and histology to radiology. The site also includes centers for nursing, nutrition, pharmacy, dentistry, and public health. The site has more than 2700 databases of medical information.

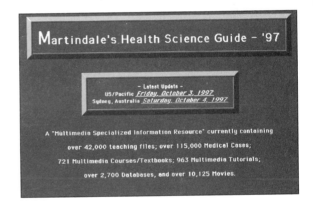

MD Gateway

http://www.mdgateway.com/

MD Gateway provides an eclectic collection of health resources for doctors and consumers, including an alphabetical listing of professional associations, medical schools, online publications, and pharmaceutical companies, in addition to sections on medical information in the library and wellness centers. Every time the page is reloaded, there is an historical health-related factoid.

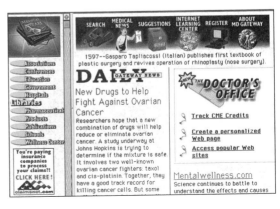

MedExchange

http://www.healself.com/dir/

MedExchange is a huge directory of health and medicine sites with thousands of articles. Among the general categories are alternative medicine, diseases and conditions, health education institutions and organizations, lifestyle, and medicine.

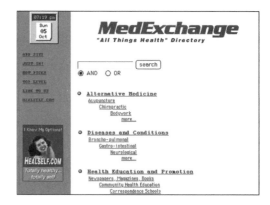

Medical Matrix

http://www.medmatrix.org

Medical Matrix has a wide variety of online resources that include major journals, textbooks, disease and conditions, and patient education. To access this site, you must complete an online registration form.

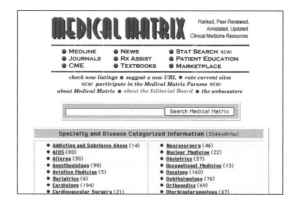

Medicine on the Net

http://www.cnet.com/Content/Features/Net/Medicine/

Medicine on the Net, from CNet, contains hundreds of medical sites that cover specific diseases, case studies, preventive care, and other health-related topics. Medicine on the Net also includes medical newsgroups where you can post and respond to thousands of messages and **Search.com,** which provides search engines and authoritative medical databases for finding medical information. In addition, for reviews of health sites, click on **Best of the Web.**

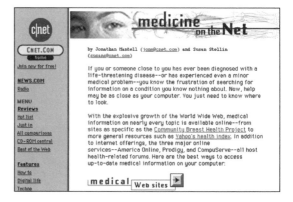

Medref

http://www.medref.com/

Medref organizes medical Web sites on the Internet to help users locate and review information regarding medical care, health problems, diseases, physicians, and medical facilities.

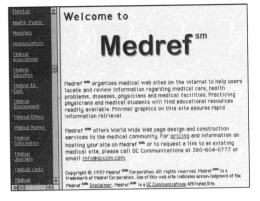

Medscape

http://www.medscape.com/

Medscape is a series of indexes that provide a wealth of health information and the latest medical headlines. Thousands of articles are available, including updated material on the latest developments in drug therapy, diagnosis, and general medical knowledge. In addition, you can use Merriam Webster's Online Medical Dictionary or learn about everyday medications. For an overview of Medscape's resources, click on the **Site Map** at the bottom of the page. To access the site's free services, you must complete an online registration form.

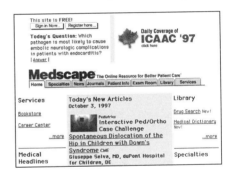

MedWeb Directories

http://www.gen.emory.edu/medweb/medweb.directories.html

MedWeb Directories, provided by Emory University Health Sciences Center, contains tons of medical and health resources gathered from the Internet. Scroll to the bottom of the page and click on **What's new** for the latest additions.

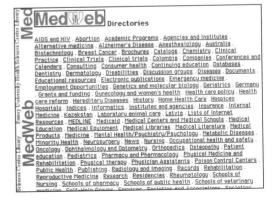

Michigan Electronic Library Health Information Resources

http://mel.lib.mi.us/health/health-index.html

The Michigan Electronic Library provides a wide assortment of Health Information Resources. Topics include aging, death and dying, drug information, osteopathic medicine, surgery, stress, and much more.

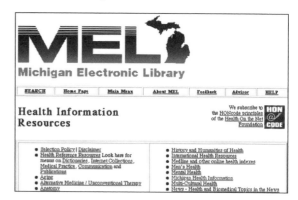

The Multimedia Medical Reference Library

http://www.med-library.com/

The Multimedia Medical Reference Library, maintained by Jonathan Tward, contains a wide variety of medical topics ranging from AIDS to urology. For an overview of the site, click on **Index.**

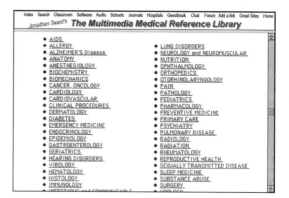

NetGuide HealthGuide

http://netguide.com/Health

NetGuide HealthGuide presents brief descriptions and links to the top-rated health sites for alternative medicine, children's health, diseases and conditions, exercise and fitness, mental health, news and advice, nutrition, and sexuality. HealthGuide also includes links to the 10 top-rated general health sites on the Net and other health sites in the **Reference Shelf** section.

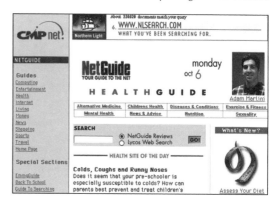

NetHealth

http://www.nethealth.com/intro.html

The NetHealth Guide to the Internet contains over 500 reviewed sites with reliable medical information on hundreds of topics ranging from addiction to x-ray and diagnostic imaging.

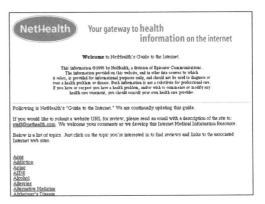

NOAH: New York Online Access to Health

http://www.noah.cuny.edu/

NOAH: New York Online Access to Health, the combined effort of the New York Public Library and other educational institutions, provides a wealth of consumer health resources ranging from aging and Alzheimer's disease to tuberculosis. The site is completely available in Spanish and has numerous health topics and search tools.

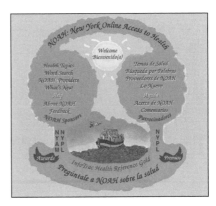

The Science Guide

http://www.scienceguide.com/

The Science Guide is a voluminous directory with many scientific topics. Click on the smaller print **Directory of Directories** to find a number of different directories. Next, click on **Medicine** to find a medical directory for topics ranging from general to vascular medicine.

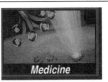

Stanford University Medical Center

http://www-med.stanford.edu/

Stanford University Medical Center provides a variety of health resources. Among them are the **Health Library** and the **HealthLink.**

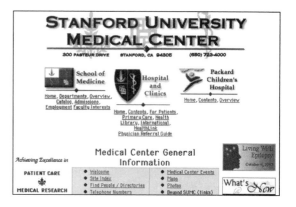

Starting Point

http://www.stpt.com/health/health.html

Starting Point is a catalog of health categories that include alternative medicine, psychology, diet and nutrition, and fitness and exercise.

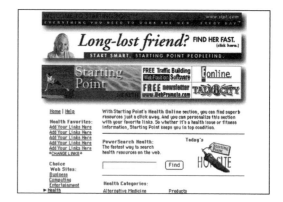

Study Web

http://www.studyweb.com/

Study Web offers a collection of more than 26,000 sites with categories for **Medicine, Mental Health,** and **Health and Nutrition.**

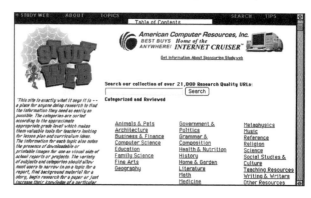

Three Rivers Free-Net

http://trfn.clpgh.org/health/

Three Rivers Free-Net contains a vast number of resources that include health news, staying healthy, special diseases and health topics, general health indexes, and health organizations.

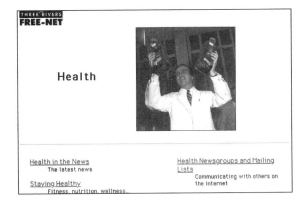

University of Michigan Health & Medical Library

http://www.med.umich.edu/1libr/1libr.htm

The University of Michigan Health & Medical Library offers a wealth of health and medical online information, along with links to other health care sites. Categories include child and adolescent health, primary and preventive care, heart information, mature matters, prescription drugs, and tests and procedures.

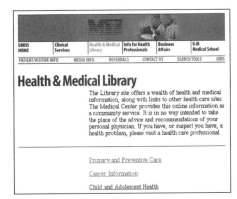

University of Virginia Health Science Library Web Resource Directory

http://www.med.virginia.edu/hs-library/info_serv/bookmark.html

The University of Virginia Health Science Library Web Resource Directory has a variety of health-related topics, including health and medical, complementary/alternative medicine, nursing, pharmacy/drug information, and consumer health. The site also connects to every major and minor search engine on the Internet, providing almost unlimited access to additional resources.

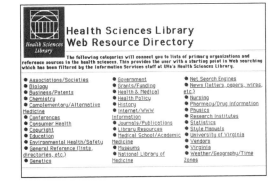

University of Washington Health Links

http://healthlinks.washington.edu/your_health/

The University of Washington Health Links provides a wide variety of sites for personal health information. Categories include AIDS, foot care, health service, lung disease, women's health care, and much more.

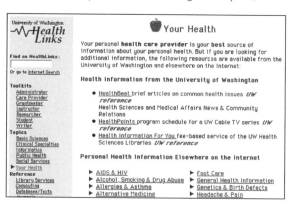

University of Wisconsin Medical School Internet Health Guide

http://www.biostat.wisc.edu/infolink/ihg/ihg.html

The University of Wisconsin Medical School Internet Health Guide has over 50 topics in **The Health Index** ranging from adolescent health to vision and eye problems. Click on one of these to find features, articles, columns, and clinical news. In addition, in the **Healthline** section you can listen to health-related articles on RealAudio.

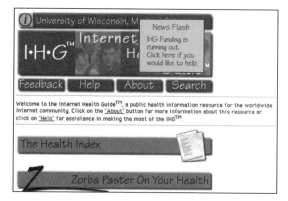

U.S. News Online Health

http://www.usnews.com/usnews/nycu/health.htm

U.S. News Online provides an annotated catalog of major health sites. The topics include general resources, agencies, associations, advocates, publications, AIDS, cancer, drugs and alcohol, mental health, and fat and fitness. In addition, you can ask your own question of a *U.S. News* health advisor or read answers to 10 health-related FAQs located on the bottom of the page.

The Virtual Hospital

http://vh.radiology.uiowa.edu/

The Virtual Hospital, designed by the University of Iowa College of Medicine, deserves the highest accolades for medical information. Among its multitude of resources you may choose **for healthcare providers** to find information by specialty, by organ system, or by type. **Beyond the Virtual Hospital** offers peer review of medical Web sites. **For patient** contains the *Iowa Health Book* and the *Iowa Family Practice Handbook.* You can browse by organ system or find an annotated list of materials. Click on **Peer reviewed World-Wide Web sites on common medical problems** to find topics ranging from pediatrics to general health.

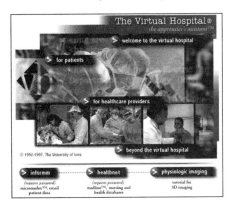

Web Guide

http://www.excite.com/apple/guide/Health_and_Fitness/

The Web Guide, from Excite for Apple Computers, contains a collection of health and fitness sites with categories ranging from advice to substance abuse.

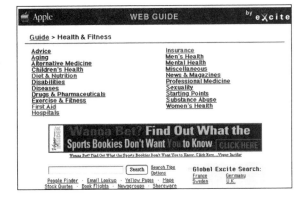

WebCrawler

http://webcrawler.com/select/med.new.html

WebCrawler, a major Internet search engine, provides a well-organized electronic encyclopedia of selected Web sites organized in 24 health topics. Topics include allergies, eye and ear, heart disease, plastic surgery, sex and health, and numerous others.

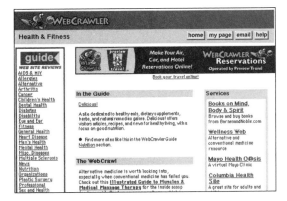

WellnessWeb

http://www.wellweb.com/

WellnessWeb, the patient's network, offers a wealth of information for complementary medicine, conventional medicine, and nutrition/fitness. For an overview of the site's resources, click on the alphabetical **Master Index.**

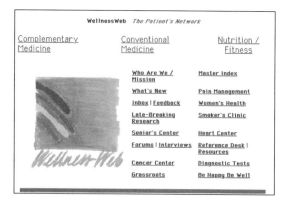

World Internet Directory

http://www.tradenet.it/links/sc/sc.html

World Internet Directory is a site containing personalized medical home pages. Scroll down the page and click on **Health.** This section contains links that range from acupuncture to medicine.

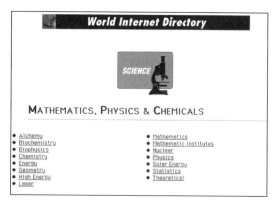

WWW Medical Information Network

http://www.geocities.com/HotSprings/3025/

WWW Medical Information Network provides premier medical information by specialty, disease, mental health, health and fitness, and disabilities.

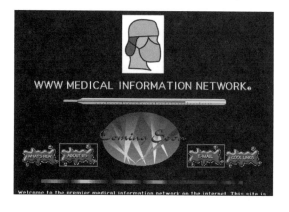

Yahoo! Health

http://www.yahoo.com/Health/

Yahoo! Health contains a well-organized health directory with tens of thousands of sites divided into more than 40 categories ranging from alternative medicine to the workplace. The medicine category features more than 3000 entries ranging from acupuncture to medical Usenet newsgroups.

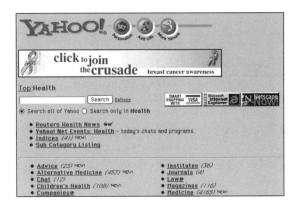

Your Health IS Your Business

http://www.siu.edu/departments/bushea/

Your Health IS Your Business, developed at the University of Southern Illinois, offers everything from health news, online journals, search tools, and topics ranging from alternative medicine to women's health. Each link has a brief description to help decide whether you want to visit it.

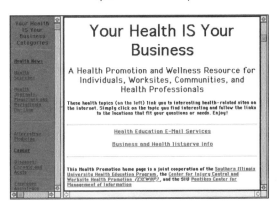

Medical Schools, Hospitals, and Organizations

CHAPTER 24

Accredited Medical Schools of the U.S. and Canada

http://www.aamc.org/meded/medschls/start.htm

Accredited Medical Schools of the U.S. and Canada is a list of medical schools and programs arranged alphabetically by state or by province.

Medical Education

Accredited Medical Schools of the U.S. and Canada

The medical schools and programs are listed alphabetically in order of state or province. It is also indicated whether each school participates in the American Medical College Application Service (AMCAS®), The University of Texas System Medical and Dental Application Center (UTSMDAC), or the Ontario Medical School Application Service (OMSAS). If you wish to receive application materials for any schools which participate in these services, please contact the appropriate addresses listed below:

AMCAS
Association of American Medical Colleges
Section for Student Services
2501 M Street, NW; Lbby-26
Washington, DC 20037-1300
E-mail: amcas@aamc.org

The University of Texas System Medical and Dental Application Center
702 Colorado, Suite 620
Austin, TX 78701

The American Hospital Directory

http://www.ahd.com

The American Hospital Directory lets you look up any hospital in the United States free of charge and see its general characteristics, services provided, financial information, utilization statistics, and other useful information.

The American Hospital Directory™

Your source for comparative hospital data

The American Hospital Directory provides comparative data for most hospitals. Information is taken from Medicare claims data, cost reports, and other public use files obtained from the federal Health Care Financing Administration.

Look up any hospital in the United States that treats Medicare patients. The directory includes many measurements of a hospital and its performance.

+ Hospital Characteristics   + Services Provided   + Utilization Statistics
+ Financial Statistics   + Accreditation Status   + Hospital Web Page

H Free Services
This is the gateway to summary data for most hospitals.
Visit as often as you like and look up as many hospitals as you like.

H Subscription Services
This is the gateway to more detailed information about hospitals.
Detailed information is only available to subscribers.

521

California Consumer HealthScope

http://www.healthscope.org/core.htm

California Consumer HealthScope, sponsored by the Pacific Business Group, compares health plans, hospitals, nursing homes, and health care services on the quality features that are important to you.

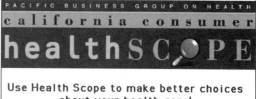

HCIA-Mercer's 100 Top Hospitals

http://www.hcia.com/newsletters/100top/

The HCIA-Mercer's 100 Top Hospitals provides a yearly list of the 100 top-rated U.S hospitals by state.

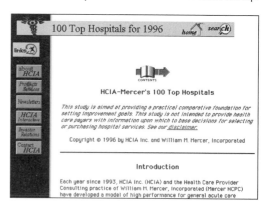

HospitalWeb

http://neuro-www.mgh.harvard.edu/hospitalweb.nclk

HospitalWeb is a series of indexes to hospitals, medical schools, and medical organizations and companies that have Web sites. Each index provides specific information on a wide variety of health-related topics and a number of search tools.

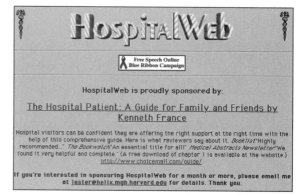

The Interactive Medical Student Lounge

http://www.geocities.com/Heartland/1756/lounge.html

The Interactive Medical Student Lounge, designed for pre-med and medical students, contains useful consumer information in the links **Medical Reference** and **Medical School** lists.

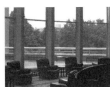

The Internet Hospital Directory

http://dialspace.dial.pipex.com/r.bowyer/hospital.htm

The Internet Hospital Directory provides a comprehensive list of hospitals in the United States. Hospitals can be located alphabetically, by county, by state, and by a regional map.

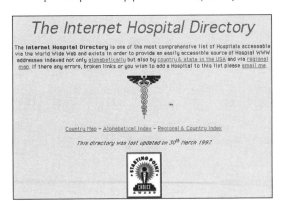

MD Gateway

http://www.mdgateway.com/

MD Gateway provides an eclectic collection of health resources for doctors and consumers, including an alphabetical listing of professional associations, medical schools, online publications, and pharmaceutical companies, in addition to sections on medical information in the library and wellness centers. Every time the page is reloaded, there is an historical health-related factoid.

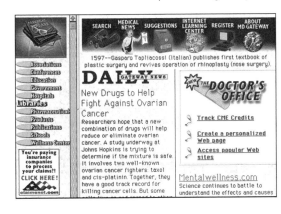

MedWeb Medical Centers and Medical Schools

http://www.gen.emory.edu/MEDWEB/keyword/
medical_centers_and_medical_schools.html

MedWeb, from Emory University Health Sciences Center, offers a giant index to medical schools and centers. Categories range from academic programs to societies and associations.

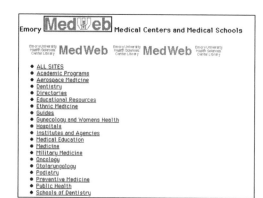

The Multimedia Medical Reference Library Medical Schools

http://www.med-library.com/schools.htm

The Multimedia Medical Reference Library Medical Schools, maintained by Jonathan Tward, is a comprehensive index of the major medical schools worldwide.

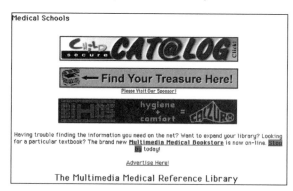

National Institutes of Health

http://www.nih.gov/

The National Institutes of Health is one of the world's foremost biomedical research centers and the federal focal point for biomedical research in the United States. Scroll down and click on **Institutes and Offices** to find a list of the 24 National Institutes of Health sites.

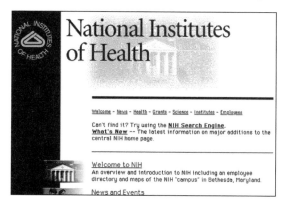

Nationwide Hospitals, Medical Groups, & Clinics Locator

http://www.cmt4911.com/usamap.htm

Nationwide Hospitals, Medical Groups, & Clinics Locator contains a list of links to hospitals, clinics, and medical groups in the United States. To find a hospital, click on a state in the map or click on a state in the list.

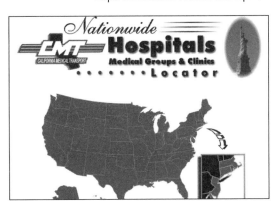

So You Want To Be A Doctor

http://www.review.com/medical/

So You Want To Be A Doctor, from the Princeton Review, features **Find-O-Rama,** which provides detailed profiles of medical schools that match your needs.

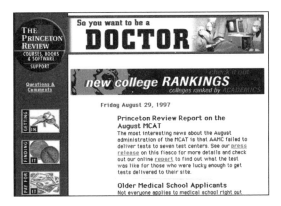

Tore B Sjøboden's Medical Schools Links

http://www.anat.dote.hu/~tore/medfak/

Tore B Sjøboden's Medical Schools Links is a worldwide list of medical school sites on the Web.

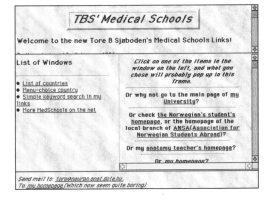

U.S. Health Science Centers and Medical Schools

U.S. Health Science Centers and Medical Schools is an alphabetical index to medical schools in the United States, as well as around the world.

http://medic.med.uth.tmc.edu/publ/00001170.htm

U.S. Health Science Centers and Medical Schools

Select here for World Medical Schools

United States:
Alabama Alaska Arizona Arkansas California Colorado Conneticut Delaware District of Columbia Florida Georgia Hawaii Idaho Illinois Indiana Iowa Kansas Kentucky Louisiana Maine Maryland Massachusettes Michigan Minnesota Mississippi Missouri Montana Nebraska Nevada New Hampshire New Jersey New Mexico New York North Carolina North Dakota Ohio Oklahoma Oregon Pennsylvania Rhode Island South Carolina South Dakota Tennessee Texas Utah Vermont Virginia Washington West Virginia Wisconsin

Alabama

♦ University of Alabama School of Medicine (Birmingham)
♦ University of South Alabama College of Medicine (Mobile)

Alaska

U.S. News Online America's Best Hospitals

U.S. News Online America's Best Hospitals presents its eighth annual (1997) ranking of America's best hospitals. A total of 1800 hospitals were evaluated and the rankings include the 135 hospitals that earned the highest scores in the 17 specialties. The site also offers an alphabetical listing of rankings, rankings of regional and metropolitan hospitals, and rankings of specialty hospitals such as pediatrics and pulmonary disease.

http://www.usnews.com/usnews/nycu/hosphigh.htm

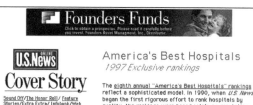

U.S. News Online The Rankings

U.S. News Online The Rankings contains rankings of graduate schools based on its annual book, *1997 America's Best Graduate Schools.* U.S. News Online includes school rankings of research-oriented medical, primary care–oriented medical, dental, nursing, pharmacy, and other health-related graduate schools. The site also provides career outlooks and the 1997 Career Planner, which contains information on finding a medicine/health career.

http://www.usnews.com/usnews/edu/beyond/bcrank.htm

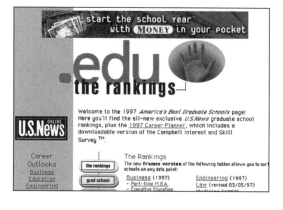

World Wide Web

http://research.med.umkc.edu/wwwsites.html

World Wide Web, maintained by the University of Missouri-Kansas City School of Medicine, provides links to virtually all of the U.S. and Canadian medical schools on the Web. The site includes links to residency programs indexed by state and specialty.

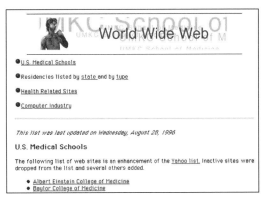

Yahoo! Directory of Dental Institutes

http://www.yahoo.com/Health/Dentistry/Institutes/

Yahoo! Directory of Dental Institutes is an alphabetical list of more than 100 dental schools on the Web.

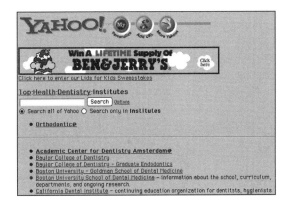

Yahoo! Directory of Diseases and Conditions

http://www.yahoo.com/Health/
Diseases_and_Conditions/Organizations/

Yahoo! Directory of Diseases and Conditions contains an alphabetical list of diseases and conditions ranging from AIDS/HIV to William's syndrome. Each disease category includes the leading professional organizations associated with it.

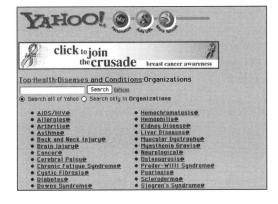

Yahoo! Directory of Medical Organizations

Yahoo! Directory of Medical Organizations is an alphabetical list of specialties and each specialty has the leading professional organizations associated with it.

http://www.yahoo.com/Health/Medicine/Organizations/

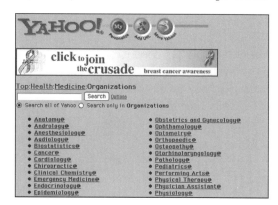

Yahoo! Directory of Medical Schools

Yahoo! Directory of Medical Schools is an alphabetical list of more than 200 medical schools on the Web.

http://www.yahoo.com/Health/
Medicine/Education/Medical_Schools/

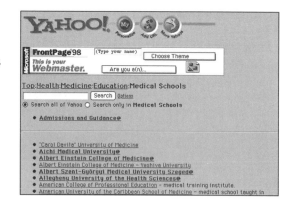

Yahoo! Yellow Pages

Yahoo! Yellow Pages is a database that provides information about the hospitals nearest you. A map and driving directions to each hospital are also provided.

http://yp.yahoo.com/yt.hm?CMD=FILL&SEC=
startfind&FAM=yahoo&FT=2&FS=8062&what=hospital

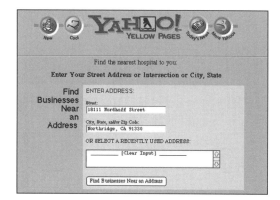

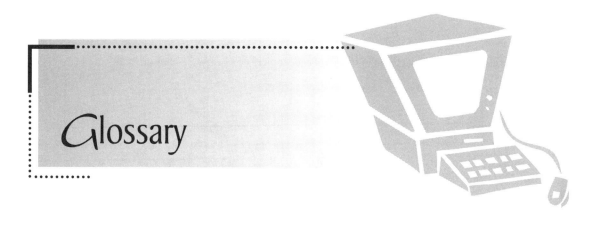

Glossary

browser Software that lets users surf the World Wide Web. Netscape and Internet Explorer are the two most popular browsers.

bps (bits per second) The measurement of data transmission speed. Presently the fastest modem transfer over phone lines is 56 kilobits per second (kbps).

database A collection of computerized information such as an index or a library catalog.

download The process of transferring computer files to your computer.

electronic mail (e-mail) Sending messages electronically over a computer network. Pine is the e-mail service most commonly used at universities and Eudora Lite is a mail application used most often by the general public.

e-mail address A name and a computer location (often referred to as a host). For example, in kberger@qmp.com, kberger is the name and qmp is the location.

FAQs Files found at Internet sites that answer frequently asked questions (FAQs). It is a good idea to check for FAQs and read them.

FTP (file transfer protocol) The basic Internet function that lets files be transferred between computers. It can be used to download files from a remote host computer, as well as upload files from your computer to a remote host computer.

flame An argumentative posting of an e-mail message or newsgroup message in response to another posting.

gopher A program that lets the user browse the Internet using menus.

hard drive The computer's main storage device.

home page The main page in a Web site with hyperlinks to other pages.

HTML (hypertext markup language) The basic language used to build hypertext electronic documents on the Web.

hyperlink A graphic, icon, or word in a file that, when clicked, automatically opens another file for viewing.

Internet A global network that links millions of computers together.

ISP (Internet service provider) An organization that charges a fee for users to dial into its computer for an Internet connection.

Java A programming language, designed by Sun Microsystems, to write programs that can be downloaded from the Internet with a Java interpreter. Many Web pages on the Internet use small Java applications or applets to display animations.

kbps (kilobits per second) A computer modem's speed rating is measured in units of 1024 bits. This is the maximum number a device can transfer in one second under the best conditions.

modem An electronic device that makes it possible for computers to communicate electronically with each other.

network Computers that share storage devices, peripherals, and applications. A network can be connected by telephone lines, satellites, or cables.

netiquette The etiquette used in cyberspace.

online A computer interacting with an online service or the Internet. For example, a person goes online to read his or her e-mail.

online service A commercial service like America Online (AOL) that gives access to electronic mail (e-mail), news service, and the Web.

plug-ins Programs built to extend a browser's capabilities. Plug-ins enable you to see and hear video, audio, and other kinds of multimedia files.

RealAudio A plug-in that lets you listen to live or prerecorded audio transmission on the Web.

usenet newsgroups Usenet stands for USEr NETwork, which provides users with news and e-mail. Newsgroups refers to electronic bulletin boards where anyone can post or read notes related to a specific topic.

URL (uniform resource locator) A site address on the Web. For example, the URL for the California State University home page is http://www.csun.edu.

World Wide Web An Internet service that lets you navigate the Internet using hypertext documents.

Index